REVIEW NEET PG 2019

KD RADADIYA
MD, Radiolodiagnosis
(Fellow – Intervention Neuroradiology at KEM Hospital, Mumbai)

Peepee Publishers and Distributors (P) Ltd.®

REVIEW NEET PG 2019

Published by
Pawaninder P. Vij and Anupam Vij

Peepee Publishers and Distributors (P) Ltd.
Head Office: 160, Shakti Vihar, Pitam Pura, Delhi-110 034 (India)

Correspondence Address:

7/31, First Floor, Ansari Road, Daryaganj
New Delhi-110 002 (India)

Ph: 41512412, 23246245, 9811156083

e-mail: peepee160@yahoo.co.in

e-mail: peepee160@gmail.com

www.peepeepub.com

join us on facebook.com/pp.publishers

First Edition: 2019

ISBN: 978-81-8445-264-8

Dedicated to

Parents (Kantaben, Jamnadas)

PG ASPIRANTS

Preface

When I was doing my preparation for PG Entrance Examination, I myself realized that many of the upcoming exam questions are asked from last year paper. So, I remained very curious to find authentic book of previous year paper. Many times book contains wrong questions, wrong answers or too lengthy non-specific explanations. In this way I find very depressed to myself. And I always thought that there would be a best book on previous year paper. It now gives me immense pleasure to share this book with all possible questions with best possible explanations.

This book is written in such a way that it can be completed in a very short time with retrograde manner. The book covers all possible MCQs of previous year exam. Its explanation is a handy reference for those who are preparing to appear in postgraduate entrance examinations and it gives a comprehensive, brief and yet lucid account of subject.

Please remember I have given the best effort to this book and hopefully you will find all relevant theories in this user-friendly book. Despite of every possible effort have been undertaken to ensure no technical or typographical errors in the book, such mistakes are bound to be present in any book. If you come across any such error or if you have any comment, suggestions, queries, you are most welcome to e-mail to us for a prompt response. All contributions will be duly acknowledged. Do share your experience while reading this book.

We pray, you have a successful career ahead.

Wish you have success, not just in next exam but throughout in your life!

Have a great life ahead.

Dr. Krushnadas Radadiya (KD RADADIYA)

Email: kdbrijpg@gmail.com

Acknowledgements

I would like to thank the following people:

Dr. Brij Teli, 3rd Year Resident, MD Medicine ***Dr. Rajesh Teli, MD Medicine***	
Sterling Hospital	**Radiology Department**
Dr. Ajit Vadher, MD Radiodiagnosis	Dr. Anjana Trivedi, MD Radiodiagnosis
Dr. Abhay Javia, DM Respiratory Medicine	Dr. Chetna Dodiya, DMRD
Dr. Gaurang Vaghani, MCH Neurosurgery	Dr. Hiral Hapani, MD Radiodiagnosis
Dr. Kaushik Kotak, MS General Surgery	Dr. Jagruti Kalola, MD Radiodiagnosis
Dr. Kamal Parikh, MD Medicine	Dr. Mahak Sood, MD Radiodiagnosis
Dr. Nilesh Makwana, MD Radiodiagnosis	Dr. Maulik Jethva, MD Radiodiagnosis
Dr. Ram Pansuriya, MD Radiodiagnosis	Dr. Mehta Aditya
Dr. Rishikesh Kalaria, DM Gastroenterology	
Dr. Roshan Mistry, DM Neurology	
Dr. Sanjay Teelala, MCH Neurosurgery	
Dr. Sonika Sharma, MD Radiodiagnosis	
Dr. Shailesh Moral, MD Pathology	
Dr. Tejas Karangia, MCH Vascular Surgery	

I would also like to thank the entire staff of Peepee Publishers and Distributors (P) Ltd.

From the Author's Desk

It now gives me immense pleasure to share this book. I have given exam this year and also at previous year. The most important thing, which I have observed during this exam, is that there are many questions, which they have asked, from same topics of previous year paper. Here I can give one example such as 'Myasthenia Gravis', in 2018 they asked 'Myasthenia Gravis is caused by' and now they asked about 'Tensilon (Edrophonium) test used in Myasthenia Gravis'. Therefore, students find **very less direct repeats** from previous year paper, but I say there are **many indirect repeats from same topic**, which had been asked in previous year. Now, we can see benefit of sincerely studying previous year paper.

This book can be best utilized in this way. First make a list of topics from this book, which have been asked in this year and read these topics thoroughly from this book and from your reference book. Revise these topics at least three times. Read these topics within few days before your NEET PG exam.

I have given so much emphasis to not to miss any question/ topic from this exam. Therefore, this book will surely guide you about how was this exam and what to read further. Which topics, you must know thoroughly and where your knowledge is lacking.

Therefore, friends read this book as reference to find out this year's exams topics and make sure not to leave any question of this book as optional. In this way you find, this book will be most helpful to you.

So, 'How's the Josh'!

Dr. KD Radadiya (Krushnadas Radadiya)

Contents

References

- Anatomy–Gray's Anatomy for Students.
- Physiology–Ganong's Review of Medical Physiology.
- Biochemistry–Lippincott's Illustrated Reviews Biochemistry.
- Pharmacology–Essentials of Medical Pharmacology by KD Tripathi, Goodman and Gillman's–The Pharmacological Basis of Therapeutics.
- Pathology–Robbins Basic Pathology.
- Microbiology–Ananthanarayan and Paniker's Textbook of Microbiology, Randhawa–Textbook of Microbiology.
- Forensic Medicine–Essentials of Forensic Medicine and Toxicology by Reddy.
- Preventive and Social Medicine–Park's Textbook of Preventive and Social Medicine.
- ENT–Diseases of Ear, Nose and Throat by Dr. PL Dhingra.
- Ophthalmology–Review of Ophthalmology by AK Khurana; Review of Ophthalmology by Ruchi Rai.
- Medicine–Harrison's Principles of Internal Medicine, 20th edition.
- Surgery–Sabiston Textbook of Surgery, Schwartz's Principles of Surgery.
- Pediatric–Ghai Essential Pediatrics, Nelson Textbook of Pediatrics, Sharma–Principle and Practice of Pediatrics.
- Obstetrics–Williams Obstetrics, DC Dutta's Textbook of Obstetrics.
- Gynecology–Shaw's Textbook of Gynecology, DC Dutta's Textbook of Gynecology.
- Anesthesia–Miller's Anesthesia.
- Orthopedic–Essential Orthopedics by J Maheshwari.
- Psychiatry–Kaplan and Sadock's Comprehensive Textbook of Psychiatry.
- Dermatology–Illustrated Synopsis of Dermatology and Sexually Transmitted Diseases by Neena Khanna.
- Radiology–Textbook of Radiology and Imaging by David Sutton, Grainger and Allison's Diagnostic Radiology.

CHAPTER 1

ANATOMY

1. Umbilical dermatome is located at which level?

A. L2 | B. T9
C. T10 | D. L3

Answer: Option C. T10

Explanation:

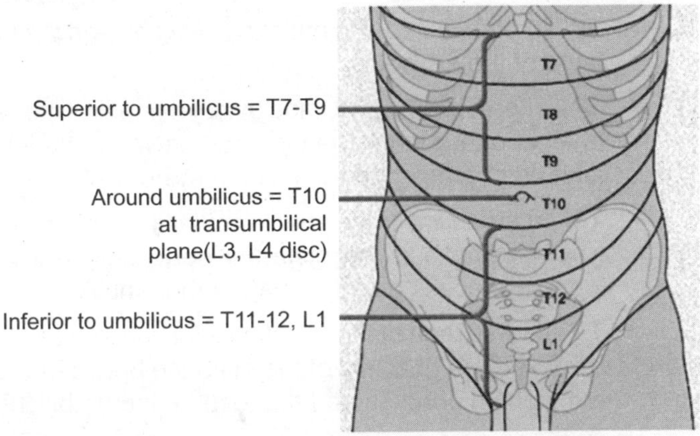

Following is a list of **spinal nerves** and points that are characteristically belonging to the dermatome of each nerve:

- **C2** - At least one cm lateral to the **occipital protuberance** at the **base of the skull**. Alternately, a point at least 3 cm behind the ear.
- **C3** - In the **supraclavicular fossa**, at the **midclavicular line**.
- **C4** - Over the **acromioclavicular joint**.
- **C5** - On the lateral (radial) side of the **antecubital fossa**, just proximally to the elbow.
- **C6** - On the dorsal surface of the **proximal phalanx** of the **thumb**.
- **C7** - On the dorsal surface of the **proximal phalanx** of the **middle finger**.

- **C8** - On the dorsal surface of the proximal phalanx of the **little finger**.
- **T1** - On the medial (ulnar) side of the **antecubital fossa**, just proximally to the **medial epicondyle of the humerus**.
- **T2** - At the apex of the **axilla**.
- **T3** - **Intersection** of the **midclavicular line** and the third **intercostal space.**
- **T4** - Intersection of the **midclavicular line** and the fourth intercostal space, located at the level of the nipples.
- **T5** - Intersection of the midclavicular line and the fifth intercostal space, horizontally located midway between the level of the nipples and the level of the **xiphoid process**.
- **T6** - Intersection of the midclavicular line and the horizontal level of the **xiphoid process**.
- **T7** - Intersection of the midclavicular line and the horizontal level at one quarter the distance between the level of the xiphoid process and the level of the **umbilicus**.
- **T8** - Intersection of the midclavicular line and the horizontal level at one half the distance between the level of the xiphoid process and the level of the umbilicus.
- **T9** - Intersection of the midclavicular line and the horizontal level at three quarters of the distance between the level of the xiphoid process and the level of the umbilicus.
- **T10** - Intersection of the midclavicular line, at the horizontal level of the umbilicus.
- **T11** - Intersection of the midclavicular line, at the horizontal level midway between the level of the umbilicus and the **inguinal ligament**.
- **T12** - Intersection of the midclavicular line and the midpoint of the inguinal ligament.
- **L1** - Midway between the key sensory points for T12 and L2.
- **L2** - On the anterior medial thigh, at the midpoint of a line connecting the midpoint of the inguinal ligament and the **medial epicondyle of the femur**.
- **L3** - At the **medial epicondyle of the femur**.
- **L4** - Over the **medial malleolus**.

- **L5** - On the **dorsum of the foot** at the third **metatarso-phalangeal joint**.
- **S1** - On the lateral aspect of the **calcaneus**.
- **S2** - At the midpoint of the **popliteal fossa**.
- **S3** - Over the **tuberosity of the ischium** or **infragluteal fold.**
- **S4** and **S5** - In the **perianal** area, less than one cm lateral to the **mucocutaneous zone.**

2. Internal capsule are which type of fibers?

A. Association fibers
B. Projection fibers
C. Commissural fibers
D. Intrahemispheric fibers

Answer: Option B. Projection fibers

Explanation:

White matter tracts in the brain, also known as **white matter fibres,** are classified into three categories:

The internal capsule is a **white matter** structure.The **corticospinal tract** constitutes a large part of the internal capsule. Other constituents of internal capsule are **optic radiation** and **corticobulbar tract.** All of these are projection fibers.

Projection tracts

- Tracts connecting the cortex with other area in the CNS, e.g., deep nuclei, **brainstem**, **cerebellum** or **spine**
- May be efferent (motor) or afferent tracts (sensory).
- White matter tracts that can be identified by fibre tracking include:
  - **Corticospinal tract** (CST)
  - **Corticobulbar tract** (CBT)
  - **Medial lemniscus** (ML)
  - **Optic radiation** (OR)

Association Tracts

- Tracts connecting different areas in the same hemisphere (also known as intrahemispheric tracts).
- DTI tractography can identify the following tracts:

- Arcuate fasciculus
- Superior and inferior occipitofrontal fasciculi
- Cingulum, uncinate and inferior longitudinal bundle

Commissural Tracts

- Tracts connecting the same cortical area in opposite hemispheres
- **Corpus callosum** (CC) is the main commissural tract
- **Anterior commissure**
- **Posterior commissure**

3. Uvula vesicae is formed by which part of prostate gland?

A. Median lobe B. Lateral lobe

C. Anterior lobe D. Posterior lobe

Answer: Option A. Median lobe

Explanation:

In men, the **prostate gland** lies outside the opening for the urethra. The median lobe of the prostate causes an elevation in the mucous membrane behind the internal urethral orifice called the uvula **vesicae of urinary bladder. The uvula can enlarge when the prostate becomes enlarged.**

INTERIOR OF THE BLADDER

Rugae:

Trigone of the bladder:

Features of Trigone:

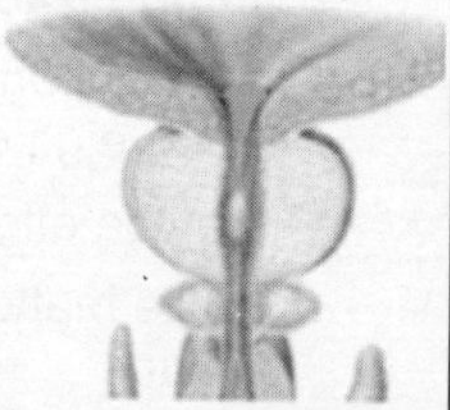

1. **Anteroinferior angle:** Internal orifice of the urethra.
2. **Two posterosuperior angles:** Openings of the ureters.
3. **Uvula vesicae:** A slight elevation in the mucous membrane immediately above and behind the internal urethral orifice.
   - Produced by **median lobe of prostate.**
4. **Interureteric ridge/crest or bar of Mercier:**
   - Forms the base of the trigone.
   - Produced by the continuation of inner longitudinal muscle coats of 2 ureters.

Contd

Contd.

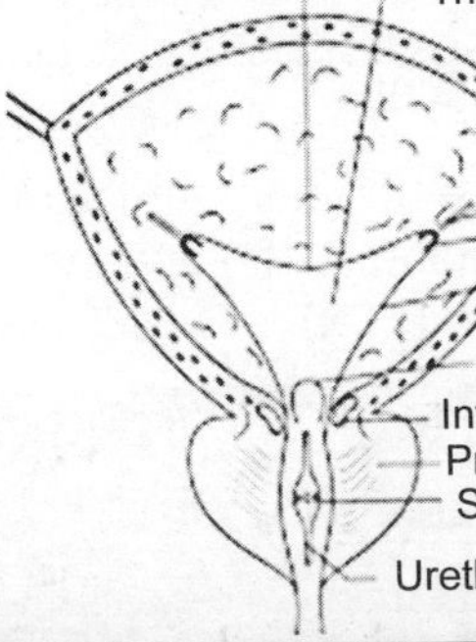

4. Right coronary artery arises from which portion of heart?

A. Posterior sinus

B. Coronary sinus

C. Right aortic sinus

D. Left aortic sinus

Answer: Option C. Right aortic sinus

Explanation:

Right coronary artery arises from right aortic sinus. It is also known as anterior aortic sinus.

- Right coronary artery (RCA) originating above the right cusp of the aortic valve, at the right aortic sinus in the heart. It travels down the right coronary sulcus, towards the crux of the heart.
- It branches into the **posterior descending artery and the right marginal artery**.
- At the origin of the RCA is the **conus artery**.
- In addition to supplying blood to the right ventricle (RV), the RCA supplies 25% to 35% of the left ventricle (LV).
- In **85%** of patients (Right Dominant), the **RCA gives off the posterior descending artery (PDA).**
- In the other **15%** of cases (Left Dominant), the **PDA is given off by the left circumflex artery**.
- The PDA supplies the inferior wall, ventricular septum, and the posteromedial papillary muscle.
- The RCA also supplies the SA nodal artery in 60% of people.

- The other 40% of the time, the SA nodal artery is supplied by the left circumflex artery.

Left coronary artery arises from left aortic sinus. It is also known as posterior aortic sinus.

It bifurcates into the anterior interventricular artery (also called the left anterior descending (LAD) and the Widow maker) and the left circumflex artery (LCx).

5. All of the following are derivative of external oblique aponeurosis, *except*:

A. Inguinal ligament
B. Pectineal ligament
C. Lacunar ligament
D. Linea semilunaris

Answer: Option D. Linea semilunaris

Explanation:

External Oblique Aponeurosis

In the middle line, it interlaces with the aponeurosis of the opposite muscle, forming the linea alba, which extends from the xiphoid process to the pubic symphysis.

That portion of the aponeurosis which extends between the anterior superior iliac spine and the pubic tubercle is a thick band, folded inward, and continuous below with the fascia lata; it is called the **inguinal ligament**.

The portion which is reflected from the inguinal ligament at the pubic tubercle is attached to the pectineal line and is called the **lacunar ligament**.

From the point of attachment of the latter to the pectineal line, a few fibers pass upward and medial ward, behind the medial crus of the superficial inguinal ring, to the linea alba; they diverge as they ascend, and form a thin triangular fibrous band which is called the **reflected inguinal ligament**.

The **pectineal ligament** (sometimes known as the **inguinal ligament of Cooper**) is an extension of the **lacunar ligament** that runs on the pectineal line of the pubic bone. The pectineal ligament is the posterior border of the **femoral ring**.

The **linea semilunaris** (also **semilunar line** or **Spigelian line**) is a curved tendinous intersection found on either side of the rectus abdominis muscle. Each corresponds with the lateral border of the rectus abdominis, extends from the cartilage of the ninth rib to the pubic tubercle, and is formed by the aponeurosis of the internal oblique at its line of division to enclose the rectus, reinforced anteriorly by the external oblique and posteriorly by the transversus abdominis above the arcuate line (also known as *linea semicircularis* or *Douglas' line*).

A hernia through the linea semilunaris is called a Spigelian hernia, which is also referred to as a spontaneous lateral ventral hernia.

6. Which of the following is structure is transmitted through the foramen depicted in given image?

A. Inferior alveolar nerve
B. Facial nerve
C. Maxillary nerve
D. Trigeminal nerve

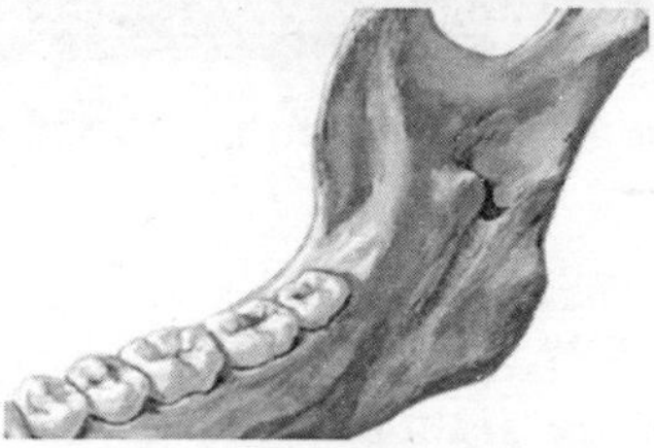

Answer: Option A. Inferior alveolar nerve

Explanation:

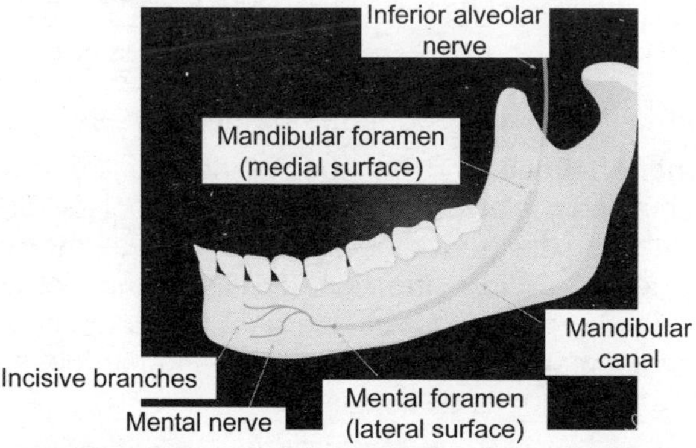

Here the above image is showing inner aspect of mandible. Arrow is depicting mandibular foramen.

The **mandibular foramen** or **inferior alveolar foramen** is located on the medial surface of the ramus of the **mandible** and is the entrance to the **mandibular canal.**

It transmits the **inferior alveolar nerve,** a branch of the **posterior division of the mandibular division** of the **trigeminal nerve** that supplies all the ipsilateral **teeth** up to the midline as well as the **inferior alveolar artery** and the vein.

Superiorly it has a small tubercle or ridge, the **lingula,** where the **sphenomandibular ligament** attaches.

7. Cholecystocaval line separates which of the following structure of liver?

A. Right and left lobe of liver

B. Gallbladder and inferior vena cava

C. Right lobe and caudate lobe

D. Left lobe and quadrate lobe

Answer: Option A. Right and left lobe of liver

Explanation:

Anatomical lobe

Liver has a larger **right** and smaller **left 'anatomical' lobes**. The line of attachment of falciform ligament on anterior and superior surfaces of liver and the fissure for ligamentus venosum and fissure for ligamentum teres on the posteroinferior surface of the liver separate the two lobes.

The right lobe also presents **quadrate lobe** and **caudate lobe.**

Functional lobes and segments of the liver

The **functional** right and left lobes of the liver are separated by an imaginary plane passing along the floor of fossa for gallbladder and the groove for inferior vena cava (**cholecysto-caval line – Cantlie's line**). On the anterosuperior surface of the liver the plane passes little right to the attachment of falciform ligament. The functional right and left lobes of the liver are of more or less equal in size.

The liver is further divided into **Couinaud segments**. Each segment is supplied by a principal branch hepatic artery and portal vein and the bile of these segments are collected by a principal branch of hepatic duct. Each functional lobe of the liver consists of four segments. The segments **I, II, III** and **IV** belong to the functional LEFT lobe and segments **V, VI, VII** and **VIII** to the functional RIGHT lobe.

The lobes can be further divided as **right anterior** (Segments V and VIII) and **right posterior** (Segments VI and VII) **sections/ sectors** in the right functional lobe and **left medial** (Segment IV) and **left lateral** (Segments II and III) **sections/sectors** in the left functional lobe. The hepatic veins lie in liver parenchyma between the sections.

Segment I corresponds to the gross anatomical caudate lobe and segment IV to the quadrate lobe.

8. Which of the following muscle is shown by arrow in below given image?

A. Supinator
B. Extensor carpi radialis longus
C. Brachioradialis
D. Extensor carpi ulnaris

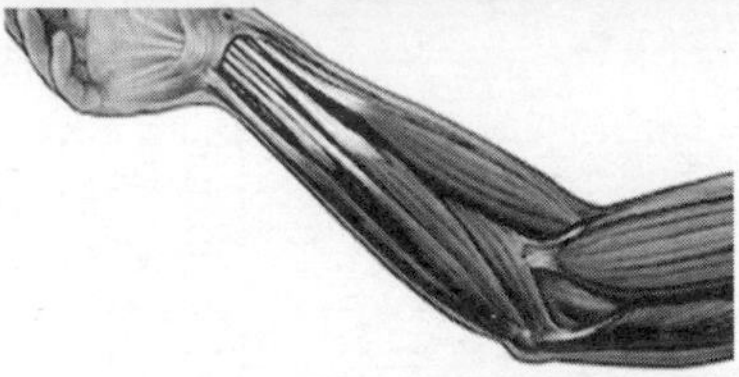

Answer: Option C. Brachioradialis

Explanation:

Here key to identify the muscle is correct identification of forearm position–supine or prone.

First forearm is placed in supine position.

Now two muscles in given options are extensor carpi radialis longus and extensor carpi ulnaris muscles, which are seen in prone position so these will not be the answer. Supinator is directed obliquely that curved around upper third of radius.

So remaining option, brachioradialis will remain our answer. Brachioradialis is located at radial/lateral aspect of forearm which can be seen clearly on above image.

Movement	Target	Target motion direction	Prime mover	Origin	Insertion
Superficial anterior compartment of forearm					
Bends wrist toward body; tilts hand to side away from body	Wrist; hand	Flexion; abduction	Flexor carpi radialis	Medial epicondyle of humerus	Base of second and third metacarpals
Assists in bending hand up toward shoulder	Wrist	Flexion	Palmaris longus	Medial epicondyle of humerus	Palmar aponeurosis; skin and fascia of palm
Assists in bending hand up toward shoulder; tilts hand to side away from body; stabilizes wrist	Wrist; hand	Flexion, abduction	Flexor carpi ulnaris	Medial epicondyle of humerus; olecranon process; posterior surface of ulna	Pisiform, hamate bones, and base of fifth metacarpal
Bends fingers to make a fist	Wrist; fingers 2-5	Flexion	Flexor digitorum superficialis	Medial epicondyle of humerus; coronoid process of ulna; shalf of radius	Middle phalanges of fingers 2–5
Deep anterior compartment of forearm					
Bends tip of thumb	Thumb	Flexion	Flexor pollicis longus	Anterior surface of radius; interosseous membrane	Distal phalanx of thumb 2–5

Contd.

Contd.

Bends fingers to make a fist; also bends wrist toward body	Wrist; fingers	Flexion	Flexor digitorum profundus	Coronoid process; anteromedial surface of ulna; interosseous membrane	Distal phalanges of fingers 2–5
Superficial posterior compartment of forearm					
Straightens wrist away from body; tilts hand to side away from body	Wrist	Extension; abduction	Extensor radialis longus	Lateral supracondylar ridge of humerus	Base of second metacarpal
Assists extensor radialis longus in extending and abducting wrist; also stabilizes hand during finger flexion	Wrist	Extension; abduction	Extensor carpi radialis brevis	Lateral epicondyle of humerus	Base of third metacarpal
Opens fingers and moves them sideways away from the body	Wrist fingers	Extension; abduction	Extensor digitorum	Lateral epicondyle of humerus	Extensor expansions; distal phalanges of fingers
Extends little finger	Little finger	Extension	Extensor digiti minimi	Lateral epicondyle of humerus	Extensor expansion; distal phalanx of finger 5
Straightens wrist away from body; tilts hand to side toward body	Wrist	Extension; abduction	Extensor carpi ulnaris	Lateral epicondyle of humerus; posterior border of ulna	Base of fifth metacarpal

Contd.

Contd.

Deep posterior compartment of forearm					
Moves thumb sideways towards body; extends thumb; moves hand sideways toward body	Wrist; thumb	Thumb: abduction, extension; wrist: abduction	Abductor pollicis longus	Posterior surface of radius and ulna; interosseous membrane	Base of first metacarpal; trapezium
Extends thumb	Thumb	Extension	Extensor pollicis brevis	Dorsal shaft of radius and ulna; interosseous membrane	Base of proximal phalanx of thumb
Extends thumb	Thumb	Extension	Extensor pollicis longus	Dorsal shaft of radius and ulna; interosseous membrane	Base of distal phalanx of thumb
Extends index finger; straightens wrist away from body	Wrist: index finger	Extension	Extensor indicis	Posterior surface of distal ulna; interosseous membrane	Tendon of extensor digitorum of index finger

Brachioradialis is a flexor at the elbow and works with **biceps brachii** and **brachialis**. Is it located in the superficial layer of the **posterior compartment of the forearm** and is particularly useful in elbow stabilisation.

Despite the bulk of the muscle being visible from the anterior surface of the forearm, it is a posterior compartment muscle and thus, its innervation derives from the posterior compartment. It is one of the three muscles forming the **mobile wad of Henry**.

Summary

- **Origin:** Proximal 2/3rd of lateral supracondylar ridge of **humerus.**
- **Insertion:** Lateral surface of distal end of radius just proximal to styloid process of radius.
- **Innervation: Radial nerve** (C5, C6).
- **Action:** Flexor of the elbow with particular use in stabilisation.

9. Which the following muscle is developed from first pharyngeal arch?

A. Stylohyoid
B. Anterior belly of digastric
C. Posterior belly of digastric
D. Cricothyroid

Answer: Option B. Anterior belly of digastric

Explanation:

See table on the next page.

10. Which nerve supplies following given area of hand?

A. Ulnar nerve
B. Median nerve
C. Radial nerve
D. Anterior interosseous nerve

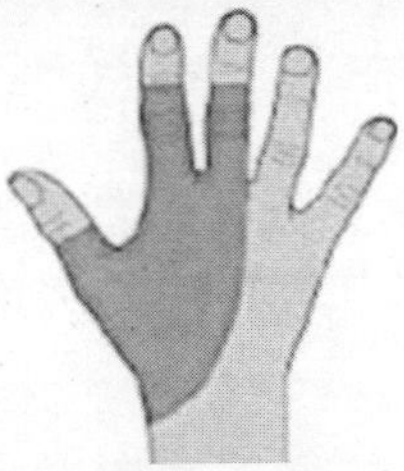

Answer: Option C. Radial nerve

Q. No. 9

Arch	Nerve	Muscles	Skeletal structures	Ligaments	Artery
First (mandibular)	Trigeminal nerve (CN V) (maxillary and mandibular branches only)	Muscles of mastication, mylohyoid; anterior belly of digastric, tensor tympani, tensor veil palatine	Malleus incus	Anterior ligament of malleus, sphenomandibular ligament	Maxillary artery
Second (hyoid)	Facial nerve (CN VII)	Muscles of facial expression, stapedius stylohyoid, posterior belly of digastric	Stapes, styloid process, lesser cornu and upper body of the hyoid bone	Stylohyoid ligament	Stapedial artery (rarely)
Third	Glassopharyngeal nerve (CN IX)	Stylopharyngeus, superior and middle pharyngeal constrictors	Greater cornu and lower part of body of the hyoid bone		Contributions to the carotid arteries
Fourth and sixth	Superior laryngeal branch of vagus nerve (CN X)— Fourth arch; recurrent laryngeal branch of vagus nerve (CN X)– sxith arch	Cricothyoid, levator veil palatine, inferior pharygeal constrictors, intrinsic muscles of larynx, striated muscles of the esophagus	Thyroid, cricoid, arytenoid, corniculate, cuneiform cartilages		The artery of the fourth arch contributes to the subclavian artery on the right and the aortic arch on the left; the artery of the sixth arch forms the ductus arteriosus and the pulmonary artery

Explanation:

Radial Nerve

- **Origin:** One of the two posterior cords of the brachial plexus.
- **Course:** Posteromedially with the axillary vessels, behind the humerus, then anteriorly towards the elbow where it divides into superficial and deep branches.
- **Terminal branches:** Posterior interosseous (deep) and superficial radial nerves.
- **Motor:** Elbow, wrist and finger extension.
- **Sensory:** Dorsal aspect of the thumb, index and middle fingers.

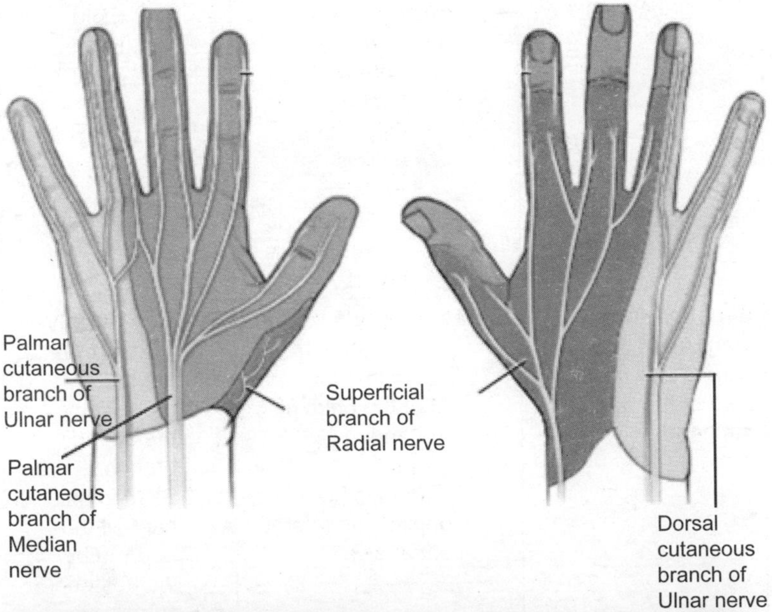

11. Which nerve supplies 1st lumbricals of hand?

A. Ulnar nerve

B. Median nerve

C. Radial nerve

D. Anterior interosseous nerve

Answer: Option B. Median nerve

Ulnar nerve	Median nerve	Radial nerve
C7, 8, T1 Medial cord	C5678T1 Medial and lateral cord	C5-T1 Posterior cord
Motor supply • **Forearm** Ulnar 1/2 on the FDP, FCU • **Intrinsic and muscles** All intrinsic muscles of the hand except 4 muscles; LOAF are supplied by the median nerve	• **Motor supply Forearm** Flexors of the forearm; pronator terers, FCR, palmaris longus, FDS • **Anterior interosseus nerve** supplies FPL and 1/2 of the FDP. • **Intrinsic hand muscles** LOAF: – Lateral 2 lumbricals – Opponens pollicis – Abductor pollicis brevis – Flexor pollicis brevis	**Motor supply** • Triceps, brachialis (small part), brachioradialis • Extensors of the forearm; by the posterior interosseus nerve – ED – EDM – ECU – ABPL – EPL – EPB – EIN
Sensory supply Medial one and 1/2 fingers and medial third of the palm of the hand	**Sensory supply** • Lateral 3 and 1/2 fingers and lateral 2/3 of the palm of the hand • The palmar cutaneous branch supplies the lateral palmar skin	**Sensory supply** • Radial 1/1/2 fingers dorsally by the superficial branch • Skin on the back of the forearm by the posterior cutaneous nerve of the forearm
Partial claw hand	**Ape hand**	**Wrist drop**
• Finger spreading test • Card test • Froment's test • Sensory distribution	• Abductor pollicis brevis test • Tinel's test • Phalen's test	• Wrist extension test

CHAPTER 2

PHYSIOLOGY

1. ADH acts on which of the following channel?

A. Aquaporin 1
B. Aquaporin 2
C. Aquaporin 3
D. Aquaporin 4

Answer: Option B. Aquaporin 2

Explanation:

Aquaporins are water channels through which water reabsorption is facilitated.

ADH (Vasopressin) acts on aquaporin-2.

This action is mediated via vasopressin V2 receptor, cyclic adenosine 5-monophosphate (cAMP) and protein kinase A.

This aquaporin-2 is stored in vesicles in the cytoplasm of principal cells. Vasopressin causes rapid insertion of these vesicles into the apical membrane of cell.

Channel	Location
Aquaporin 1	Luminal membrane of PCT
Aquaporin 2	Luminal membrane of CD
Aquaporin 3	Basolateral membrane of CD
Aquaporin 4	Basolateral membrane of MCD

2. Golgi tendon organ is stimulated by which of the following muscle feature?

A. Muscle density
B. Muscle strength
C. Muscle tension
D. Muscle length

Answer: Option C. Muscle tension

Explanation:

Golgi tendon organ is stimulated by increase tension in the muscle.

GOLGI TENDON ORGAN

Location

Located at the musculotendinous junction (90%) and in the tendon itself (10%).

Each organ is attached with *less than 25 extrafusal fibers* (>25 fiber are present in 5% of Golgi tendon organ) (*Ganong:* **3–25 fiber, Guyton:** 10–15 fiber) from a small number of *motor units* (<15 motor unit). Unlike muscle spindle, these fibers are *in series* with extrafusal fibers of muscle.

Stimulated by: Increase Tension at Muscle Tendon

They are stimulated by both passive stretch and active contraction of the muscle. That increases muscle tension.

The threshold of the Golgi tendon organs is low.

Afferent: Ib fiber (myelinated).

Efferent supply to muscle spindle: Absent.

Central connection: Ib fibers on α-motor neurons via an inhibitory interneuron in spinal cord.

Functions: Inverse stretch reflex

Active muscle contraction stimulates the Golgi tendon organs and group Ib afferent fibers.

The group Ib afferents stimulates inhibitory interneurons in the spinal cord. These interneurons inhibit α-motor neurons and cause relaxation of the muscle that was originally contracted.

At the same time, antagonistic muscles are excited (contraction). This is *inverse stretch* (myotatic) reflex. It is a bisynaptic reflex.

3. Peripheral chemoreceptors are sensitive to hypoxia through which of the following channel?

A. O2 sensitive Sodium channel

B. O2 sensitive Calcium channel

C. O2 sensitive potassium channel

D. O2 sensitive chloride channel

Answer: Option C. O2 sensitive potassium channel

Explanation:

Peripheral chemoreceptor are the type I glomus cells which have O_2-sensitive K^+ channels. These channels are highly sensitive to hypoxia.

Peripheral Chemoreceptors

Respond to: An increase in CO_2 ($\uparrow PaCO_2$) and H^+ (acidosis) and a decrease in O_2 ($\downarrow PaO_2$) in arterial blood.

Sensor cell: The type I glomus cells inside chemo receptors are the sensor cells, which respond directly to hypoxia. They have O_2sensitive K^+ channels.

- The main neurotransmitter release by glomus cell is ATP (main), Ach and dopamine.

Blood flow: Both chemoreceptors have highest blood flow in body (2000 mL/min/100 gm of tissue).

Because of this, O_2 needs of these cells can be met by dissolve O_2 only (does not respond to anemic hypoxia).

Central Chemoreceptors

The central chemoreceptors (neurons) project directly to the respiratory centers.

They respond to increase H^+ ion of CSF. But increase blood H^+ ions (acidosis) fail to stimulates central chemoreceptor (because BBB does not allow charged ions).

Blood CO_2 can influence these centra chemoreceptors indirectly by getting converted into H^+. *By virtue of this, CO_2 is able to act on both central (70–80% of the effect of CO_2) as well as on peripheral (20–30% of the effect of CO_2) chemoreceptors.*

Hypoxia cannot stimulate central chemoreceptors; rather they are depressed by hypoxia.

4. In which of the following conditions Bainbridge reflex is initiated?

A. Increase in peripheral resistance

B. Increase in arterial pressure

C. Left ventricle engorgement

D. Right atrium engorgement

Answer: Option D. Right atrium engorgement

Explanation:

Receptor for Bainbridge reflex is mediated by activation of stretch receptor, mainly located at veno-atrial junctions of right atrium and these receptor are activated by stretch on right atrium or right atrial engorgement.

Bainbridge Reflex

Bainbridge reported that infusing blood or saline into dogs accelerated their heart rate. This change in heart rate (HR) is independent of BP.

Receptor: Stretch receptors in both atrial walls. These receptors are located principally in the venoatrial junctions: in the right atrium at its junctions with the venae cavae and in the left atrium at its junctions with the pulmonary veins.

Activation of receptor: Stretch on right atrium (increase in venous return) activates these receptors (so-called *low pressure baroreceptors*).

Low pressure baroreceptor are of two types: Those that discharge primarily during atrial systole (type A), and those that discharge primarily late in diastole, at the time of peak atrial filling (type B).

Afferent: Vagal afferent. Bilateral transection of the vagi abolish this response.

Center: Brainstem.

Efferent: Parasympathetic (decrease) and sympathetic (increase).

Response: Increase in HR. The response is highly selective to heart. Reflex increase in HR is large but changes in ventricular contractility are generally negligible. Furthermore, there is no increase in sympathetic activity in the peripheral arterioles.

5. The most important determinant of tubuloglomerular feedback system is:

A. Control of glomerular filtration rate

B. Sodium concentration

C. Blood pressure

D. Control of plasma volume

Answer: Option A. Control of Glomerular filtration rate

Explanation:

Tubuloglomerular feedback system is a main mechanism for the autoregulation of Glomerular filtration rate.

Sensor cell for TGF is macula densa. The macula densa is a collection of densely packed epithelial cells at the junction of the thick ascending limb (TAL) and distal convoluted tubule (DCT), which senses Na/Cl. The tubuloglomerular feedback is mediated by sensing NaCl concentration in macula densa (AI-2006). According to this GFR will increase or decrease. In response increased sodium chloride (salt) concentration at the macula densa, there is reduction of glomerular filtrate rate. In response to decreased salt concentration at the macula densa, there is increased GFR.

TUBULOGLOMERULAR FEEDBACK

To perform the function of autoregulation, the kidneys have a feedback mechanism that links changes in NaCl concentration at the macula densa with the control of renal arteriolar resistance.

Decreased macula densa NaCl causes dilation of afferent arterioles and increased renin release.

The sensor for TGF is the macula densa. It senses the amount of Na^+ and Cl^- in it.

The Na^+ and Cl^- enter the macula densa cells via the Na-K-2Cl cotransporter in their apical membranes.

The increased Na^+ and Cl^- causes increased Na-K- ATPase activity and the resultant increased ATP hydrolysis. ATP hydrolysis causes more adenosine to be formed in macula densa cell.

Adenosine acts via adenosine A1 receptors on the macula densa cells to increase their release of Ca^{2+} to the vascular smooth muscle in the afferent arterioles. This causes afferent vasoconstriction and a resultant decrease in GFR.

Opposite mechanism is seen in case of decrease NaCl in macula densa.

Although a change in NaCl transport is a key modulator of the macula densa pathway, the pathway depends more on the luminal concentration of Cl^- than Na.

Factors that *decrease* TGF sensitivity include:

- Atrial natriuretic peptide
- Nitric oxide
- cAMP
- PGI2
- High-protein diet

Factors that *increase* TGF sensitivity include:

- Adenosine
- Thromboxane
- 5-HETE
- Angiotensin II
- Prostaglandin E2
- Aldosterone

6. Which of the following is false regarding decerebrate rigidity?

A. Flexion of upper limb, extension of lower limb

B. Lesion between superior and inferior colliculi produces rigidity

C. Cutting the dorsal root will abolish rigidity

D. Both upper and lower limbs are extended

Answer: Option A. Flexion of upper limb, extension of lower limb

Explanation:

Flexion of upper limb and extension of lower limb is seen in decorticate rigidity which is seen in decortications (removal of the cerebral cortex).

Decerebrate Rigidity (Mid-Collicular Transection)

Two brainstem centers that are very important to the maintenance of muscle tone in antigravity muscles (primarily extensors) are the pontine reticular formation (medial reticulospinal tract), and Deiter's nucleus (lateral vestibulospinal tract).

Both centers have an excitatory influence on extensors.

Stimulation of cells in the pontine reticular formation has a very powerful excitatory effect on extensors, but its activity is normally modulated (inhibited) by central (cortical) projections.

If the spinal cord is cut above the level of the pontine reticular formation (mid collicular–A complete transection of the brainstem between the superior and inferior colliculi), the inhibitory influence is removed and there is an exaggerated activation of muscle tone in extensors (antigravity muscles).

This produces a rigid posture which is referred to as decerebrate rigidity.

In humans arms and legs are extended, back is arched, head dorsiflexed, and feet ventroflexed (curling of toes lifts against gravity). This stiff posture does not permit joints to bend and the body is capable of standing upright.

Gamma rigidity–Cutting the dorsal roots abolishes decerebrate rigidity. Cutting the Ia spindle afferents interrupts the myotatic stretch reflex. This demonstrates that the decerebrate rigidity was primarily due to the hypersensitivity of muscle spindles resulting from descending excitation of gamma motoneurons. Removal of the gamma contribution abolishes the rigidity. ***Therefore, decerebrate rigidity is considered primarily a gamma rigidity***.

Alpha rigidity–A selective increase in alpha motoneuron activity can produce what is referred to as alpha rigidity. This can be demonstrated after reversing decerebrate rigidity caused by gamma excitability (cutting the dorsal roots) and increasing the excitation of alpha motoneurons.

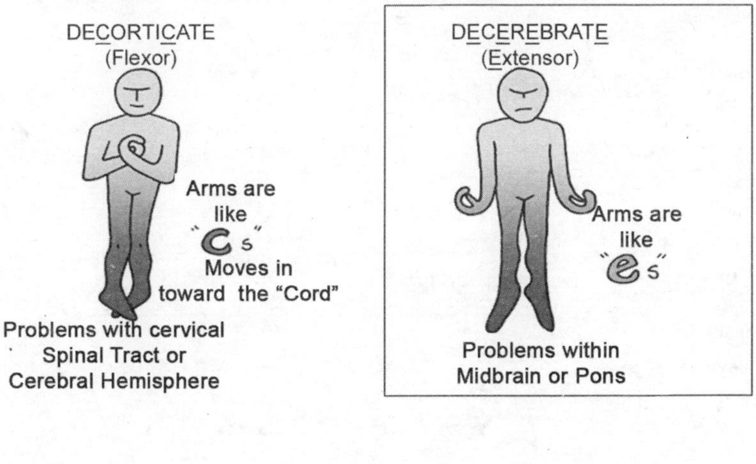

7. Which of the following is not a dietary fiber?

A. Inulin
B. Lignin
C. Gum
D. Cellulose

Answer: Option C. Gum

Explanation:

Mainly Dietary fiber consists of non-starch polysaccharides and other plant components such as cellulose, resistant starch, resistant dextrins, inulin, lignins, chitins, pectins, beta-glucans and oligosaccharide.

Gums (also a fiber) are polysaccharides of mainly natural origin, capable of causing a large increase in a solution's viscosity, even at small concentrations. They are mostly botanical gums, found in the woody elements of plants or in seed coatings. **But they are used in the food industry as thickening agents, gelling agents, emulsifying agents, and stabilizers, and in other industries as adhesives, binding agents, crystal inhibitors, clarifying agents, encapsulating agents, flocculating agents, swelling agents, foam stabilizers, etc.**

Note: Gum fiber supplements are relatively new to the market. Often sold as a powder, vegetable gum fibers dissolve easily with no aftertaste. In preliminary clinical trials, they have proven effective for the treatment of irritable bowel syndrome. Examples of vegetable gum fibers are guar gum and gum arabic.

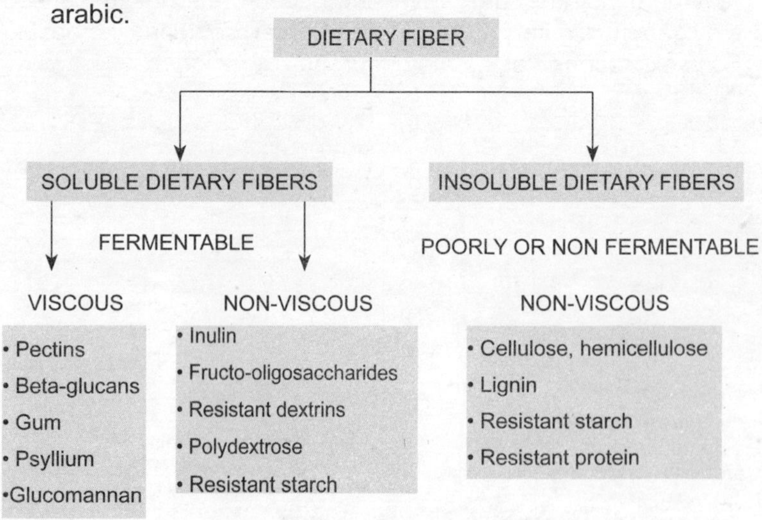

Recent definition of dietary fibers according to British Nutrition Foundation (2018)

Dietary fibers refers to a group of substances in plant foods which cannot be completely broken down by human digestive enzymes. This includes waxes, lignin and polysaccharides such as cellulose and pectin. Originally it was thought that dietary fiber was completely indigestible and did not provide any energy. It is now known that some fiber can be fermented in the large intestine by gut bacteria, producing short chain fatty acids and gases.

Effects

- Increases food volume without increasing caloric content to the same extent as digestible carbohydrates, providing satiety which may reduce appetite.
- Lowers total and LDL cholesterol, which may reduce the risk of cardiovascular disease.
- Regulates Post-prandial blood sugar, which may reduce glucose and insulin levels in diabetic patients and may lower risk of diabetes.
- Speeds the passage of foods through the digestive system, which facilitates regular defecation.
- Attracts water and forms a viscous gel during digestion, slowing the emptying of the stomach and intestinal transit, shielding carbohydrates from enzymes, and delaying absorption of glucose, which lowers variance in blood sugar levels.
- Adds bulk to the stool, which alleviates constipation thereby protect from colonic cancer and reduces incidence of irritable bowel syndrome and diverticulitis.
- Balances intestinal pH and stimulates intestinal fermentation production of short-chain fatty acids.

8. Which of the following centre is responsible for forced respiration outburst during excecise?

A. Pneumotaxic centre

B. Apneustic centre

C. Ventral respiratory group

D. Dorsal respiratory group

Answer: Option C. Ventral respiratory neurons

Explanation:

A part of **Ventral respiratory group (VRG)**, known as Pre-Bötzinger complex is the rhythm generator of respiration. The abrupt increase in ventilation at the start of exercise is due to psychic stimuli and afferent impulses from proprioceptors in muscles, tendons and joints. Increase body temperature and K^+ level also play a role in later part. All of these act through stimulation of VRG.

Pre-Bötzinger complex (pre-BÖTC): Known as pacemaker cells of respiration or, central pattern generator.

Located on either side of the medulla between the nucleus ambiguus and the lateral reticular nucleus.

These neurons discharge rhythmically, and they produce rhythmic discharges in phrenic motor neurons.

DRG AND VRG

Dorsal and ventral groups of respiratory neurons (DRG and VRG) are present in the medulla. However, lesions of these neurons do not abolish respiratory activity, and they apparently project to the pre-Bötzinger pacemaker neurons.

DRG contains mainly I (inspiratory neurons) neurons and is part of the nucleus of the solitary tract (or nucleus tractus solitarius, NTS).

The afferent input from arterial chemoreceptors and lung mechanoreceptor synapses on neurons in the NTS near the DRG.

So, major function of DRG is integration of sensory information from respiratory system.

VRG is a column of neurons that fire action potentials in phase with respiration.

It includes neurons depolarizing during inspiration (I neurons) and expiration (E neurons).

All of these respiratory centers are bilaterally symmetrical on the right and left sides of the brainstem.

Pneumotaxic Center – Control rate of breathing.

Located in the medial parabrachial and Kölliker-Fuse nuclei of the dorsolateral pons. Contains both E neurons and I.

The normal function of the pneumotaxic center is unknown, but it may play a role in smooth switching between inspiration and expiration ("fine-tune" the breathing).

A strong pneumotaxic signal can increase the rate of breathing 30–40 breaths per minute, whereas a weak pneumotaxic signal may reduce the rate to only 3–5 breaths per minute.

Apneustic Center – Control depth of respiration.

An area in the caudal (lower part) pons, control depth of breathing by stimulating inspiratory neurons of pre-Bötzinger complex. *The center is tonically active.* This center may act as an integration site for afferent information. The specific group of neurons that function, as the apneustic center has not been identified.

Thus, the term, pneumotaxic and apneustic are primarily used because of their historical significance. Not required for eupnoea.

9. FRC is defined as the volume of air, which remains in lung after:

A. Normal inspiration
B. Normal expiration
C. Full inspiration
D. Full expiration

Answer: Option B. Normal expiration

Explanation:

Functional Residual Capacity (FRC) is the volume of air present in the lungs at the end of normal expiration. At FRC, the opposing elastic recoil forces of the lungs and chest wall are in equilibrium and there is no exertion by the diaphragm or other respiratory muscles.

FRC is the sum of Expiratory Reserve Volume (ERV) and Residual Volume (RV) and measures approximately 2100 mL in a 70 kg, average-sized male (or approximately 30 ml/kg).

It cannot be estimated through spirometry, since it includes the residual volume. In order to measure RV precisely, one would need to perform a test such as nitrogen washout, helium dilution or body plethysmography.

A lowered or elevated FRC is often an indication of some form of respiratory disease. For instance, in emphysema, FRC is increased, because the lungs are more compliant and the equilibrium between the inward recoil of the lungs and outward recoil of the chest wall is disturbed. As such, patients with emphysema often have noticeably broader chests due to the relatively unopposed outward recoil of the chest wall. Total lung capacity also increases, largely as a result of increased functional residual capacity.

In healthy humans, FRC changes with body posture. Obese patients will have a lower FRC in the supine position due to the added tissue weight opposing the outward recoil of the chest wall.

Positioning plays a significant role in altering FRC. It is highest when in an upright position and decreases as one moves from upright to supine/prone or Trendelenburg position. The greatest decrease in FRC occurs when going from 60° to totally supine at 0°. Interestingly, there is no significant change in FRC as position changes from 0° to Trendelenburg of up to -30°. However, beyond -30°, the drop in FRC is considerable.

See Table and Figure on the next page.

10. Antegrade relaxation of intestine during peristalsis is caused by which of the following substance?

A. Serotonin

B. Vasoactive Intestinal Peptide

C. Acetyl choline

D. Substance P

Answer: Option B. Vasoactive Intestinal Peptide

Explanation:

Antegrade relaxation of intestine during peristalsis is caused by **Vasoactive Intestinal Peptide** Nitric Oxide and ATP. Retrograde contraction of intestine during peristalsis is caused by substance P and Ach.

Peristalsis

This is a reflex contraction of the gut wall to stretch (e.g. by food). It is present throughout the GIT **(from the esophagus to the rectum)**. Stretching the gut wall causes a wave of contraction and relaxation, viz. an area of circular contraction behind the stretch and an area of relaxation in front of it.

Q. No. 9

Lung volumes	**Note:** A capacity is a sum of ≥ 2 physiologic volumes.
Inspiratory reserve volume	Air that can still be breathed in after normal inspiration
Tidal volume	Air that moves into lung with each quiet inspiration, typically 500 mL
Expiratory reserve volume	Air that can still be breathed out after normal expiration
Residual volume	Air in lung after maximal expiration; RV and any lung capacity that include RV cannot be measured by spirometry
Inspiratory capacity	IRV + TV Air that can be breathed in after normal exhalation
Functional residual capacity	RV + ERV Volume of gas in lungs after normal expiration
Vital capacity	TV+IRV+ERV Maximum volume of gas that can be expired after a maximal inspiration
Total lung capacity	IRV+TV+ERV+RV Volume of gas present in lungs after a maximal inspiration

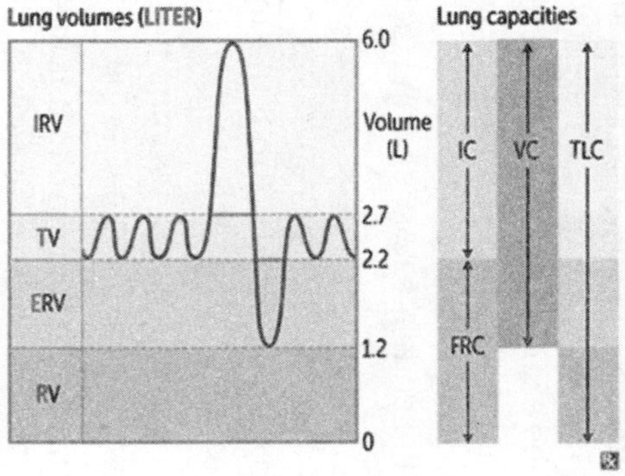

Cause/mechanism: Peristalsis occurs due to the integrated activity of the intrinsic system i.e. the enteric nervous system; however, the input from the extrinsic autonomic nervous system can increase/decrease it. If a segment of intestine is removed and the cut ends are joined in their original position, peristalsis still occurs. However, if the ends are reversed and then joined, peristalsis does not occur.

Possible sequence of events: Stretch→releases *serotonin,* which stimulates the myenteric plexus. From the myenteric plexus, cholinergic neurons go two directions:

(i) In a retrograde direction to activate neurons that release *substance P and acetylcholine* these cause the *contraction.*

(ii) In an anterograde direction to activate neurons that release *NO, VIP and ATP* these cause the relaxation in front of the stimulus.

MIGRATING MOTOR COMPLEX (MMC)

The motor and electrical activities of smooth muscle in GIT that *occur* during *fasting* (between periods of digestion) are called *migrating motor complex* or *MMC.* They are so called because the motor activity starts from the *stomach* and migrates to the *distal ileum.*

Control: Motilin hormone controls MMC. Motilin secreted by Mo cell of stomach and duodenum, jejunum, ileum and colon. Maximum duodenum-Jejunum.

MMC rate:

During the period of *fasting,* MMCs regular rate of approximately **5 cm/min**. They are completely *inhibited* by a *meal;* they *resume 90–120 minutes* **after the meal** and *occur at interval* of about *90 minutes* till the next meal.

11. Which of the following nerve fibers are slowest in conduction of nerve impulse?

A. Proprioceptive

B. Somatic motors

C. Preganglionic sympathetic

D. Postganglionic sympathetic

Answer: Option D. Postganglionic sympathetic

<table>
<tr><th colspan="9">Sensory fiber types</th></tr>
<tr><th>Type</th><th>Erlanger-Gasser Classification</th><th>Diameter (µm)</th><th>Myelin</th><th>Conduction velocity (m/s)</th><th>Associated sensory receptors</th><th>Proprio-ceptors</th><th>Mechano-ceptors</th><th>Nociceptors and thermo-receptors</th></tr>
<tr><td>Ia</td><td>Aα</td><td>13-20</td><td>Yes</td><td>80–120</td><td>Primary receptors of muscle spindle (annulospiral ending)</td><td rowspan="3">√</td><td rowspan="2"></td><td rowspan="3"></td></tr>
<tr><td>Ib</td><td>Aα</td><td>13-20</td><td>Yes</td><td>80–120</td><td>Golgi tendon organ</td></tr>
<tr><td>II</td><td>Aβ</td><td>6-12</td><td>Yes</td><td>33–75</td><td>Secondary receptors of muscle spindle (flower-spray ending). All cutaneous mechanoreceptors</td><td rowspan="2">√</td></tr>
<tr><td>III</td><td>Aδ</td><td>1-5</td><td>Thin</td><td>3–30</td><td>Free nerve endings of touch and pressure
Nociceptors of lateral spinothalamic tract
Cold thermoreceptors</td><td rowspan="2"></td><td rowspan="2">√</td></tr>
<tr><td>IV</td><td>C</td><td>0.2-1.5</td><td>No</td><td>0.5-2.0</td><td>Nociceptors of anterior spinothalamic tract
Warmth receptors</td><td></td></tr>
</table>

Explanation:

Postganglionic sympathetic is type C fiber and they are slowest conducting nerve fibers with velocity around 0.5–2.0 m/s.

Sensory

Different sensory receptors innervate different types of nerve fibers. Proprioceptors are innervated by type Ia, Ib and II sensory fibers, mechanoreceptors by type II and III sensory fibers and nociceptors and thermoreceptors by type III and IV sensory fibers.

Motor

Lower motor neurons have two kind of fibers:

Motor fiber types					
Type	**Erlanger-Gasser Classification**	**Diameter (μm)**	**Myelin**	**Conduction velocity (m/s)**	**Associated muscle fibers**
α	Aα	13-20	Yes	80–120	Extrafusal muscle fibers
β	Aβ				
γ	Aγ	5-8	Yes	4–24	Intrafusal muscle fibers

Autonomic

The autonomic nervous system has two kinds of peripheral fibers:

Fiber types				
Type	**Erlanger-Gasser Classification**	**Diameter (μm)**	**Myelin**	**Conduction velocity (m/s)**
Preganglionic fibers	B	1–5	Yes	3–15
Postganglionic fibers	C	0.2–1.5	No	0.5–2.0

12. Which of the following hormone is released by corpus luteum after ovulation?

A. Progesterone

B. Estrogen

C. LH

D. Inhibin

Answer: Option A. Progesterone

Explanation:

Ovarian phases	Uterine (endometrial) phase	Events
Follicular phase (Days 1–14)	Menstrual phase (Days 1–5)	Withdrawal of the hormonal support of the endometrium at this time causes necrosis and menstruation. Low estrogens and progesterone
	Proliferative phase (Days 6–14)	This phase is dominated by the effects of estrogen, which include the replacement of the endometrial cells lost during menses
Ovulation (Day 14)		Characterized by the LH surge, which actually induces ovulation
Luteal phase (Days 15–28)	Secretory phase (Days 15–28)	Dominated by the elevated plasma levels of **progesterone**, which, along with the secreted estrogen, prepares the uterus for implantation

Uterine cycle: Refers to cyclic changes in the endometrium during active reproductive period. These cyclic changes are brought about by the cyclic production of oestrogens and progesterone by the ovaries.

Proliferative phase (estrogen phase)

- FSH secretion is slightly elevated during this phase, causing proliferation of granulosa cells of ovaries, which produces *estrogen*.
- New endometrium then regrows (stromal cells and epithelial cells proliferate) under the influence of estrogens from the developing follicle.

- Increase endometrium thickness continue from 5th to the 14th days of the menstrual cycle.
- Before ovulation, uterine glands are also enlarged. The endometrial glands, especially those of the cervical region, secrete thin, stringy mucus.

Ovulation

- When estrogens rise above a certain level, they no longer inhibit the release of LH and FSH. Instead, they stimulate the release of LH and FSH (negative feedback loop to positive feedback loop).
- This causes a surge in the release of LH and FSH. Only the LH surge is essential for the induction of ovulation and formation of the corpus luteum.

Luteal phase (progestational phase)

- After **ovulation,** the endometrium becomes more highly vascularized and slightly edematous under the influence of estrogen and progesterone from the corpus luteum.
- Once formed, the luteal cells are stimulated by LH to secrete considerable progesterone and some estrogen. Progesterone inhibits LH secretion (negative feedback).
- Progesterone causes marked swelling and secretory development of the endometrium.
- The uterine glands become coiled and tortuous and they begin to secrete a clear fluid.
- In addition, the cytoplasm of the stromal cells increases, lipid and glycogen deposits (**subnuclear vacuolation**) increase greatly in the stromal cells, and the blood supply to the endometrium further increases.

Menstruation

- Progesterone from corpus luteum inhibits the secretion of LH and contributes to the demise of the corpus luteum, because the corpus luteum depends on LH for its continued stimulation.
- When the corpus luteum regresses, lower plasma levels of progesterone (and estradiol) no longer support the endometrium.

- Foci of necrosis appear in the endometrium, and these coalesce. In addition, spasm and degeneration of the walls of the spiral arteries take place, leading to spotty hemorrhages that become confluent and produce the menstrual flow.
- At the end of menstruation, all but the deep layers of the endometrium have sloughed.

13. Which of the following is true about physiological changes in old age?

A. Reduced V/Q mismatch

B. Reduced elastic recoil

C. Increase in mucociliary increase

D. Increase in lung compliance

Answer: Option D. Increase in lung compliance

Explanation:

RESPIRATORY SYSTEM

Lung Volume

A linear decrease of vital capacity is found that amounts to a decrement of about 26 ml per year for men and 22 ml per year for women starting at age 20. The total lung capacity remains constant, however, and thus the residual volume increases with age. The ratio of residual volume to total lung capacity (RV/TLC) is about 20 percent at age 20 and increases to 35 percent by age 60, with most of this increase in RV/TLC occurring after age 40. In most studies the functional residual capacity also increases, although not as rapidly as the residual volume.

Gas Exchange

Although alveolar oxygen tension remains constant with age, arterial oxygen pressure shows a progressive decrease, thus increasing the alveolar arterial oxygen difference (A-a). Most of this decrease in arterial oxygen pressure results from a mismatch of ventilation and perfusion. The elastic recoil of the lungs decreases with age and thus there is a greater tendency for airways to collapse. This is measured as an increase in "closing volume" which increases linearly above the age of

20. Airway closure occurs predominantly in the dependent zones of the lung and in the upright position this will result in a **ventilation-perfusion mismatch** because more perfusion occurs in the lower lobes. Although an age-related decrease in carbon monoxide diffusing capacity has been shown, it is unclear whether this contributes to the reduction in arterial oxygen pressure.

Flow Rates

There is a 20 percent to 30 percent decrease in maximum voluntary ventilation, forced expiratory volume in one second, maximal expiratory flow rate and maximum midexpiratory flow during adult life. The basis for these changes is not known but again may relate to a decrease in the elastic recoil properties of the lung. This would result in both a decreased ability to generate normal expiratory pressures as well as increased resistance to expiration due to abnormally early airway collapse.

Infections

It is well-known that elderly patients have a pronounced increase in incidence of pneumonia, both bacterial and viral, compared with younger persons. Although much of this may be due to a general depression of immune system function, other more specific factors may play a role. Pneumonia generally results from aspiration of oropharyngeal secretions and such aspiration appears more frequent in the elderly. Perhaps of even greater importance, **the normal mechanical clearing of the tracheobronchial tree by the mucociliary apparatus is significantly slower in older persons than in their younger counterparts**. Finally, due perhaps to poor oral hygiene, decreased flow of saliva or difficulty with swallowing, older persons have a higher rate of colonization of their oropharynx with Gram-negative bacilli than do younger persons.

https://www.ncbi.nlm.nih.gov/pmc/articles/PMC1273316/pdf/westjmed00220-0011.pdf

Compliance and elasticity

It is important to remember that compliance is inversely proportional to elasticity, or, elastic recoil. In old age elastic recoil of lung will be reduced and compliance increases. Compliance denotes the ease with which something can be stretched or distorted; elasticity refers to the tendency for something to oppose stretch or distortion, as well as to its ability to return to its original configuration after the distorting force is removed. So, in emphysema: Loss of elastic tissue (less elastic recoiling force) leads to increase compliance.

Compliance increased: *Old age*, Emphysema, asthma and at a minor degree in chronic bronchitis.

Compliance decreased: Pulmonary congestion, pulmonary fibrosis, pulmonary edema, consolidation, atelectasis and pleural effusion.

CHAPTER 3

BIOCHEMISTRY

1. Which of the following is true about type I diabetes?

A. Reduced protein catabolism

B. Increased glucose uptake

C. Increased lipolysis

D. Reduced hepatic glucose output

Answer: Option C. Increased lipolysis

Explanation:

Hyperglycemia in diabetes is mainly due to decreased glucose uptake in muscle and adipose tissue by Glut-4. There is also increased hepatic gluconeogenesis, glycogenlysis and eventually lipolysis result in diabetic ketoacidosis.

Profound metabolic changes occur in people with type 1 diabetes mellitus during insulin deprivation.

These include an increase in basal energy expenditure and reduced mitochondrial function. In addition, protein metabolism is significantly affected during insulin deprivation.

High level of glucagon seen in poorly controlled type 1 diabetic people contributes to their increased energy expenditure and thus to their catabolic state.

High glucagon is likely to increase gluconeogenesis, which is an energy consuming reaction that may also contribute to a hypermetabolic state in T1DM during insulin deprivation.

High glucagon levels, unopposed by insulin, enhance hepatic glucose production which is a key contributor to hyperglycemia, glycosuria, and energy wasting. Thus hyperglucagonemia seems to be a pivotal catabolic factor in T1DM during insulin deprivation.

2. Which of the following protein is not synthesized by liver?

A. Plasma hormone
B. Albumin
C. Acute phase protein
D. Immunoglobulin

Answer: Option D. Immunoglobulin

Explanation:

Immunoglobulins, also known as antibodies, are glycoprotein molecules produced by **plasma cells (white blood cells) not by the liver**.

Major plasma proteins

- **Human serum albumin**, osmolyte and carrier protein
- **α-fetoprotein**, the fetal counterpart of serum albumin
- **Soluble plasma fibronectin**, forming a blood clot that stops bleeding
- **C-reactive protein**, opsonin on microbes
- **Acute phase protein.**

Factors in hemostasis and fibrinolysis

- **Stimulators of coagulation:**
  - **All factors in the coagulation cascade. While the endothelium does produce some factor VIII, the majority of factor VIII is produced in the liver.**
- **Inhibitors of coagulation:** Inactivate an enormous variety of proteinases.
  - **α2-macroglobulin**
  - **α1-antitrypsin**
  - **Antithrombin III**
  - **Protein S**
  - **Protein C**
- **Fibrinolysis:** Breakdown of **fibrin** clots
  - o **Plasminogen**
- **Inhibitors of fibrinolysis**
  - o **α2-antiplasmin**

- **Complement components C1-9, Complement component 3 (C3).**

Carrier proteins

- **Albumin**, carries thyroid hormones and other hormones, particularly fat soluble ones, fatty acids to the liver, unconjugated bilirubin, many drugs and Ca2+
- **Ceruloplasmin**, carries copper
- **Transcortin**, carries cortisol, aldosterone and progesterone
- **Haptoglobin**, carries free hemoglobin released from erythrocytes
- **Hemopexin**, carries free heme released from hemoglobin
- **IGF binding protein**, carries insulin-like growth factor 1
- **Major urinary proteins**, carries pheromones in rodents
- **Retinol binding protein**, carries retinol
- **Sex hormone-binding globulin**, carries sex hormones, specifically testosterone and estradiol
- **Thyroxine-binding globulin**, carries the thyroid hormones thyroxine (T4) and 3,5,3'-triiodothyronine (T3)
- **Transthyretin**, carries the thyroid hormone thyroxine (T4)
- **Transferrin**, carries iron ions in the ferric form (Fe^{3+})
- **Vitamin D-binding protein**, carries vitamin D.

Hormones

- **Insulin-like growth factor 1**, a polypeptide protein hormone which plays an important role in childhood growth and continues to have anabolic effects in adults
- **Thrombopoietin**, a glycoprotein hormone that regulates the production of platelets by the bone marrow
- **Hepcidin**, a peptide hormone that regulates iron homeostasis.

Prohormones

- **Angiotensinogen**, when converted to angiotensin causes vasoconstriction and release of aldosterone, in effect increasing blood pressure.

Apolipoproteins

- Almost all **apolipoprotein**, except apo B48 (produced by intestine)

3. A 25 years old alcoholic male patient presented with dyspnoea with bilateral pedal edema. His pulse rate was 130/min and on auscultation revealed bilateral basal crepitation. Which of the following vitamin deficiency associated with these findings?

A. Vitamin B2 B. Vitamin B6

C. Vitamin B1 D. Vitamin K

Answer: Option C. Vitamin B1

Explanation:

Here above alcoholic patient presented with symptoms and signs of congestive cardiac failure. Thiamine deficiency may presents with features of cardiac failure (called as wet beriberi) and alcohol is a predisposing factor for thiamine deficiency.

THIAMINE (ANEURINE)

Sources

- Aleurone layer of cereals. Hence whole wheat flour and unpolished hand pound rice has better nutritive value. Yeast is also a good source of thiamine.

Active Form of Thiamine

Thiamine Pyrophosphate (TPP) also called Thiamine diphosphate (TDP).

Coenzyme Role of Thiamine Pyrophosphate

Thiamine generally function in the decarboxylation reaction of alpha keto acids and branched chain amino acids.

- **Pyruvate Dehydrogenase** which convert Pyruvate to Acetyl CoA
- **Alpha KetoGlutarate Dehydrogenase** in Citric Acid Cycle which convert α KetoGlutarate to Succinyl CoA
- **Branched Chain Ketoacid Dehydrogenase** which catalyses oxidative decarboxylation of Branched Chain Amino acids

- **Trans Ketolase** in **Pentose Phosphate Pathway**. This is the biochemical basis of assay of Thiamine status of the body.
- **Deficiency of Vitamin B1 (Thiamine)** Beriberi.

Two types

1. **Wet beriberi:** Marked peripheral vasodilatation, resulting in high output cardiac failure with dyspnoea, tachycardia, cardiomegaly, pulmonary and peripheral edema.
2. **Dry beriberi:** Involves both peripheral and central nervous system.

Peripheral nervous system

- Typically a symmetric motor and sensory neuropathy with pain, paraesthesia and loss of reflexes. The legs are affected more than the arms.

Central nervous system

Wernicke's Encephalopathy–in alcoholics with chronic thiamine deficiency

- Horizontal Nystagmus
- Ophthalmoplegia
- Truncal ataxia
- Confusion
- Wernicke-Korsakoff Syndrome
- Along with features of Wernicke's Encephalopathy
- Amnesia
- Confabulatory psychosis.
- *Acute pernicious (fulminating) beriberi (shoshin beri-beri), in which heart failure and metabolic abnormalities predominate.*
- **Biochemical assessment of thiamin deficiency.**

3. **Erythrocyte transketolase activity is reduced.**
4. **Urinary thiamine excretion.**

Thiamine toxicity

- There is no known toxicity of thiamine Recommended Daily Allowance (RDA) of Vitamin B1
- 1–1.5 mg/day

Thiamine and nerve conduction

Thiamine triphosphate has a role in nerve conduction; it phosphorylates, and so activates, a chloride channel in the nerve membrane.

4. Which of the following amino acid is required for conversion of norepinephrine to epinephrine?

A. Cysteine B. Arginine

C. Methionine D. Glycine

Answer: Option C. Methionine

Explanation:

Conversion of norepinephrine to epinephrine is a transmethylation reaction which is caused by S-Adenosyl Methionine.

Phenylethanolamine N-methyltransferase (PNMT) is an enzyme found primarily in the adrenal medulla that converts norepinephrine (noradrenaline) to epinephrine (adrenaline).

Examples of transmethyl reactions:

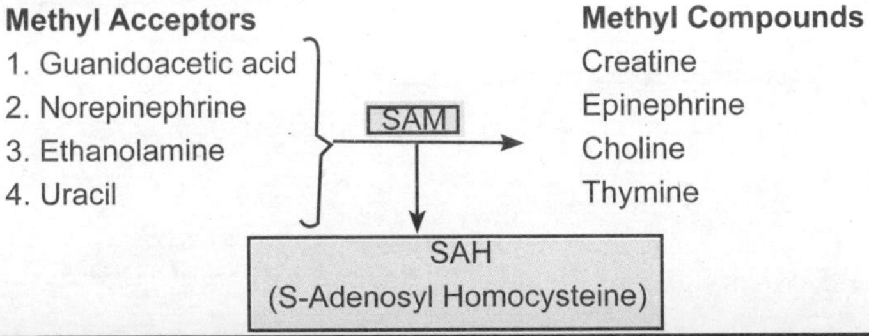

5. Which of the following amino acid is related with formation of urea, nitric oxide, creatinine?

A. Glutamate B. Aspartate

C. Arginine D. Glycine

Answer: Option C. Arginine

Explanation:

Arginine is included in group of basic aminoacid.

It is a semi essential glucogenic aminoacid.

Arginine is involved in synthesis of:

- Urea (At terminal step of urea cycle, arginine splits to urea and ornithine)
- Creatinine
- Nitric oxide (Arginine splits into Nitric oxide and citruline by enzyme nitric oxide synthetase)
- Agmantine (an aminoguanidine).

6. Which of the following is amino acid associated with linkage of Krebs's cycle with urea cycle?

A. Arginine
B. Alanine
C. Fumarate
D. Aspartate

Answer: Option D. Aspartate

Explanation:

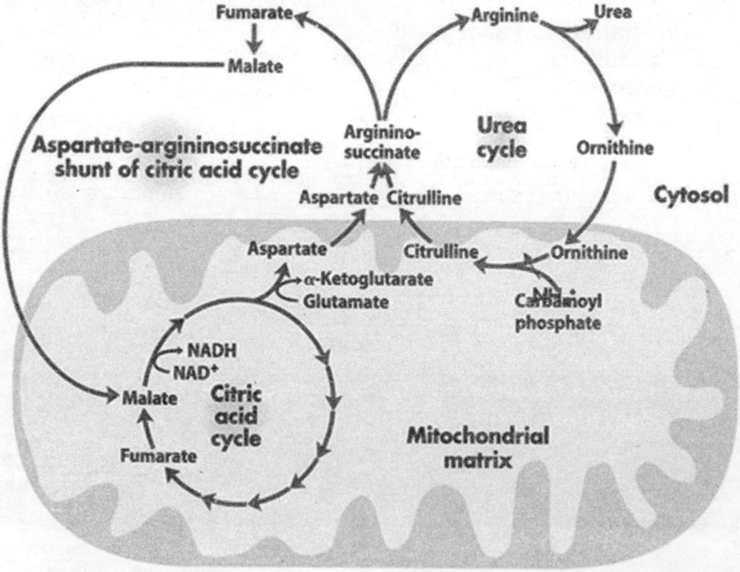

Aspartate is amino acid associated with linkage of Krebs cycle with urea cycle.

It is well known from given image that the fumarate that is released from argininosuccinate is converted into malate and then to oxaloacetate by making use of the TCA cycle enzymes, fumarase and malate dehydrogenase, respectively.

This oxaloacetate then undergoes transamination with glutamate to regenerate aspartate, which is then re-used by the urea cycle.

In urea cycle a condensation reaction occurs between the amino group of aspartate and the carbonyl group of citrulline to form argininosuccinate.

This reaction is ATP dependent and is catalyzed by argininosuccinate synthetase.

Now argininosuccinate undergoes cleavage by argininosuccinase to form arginine and fumarate.

And arginine is cleaved by arginase to form urea and ornithine. The ornithine is then transported back to the mitochondria to begin the urea cycle again.

7. Which is of the following is not a ribozyme?

A. Ribonuclease P B. Poly A polymerase

C. Peptidyl transferase D. RNase p

Answer: Option B. Poly A polymerase

Explanation:

Poly A Polymerase (PAP) is a template-independent polymerase that belongs to the **DNA** polymerase beta (polβ) family of enzymes. It functions as part of the cleavage/polyadenylation complex.

Ribozymes are essentially **RNA** molecules that are capable of catalyzing a chemical reaction.

Ribozymes are non-proteinaceous enzymes.

Ribonuclease P (*RNase P*) is a type of ribonuclease which cleaves RNA. RNase P is unique from other RNases in that it is a ribozyme – a ribonucleic acid that acts as a catalyst in the same way that a protein-based enzyme would. Its function is to cleave off an extra, or precursor, sequence of RNA on tRNA molecules.

Ribozyme is RNA with catalytic activity, ***e.g. Sn RNA in Spliceosom.*** *Below are the examples:*

- RNase P
- Peptidyl transferase 23S rRNA
- GIR1 branching ribozyme
- Leadzyme
- Group I and Group II introns
- Hairpin ribozyme
- Hammerhead ribozyme
- HDV ribozyme
- VS ribozyme
- Mammalian CPEB3 ribozyme
- CoTC ribozyme
- glmS ribozyme

Function:

The most common activities of natural or in vitro-evolved ribozymes are the cleavage or ligation of RNA and DNA and peptide bond formation. Within the ribosome, ribozymes function as part of the large subunit ribosomal RNA to link amino acids during protein synthesis. They also participate in a variety of RNA processing reactions, including RNA splicing, viral replication and transfer RNA biosynthesis.

8. Which of the following enzyme is not the source of cytosolic NADPH?

A. G6PD
B. Malic enzyme
C. Iso citrate dehydrogenase
D. ATP citrate lyase

Answer: Option D. ATP citrate lyase

Explanation:

ATP citrate lyase is an enzyme that in animals represents an important step in fatty acid biosynthesis.

NADPH

- **Main source of NADPH is HMP pathway** (pentose phosphate pathway) (G6PD enzyme).
- **Malic enzyme.**
- **The extra mitochondrial isocitrate dehydrogenase.**

- **Glutamate dehydrogenase.**
- **Nicotinamide nucleotide transhydrogenase.**

Nicotinamide adenine dinucleotide phosphate, abbreviated **NADP⁺** or, in older notation, **TPN** (triphosphopyridine nucleotide), is a cofactor used in anabolic reactions, such as lipid and nucleic acid synthesis, which require NADPH as a reducing agent.

NADPH is the reduced form of $NADP^+$. $NADP^+$ differs from NAD+ in the presence of an additional phosphate group on the 2′ position of the ribose ring that carries the adenine moiety.

The isocitrate dehydrogenase mechanism appears to be the major source of NADPH in fat and possibly also liver cells. Also, in mitochondria, NADH kinase produces NADPH and ADP, using NADH and ATP as substrates.

Uses of NADPH

NADPH provides the reducing equivalents for biosynthetic reactions and the oxidation-reduction involved in protecting against the toxicity of reactive oxygen species (ROS), allowing the regeneration of glutathione (GSH). **Prevent oxidative Damage—RBC, Lens by keeping glutathione in the reduced state.**

NADPH is also used for anabolic pathways, such as cholesterol synthesis and fatty acid chain elongation.

The NADPH system is also responsible for generating free radicals in immune cells. These radicals are used to destroy pathogens in a process termed the respiratory burst. It is the source of reducing equivalents for cytochrome P450 hydroxylation of aromatic compounds, steroids, alcohols and drugs.

9. In a patient with Lecithin–cholesterol acyltransferase (LCAT) deficiency, which of the following substance is reduced after fatty meal?

A. LDL B. Chylomicrons

C. HDL D. VLDL

Answer: Option C. HDL

Explanation:

Lecithin cholesterol acyltransferase catalyzes the formation of cholesterol esters in lipoproteins.

A deficiency of LCAT causes accumulation of unesterified cholesterol in certain body tissues. Cholesterol effluxes from cells as free cholesterol and is transported in HDL as esterified cholesterol. LCAT is the enzyme that esterifies the free cholesterol on HDL to cholesterol ester and allows the maturation of HDL. LCAT deficiency does not allow for HDL maturation resulting in its rapid catabolism of circulating apoA-1 and apoA-2. **Resulting in reduction of HDL.**

Lecithin cholesterol acyltransferase deficiency (**LCAT deficiency**) is a disorder of lipoprotein metabolism. The disease has two forms:

- Familial LCAT deficiency, in which there is complete LCAT deficiency, and
- **Fish-eye disease**, in which there is a partial deficiency.

Complete LCAT Deficiency or Norum's Disease

- Corneal opacity
- Hemolytic anemia
- Progress to ESRD

Biochemical abnormalities

- Very low levels of HDL-C
- Reduction in HDL, Cholesterol and Lysolecithin
- Rise in free cholesterol
- Rise in lecithin.

Partial LCAT deficiency (Fish-eye disease)

Same features as classic LCAT deficiency, but no Hemolytic Anemia and do not progress to ESRD.

10. Which of the following enzyme is deficient in a patient with Menkes disease?

A. Prolyl oxidase
B. Lysyl oxidase
C. Prolyl hydroxylase
D. Lysyl hydroxylase

Answer: Option B. Lysyl Oxidase

Explanation:

Menke's (kinky hair kinky vessel syndrome or Steely, trichopoliodystrophy) Syndrome caused by deficiency of lysyl oxidase.

It is an X-linked recessive disorder that caused by mutation in *ATP7A gene* that result in defective Copper binding P-type ATPase and derangement in copper handling. Copper is not mobilized from Intestine.

It results in low copper levels and subsequently, deficiency in copper-dependent mitochondrial enzymes.

Diseases Associated with Collagen

Disease	Type of collagen	Gene or enzyme
Menke's disease	Lysyl oxidase	Lysyl oxidase
Osteogenesis Imperfecta Osteoporosis Ehlers-Danlos Syndrome (Type VII EDS)	Type I	COL1A1 and COL1A2
Chondrodysplasias Osteoarthritis	Type II	COL2A1
Ehlers-Danlos syndrome (Type IV EDS)	Type III	COL3A1
Alport syndrome (including both autosomal and X-linked forms)	Type IV	COL4A3 to COL4A6
Classical EDS	Type V	COL 5A1, COL 5A2
Hypermobile EDS (Type III EDS)	Type III	COL3A1 Tenascin XB (TNXB)
Epidermolysis bullosa, dystrophic	Type VII	COL7A1
Schmid metaphysial chondrodysplasia	Type X	COL10A1
Ehlers-Danlos syndrome (Type VI EDS) (Kyphoscoliotic EDS) Scurvy	Lysyl hydroxylase	Lysyl hydroxylase

11. Which of the following enzyme defect is associated with high glutamine in serum, CSF and urine?

A. Arginase

B. Lyase

C. Ornithine transcarbamylase

D. Carbamoyl phosphate synthetase I (CPS I)

Answer: Option C. Ornithine transcarbamylase

Ornithine transcarbamylase enzyme defect is associated with high glutamine in serum, CSF and urine.

Ornithine transcarbamylase (**OTC**) (also called **ornithine carbamoyltransferase**) is an enzyme that catalyzes the reaction between carbamoyl phosphate (CP) and ornithine (Orn) to form citrulline (Cit) and phosphate (P_i).

If a person is deficient in OTC, ammonia levels will build up, and this will cause neurological problems. Levels of the amino acids glutamate and alanine will be increased (as these are the amino acids that receive nitrogen from others).

Features of OTC deficiency

The typical initial symptoms of a child with hyperammonemia are non-specific: failure to feed, loss of thermoregulation with a low core temperature, and somnolence. Symptoms progress from somnolence to lethargy and coma. Abnormal posturing and encephalopathy are often related to the degree of central nervous system swelling and pressure upon the brainstem. About 50% of neonates with severe hyperammonemia have seizures.

Hyperventilation, secondary to cerebral edema, is a common early finding in a hyperammonemic attack, which causes a respiratory alkalosis. Hypoventilation and respiratory arrest follow, as pressure increases on the brainstem. In milder (or partial) urea cycle enzyme deficiencies, ammonia accumulation may be triggered by illness or stress at almost any time of life, resulting in multiple mild elevations of plasma ammonia concentration.

Levels of urea cycle intermediates may be decreased, as carbamoyl phosphate cannot replenish the cycle. The carbamoyl phosphate instead goes into the uridine monophosphate synthetic pathway. Here, orotic acid (one step of this alternative pathway) levels in the blood are increased.

Treatment for the high ammonia levels is to give ***sodium benzoate***, which combines with glycine to produce hippurate, at the same time removing an ammonium group. Biotin also plays an important role in the functioning of the OTC enzyme.

12. Ammonia toxicity causes depletion which of the following amino acid in TCA cycle?

A. Fumarate
B. Malate
C. Alpha keto glutarate
D. Oxalo succinate

Answer: Option C. Alpha keto glutarate

As the concentration of ammonia rises, there is increase in formation of glutamate from keto glutarate. Eventually reduction of alpha keto glutarate.

Ammonia is highly toxic. Normally blood ammonium concentration is < 50 μmol/L, and an increase to only 100 μmol/L can lead to disturbance of consciousness. A blood ammonium concentration of 200 μmol/L is associated with coma and convulsions.

200 μmol/L is far too low a concentration of ammonium to affect plasma pH or the normal transport of sodium and potassium ions across nerve cell membranes.

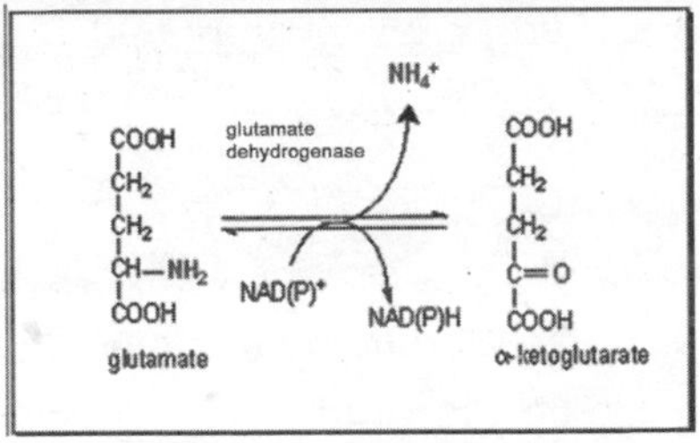

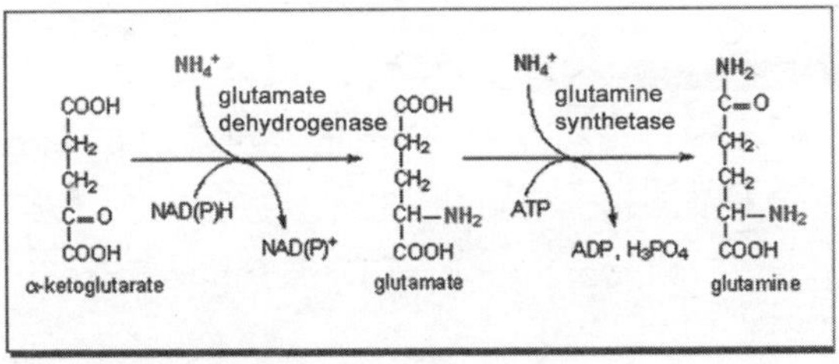

The explanation of the toxicity of such (relatively) low concentrations of ammonium lies with the enzyme glutamate dehydrogenase. This enzyme catalyses the oxidative deamination of glutamate to ammonium and keto glutarate; the reaction is readily reversible, and the direction of reaction (towards deamination of glutamate or glutamate formation) depends on the relative concentrations of the various substrates. As the concentration of ammonium rises, so the reaction proceeds in the direction of formation of glutamate from keto glutarate.

The effect of forming glutamate from keto glutarate is to deplete the mitochondrial pool of keto glutarate, which is a key intermediate in the citric acid cycle. As a result, the rate of citric acid cycle activity falls, so reducing very considerably the rate of formation of ATP.

It is this lack of ATP that affects ion transport across nerve cell membranes, so resulting in disturbance, then loss, of consciousness.

Ammonium is produced in most cells of the body, as a result of deamination of amino acids and amines. It is exported into the bloodstream as glutamine, formed by the actions of glutamate dehydrogenase, to form glutamate from keto glutarate and ammonium, then glutamine synthetase, forming glutamine from glutamate and ammonium.

13. Which of the following fatty acid deficiency associated with retinitis pigmentosa?

A. Eicosa pentaenoic acid
B. Arachidonic acid
C. Docosa Hexanoic acid
D. Palmitic acid

Answer: Option C. Docosa Hexanoic acid

Low Docosa Hexanoic acid (DHA) is associated with increased risk of Retinitis Pigmentosa.

DOCOSA HEXAENOIC ACID (DHA)

- *Sources:* Human milk, Fish liver oils, Algal oils.
- Synthesized in the body from α Linolenic acid.
- Highest concentration of DHA found in retina, cerebral cortex, sperms.
- *Functions:* Needed for the development of fetal brain and retina.
- DHA is supplied transplacentally and through breast milk.

Retinitis pigmentosa (RP) is one of the most common forms of inherited retinal degeneration. There is no cure of it. **Docosa Hexanoic acid** and Vitamin A palmitate supplements may be useful to slow worsening.

CHAPTER

4 PHARMACOLOGY

1. Highest bioavailability is for which of the following fluoroquinolone?

A. Norfloxacin

B. Gemifloxacin

C. Ciprofloxacin

D. Levofloxacin

Answer: Option B. Levofloxacin

Explanation:

Oral bioavailability of levofloxacin is nearly 100%; oral and I.V. Doses are similar. From above given options, levofloxacin has highest bioavailability.

Levofloxacin: It is the active levo(s) isomer of ofloxacin having improved activity against Strep. pneumoniae and some other gram-positive and gram-negative bacteria. Anaerobes are moderately susceptible.

Oral bioavailability of levofloxacin is nearly 100%; oral and I.V. doses are similar. It is mainly excreted unchanged, and a single daily dose is sufficient because of slower elimination and higher potency.

Theophylline, warfarin, cyclosporine and zidovudine pharmacokinetics has been found to remain unchanged during levofloxacin treatment. The primary indication of levofloxacin is community acquired pneumonia and exacerbations of chronic bronchitis in which upto 90% cure rate has been obtained. High cure rates have been noted in sinusitis, pyelonephritis, prostatitis and other UTI, as well as skin/soft tissue infections.

Pharmacokinetics of fluoroquinolones

		CIPROFL	NORFL	PEFL	OFL	LEVOFL	GEMI	PRULI	MOXI
1.	Oral bioavailability (%)	68-80	35-45	90-100	85-95	~100	70	90	85
2.	Plasma protein binding (%)	20-35	15	20-30	25	25	55-73	45	40
3.	Vol. of distribution (L/Kg)	3-4	2	2	1.5	1.3	–	–	2
4.	Percent metabolized	20	25	85	5-10	5	–	>90	70-80
5.	Elimination t1/2 (hr)	3-5	4-6	8-14	5-8	8	7	10-12	10-15
6.	Routes of administration	Oral, I.V.	Oral	Oral, I.V.	Oral, I.V.	Oral, I.V.	Oral	Oral	Oral, I.V.
7.	Dose (mg) : Oral	250-750 (BD)	400 (BD)	400 (BD)	200-400 (BD)	500 (OD)	320 (OD)	600 (OD)	400 (OD)
	: IV	100-200	–	400	200	500	–	–	400

2. Drug useful in smoking cessation:

A. Varenicline B. Acamprosate

C. Amitryptiline D. Bucarciline

Answer: Option A. Varenicline

Explanation:

Varenicline, a synthetic drug is an effective agent for smoking cessation.

Treatment of smoking cessation/quitting tobacco chewing

Majority of smokers (and tobacco chewers) wish to quit smoking/chewing, but fail to do so because of nicotine dependence.

The most important measure to help smokers quit is counseling and motivation.

This may be supplemented by pharmacotherapy.

The goals of such pharmacotherapy are:

- To reduce the craving for the satisfying (reward) effects of nicotine.
- To suppress the physical withdrawal symptoms of nicotine.

The drugs currently utilized for the above goals are:

- Nicotine replacement
- Partial agonists of α4β2 subtype NRs (Varenicline)
- Antidepressants (Bupropion)

Varenicline

This NR selective partial agonist has been marketed as oral tablets to help smoking cessation. Recent evidence has shown that the reward (reinforcing) action of nicotine is exerted through the α4β2 subtype of neuronal NRs, which are mainly localized in nucleus accumbens and other mesolimbic areas.

Activation of these NRs by nicotine induces DA release, which produces feelings of satisfaction/reward and has reinforcing effect.

Since varenicline is a partial agonist at these receptors, it provides some level of nicotine substitution, but blocks the reward effect of smoking. Clinically it has been found to reduce craving as well as nicotine withdrawal symptoms in those who stop smoking. Abstinence rates at one year of cessation are comparable to those of nicotine replacement and of bupropion.

Side effects noted are mood changes, irrational behavior, appetite and taste disturbances, sleep disorder and agitation. Warning has been issued that it may promote suicidal thoughts.

3. Mechanism of action of Oseltamivir is:

A. Neuraminidase inhibition

B. Protein synthesis inhibitor

C. Thymidylate synthetase inhibitor

D. Protease inhibition

Answer: Option A. Neuraminidase inhibition

Explanation:

Oseltamivir acts by inhibiting influenza virus neuraminidase enzyme which is needed for release of progeny virions from the infected cell. Spread of the virus in the body is thus checked. Resistance can develop by mutation of the viral neuraminidase enzyme.

CLASSIFICATION OF ANTI VIRAL DRUGS

1. **Anti-Herpes virus:** Idoxuridine, Trifluridine, Acyclovir, Valacyclovir, Famciclovir, Ganciclovir, Valganciclovir, Cidofovir, Foscarnet, Fomivirsen.
2. **Anti-Influenza virus:** Amantadine, Rimantadine, Oseltamivir, Zanamivir.
3. **Anti-Hepatitis virus/Non-selective antiviral drugs.**

   Primarily for hepatitis B: Lamivudine, Adefovir dipivoxil, Tenofovir.

   Primarily for hepatitis C: Ribavirin, Interferon.
4. **Anti-Retrovirus:**

   (a) *Nucleoside reverse transcriptase inhibitors (NRTIs):* Zidovudine (AZT), Didanosine, Stavudine,Lamivudine, Abacavir, Emtricitabine, Tenofovir (Nt RTI).

   (b) *Nonnucleoside reverse transcriptase inhibitors (NNRTIs):* Nevirapine, Efavirenz, Delavirdine.

(c) *Protease inhibitors:* Ritonavir, Atazanavir, Indinavir, Nelfinavir, Saquinavir, Amprenavir, Lopinavir.

(d) *Entry (Fusion) inhibitor:* Enfuvirtide.

(e) *CCR5 receptor inhibitor:* Maraviroc.

(f) *Integrase inhibitor:* Raltegravir.

Oseltamivir

This newer anti-influenza virus drug is a sialic acid analogue with broad spectrum activity covering influenza A (amantadine sensitive as well as resistant), H5N1 (bird flu), nH1N1 (swine flu) strains and influenza B.

It is an ester prodrug that is rapidly and nearly completely hydrolysed during absorption in intestine and by liver to the active form oseltamivir carboxylate with an oral bioavailability of ~ 80%. The active metabolite is not further metabolized and is excreted by the kidney with a t½ of 6–10 hours.

In many areas oseltamivir-resistant H1N1 (seasonal influenza) and H5N1 have been encountered, though swine flu (nH1N1) is still mostly sensitive. Some oseltamivir-resistant strains remain susceptible to zanamivir and vice versa.

Oseltamivir is indicated both for prophylaxis as well as treatment of influenza A, swine flu, bird flu and influenza B. Started at the onset of symptoms, it is the most effective drug; reduces the severity, duration and complications of the illness. Prophylactic use for 5–10 days prevents illness in contacts of influenza patients.

4. Mannitol is used in which of the following condition?

A. Acute renal failure

B. Pulmonary edema

C. Congestive heart failure

D. Acute congestive glaucoma

Answer: Option D. Acute congestive glaucoma

Explanation:

Mannitol reduces intraocular tension in acute congestive glaucoma by its osmotic action (it encourages movement of water from aqueous humour).

Mannitol is a nonelectrolyte of low molecular weight (182) that is pharmacologically inert—can be given in large quantities sufficient to raise osmolarity of plasma and tubular fluid. It is minimally metabolized in the body; freely filtered at the glomerulus and undergoes limited reabsorption: therefore excellently suited to be used as osmotic diuretic. Mannitol appears to limit tubular water and electrolyte reabsorption in a variety of ways:

- Retains water isoosmotically in PT—dilutes luminal fluid which opposes NaCl reabsorption.
- Inhibits transport processes in the thick AscLH by an unknown mechanism. Quantitatively this appears to be the largest contributor to the diuresis.
- Expands extracellular fluid volume (because it does not enter cells, mannitol draws water from the intracellular compartment)—increases G.F.R. and inhibits renin release.
- Increases renal blood flow, especially to the medulla—medullary hypertonicity is reduced (due to washing off)—corticomedullary osmotic gradient is dissipated—passive salt reabsorption is reduced.

Though the primary action of mannitol is to increase urinary volume, excretion of all cations (Na^+, K^+, Ca^{2+}, Mg^{2+}) and anions (Cl^-, HCO_3^-, PO_4^{3-}) is also enhanced.

Uses

Its indications are:

1. Increased intracranial or intraocular tension (acute congestive glaucoma, head injury, stroke, etc.): by osmotic action it encourages movement of water from brain parenchyma, CSF and aqueous humour; 1–1.5 g/kg is infused over 1 hour as 20% solution to transiently raise plasma osmolarity. It is also used before and after ocular/brain surgery to prevent acute rise in intraocular/intracranial pressure.
2. To maintain GFR and urine flow in impending acute renal failure, e.g. in shock, severe trauma, cardiac surgery, haemolytic reactions: 500–1000 ml of the solution may be infused over 24 hours. However, prognostic benefits in conditions other than cardiac surgery are still unproven. If acute renal failure has already set in, kidney is incapable of forming urine even after an osmotic load; mannitol is

contraindicated: it will then expand plasma volume pulmonary edema and heart failure may develop.

3. To counteract low osmolality of plasma/ECF due to rapid haemodialysis or peritoneal dialysis (dialysis disequilibrium). Mannitol along with large volumes of saline was infused I.V. to produce 'forced diuresis' in acute poisonings in the hope of enhancing excretion of the poison. However, this has been found to be ineffective and to produce electrolyte imbalances. Not recommended now.

Mannitol is contraindicated in acute tubular necrosis, anuria, pulmonary edema; acute left ventricular failure, CHF, cerebral haemorrhage. The most common side effect is headache. Nausea and vomiting may occur; hypersensitivity reactions are rare.

Mannitol is never used for the treatment of chronic edema or as a natriuretic.

5. Drug of choice in a patient with Mastitis:

A. Metronidazole B. Amoxicilin

C. Cloxacilin D. Ampicillin

Answer: Option C. Cloxacilin

Explanation:

Flucloxacillin or dicloxacillin are the antibiotics of choice for mastitis according to the Therapeutic Guidelines. Both antibiotics are compatible with breastfeeding. IV antibiotics should be continued for at least 48 hours or until substantial clinical improvement is seen.

Mastitis is inflammation of the breast or udder, usually associated with breastfeeding. Symptoms typically include local pain and redness. There is often an associated fever and general soreness. Onset is typically fairly rapid and usually occurs within the first few months of delivery. Complications can include abscess formation.

Risk factors include poor latch, cracked nipples, use of a breast pump and weaning. The bacteria most commonly involved are Staphylococcus and Streptococci. Diagnosis is typically based on symptoms. Ultrasound may be useful for detecting a potential abscess.

Prevention is by frequently and properly breastfeeding. Breastfeeding should typically be continued, as emptying the breast is important for healing. Breast abscess is the most common complication of mastitis. It can be prevented by early treatment of mastitis and continued breastfeeding. Once an abscess occurs, surgical drainage or needle aspiration is needed. Breastfeeding can usually continue in the presence of a treated abscess.

6. What is the mechanism of action of Tubocurarine?

A. Non-competitive inhibitor Ach receptor

B. Competitive inhibitor of Ach receptor

C. Causes persistent depolarization

D. Block Ach synapses and release of Ach

Answer: Option B. Competitive inhibitor of Ach receptor

Explanation:

D-tubocurarine is a non-depolarizing muscle relaxants act predominantly at the nicotinic receptor site and block these receptors by competing with acetylcholine (competitive antagonism). This antagonism is surmountable which acetylcholinesterase inhibitors can reverse.

Most of the competitive blockers have two or more quaternary N^+ atoms which provide the necessary attraction to the ACh binding sites, but the bulk of the antagonist molecule does not allow conformational changes in the subunits needed for opening the channel. ACh released from motor nerve endings is not able to combine with its receptors to generate end plate potential (EPP). d-TC thus reduces the frequency of channel opening but not its duration or the conductance of a channel once it has opened. When the magnitude of EPP falls below a critical level, it is unable to trigger propagated muscle action potential (MAP) and muscle fails to contract in response to nerve impulse. At very high concentrations, curare like drugs enter the Na^+ channels and directly block them to produce more intense non-competitive neuromuscular block that is only partly reversed by neostigmine. The competitive blockers also block prejunctional nicotinic receptors located on motor nerve endings.

PERIPHERALLY ACTING MUSCLE RELAXANTS

I. Neuromuscular blocking agents

A. Non-depolarizing (Competitive) blockers

- *Long acting:* d-Tubocurarine, Pancuronium, Doxacurium, Pipecuronium.
- *Intermediate acting:* Vecuronium, Atracurium, Cisatracurium, Rocuronium, Rapacuronium.
- *Short acting:* Mivacurium.

B. Depolarizing blockers

Succinylcholine (SCh., Suxamethonium), Decamethonium (C-10).

II. Directly acting agents

- Dantrolene sodium
- Quinine

Note:

1. Decamethonium is not used clinically.
2. Aminoglycoside, tetracycline, polypeptide antibiotics interfere with neuromuscular transmission at high doses, but are not employed as muscle relaxants.

7. What of the following statement is true about pegylated Filgrastim?

A. It has a short duration of action

B. It reduces neutropenia

C. It is given orally

D. GM CSF activation

Answer: Option B. It reduces neutropenia

Explanation:

Pegfilgrastim is a PEGylated form of the recombinant human granulocyte colony-stimulating factor (GCSF) analog filgrastim. It serves to stimulate the production of white blood cells (neutrophils).

Pegfilgrastim treatment can be used to stimulate bone marrow to produce more neutrophils to fight infection in patients undergoing chemotherapy.

Pegfilgrastim has a human half-life of 15 to 80 hours, much longer than the parent filgrastim (3–4 hours).

It is injected S.C. or I.V. (5 μg/kg) daily, till neutrophil count normalizes, may be used to shorten recovery time from neutropenia.

8. Which of the following drug is used in a differentiation of myasthenia gravis from cholinergic crisis?

A. Pyridostigmine
B. Methacholine
C. Neostigmine
D. Edrophonium

Answer: Option D. Edrophonium

Explanation:

The two types of weakness require opposite treatments.

They can be differentiated by edrophonium test—Inject edrophonium (2 mg. I.V.).

Improvement is there myasthenic crisis. No improvement or worsening – cholinergic crisis.

DIAGNOSTIC TESTS FOR MYASTHENIA GRAVIS

(a) **Ameliorative test:** Initially **edrophonium** 2 mg is injected I.V. as a test dose. If nothing untoward happens, the remaining 8 mg is injected after 30–60 sec. Reversal of weakness and short-lasting improvement in the strength of affected muscles occurs only in myasthenia gravis and not in other muscular dystrophies.

In case edrophonium is not available, the test can be performed with 1.5 mg I.V. neostigmine. Atropine pretreatment may be given to block the muscarinic effects of neostigmine.

(b) **Provocative test:** Myasthenics are highly sensitive to d-tubocurarine; 0.5 mg I.V. causes marked weakness in them but is ineffective in non-myasthenics. This test is hazardous: facilities for positive pressure respiration must be at hand before performing it. This test is better not performed.

(c) Demonstration of anti-NR antibodies in plasma or muscle biopsy specimen is a more reliable test.

9. Antiemetic of choice for chemotherapy induced vomiting:

A. Cyclizine
B. Tegaserod
C. Domperidone
D. Granisetron

Answer: Option D. Granisetron

Explanation:

$5\text{-}HT_3$ ANTAGONISTS Ondansetron, Granisetron, Palonosetron, Ramosetron

Distinct class of antiemetic drugs developed to control cancer chemotherapy/radiotherapy induced vomiting, and highly effective in disease/drug associated vomiting as well.

It blocks the depolarizing action of 5-HT exerted through $5\text{-}HT_3$ receptors on vagal afferents in the G.I.T. as well as in NTS and CTZ. Cytotoxic drugs/radiation produce nausea and vomiting by causing cellular damage→release of mediators including 5-HT from intestinal mucosa→activation of vagal afferents in the gut →emetogenic impulses to the NTS and CTZ. Ondansetron blocks emetogenic impulses both at their peripheral origin and their central relay. It does not block dopamine receptors. Apomorphine or motion sickness induced vomiting is not suppressed.

Granisetron

It is 10 times more potent than ondansetron and probably more effective during the repeat cycle of chemotherapy. The weak $5\text{-}HT_4$ blockade seen in ondansetron has not been detected in granisetron. Its plasma t½ is longer (8–12 hours) and it needs to be given only twice on the day of chemotherapy. Side effect profile is similar to ondansetron.

10. Which of the following causes vasodilatation and inhibits platelet aggregation?

A. PG I2
B. PG E1
C. PG F2
D. PG E2

Answer: Option A. PG I2

Explanation:

A summary of the actions of major prostaglandins, prostacyclin and thromboxane

	Organ	Prostaglandin E_2 (PGE_2)	Prostaglandin F_{2a} (PGF_{2a})	Prostacyclin (PGI_2)	Thromboxane A_2 (TXA_2)
1.	Blood vessels	Vasodilatation, ↓ BP	Vasodilatation (mostly), larger veins constrict, little effect on BP	Vasodilatation (marked and widespread), ↓ ↓ BP	Vasoconstriction
2.	Heart	Weak inotropic, reflex cardiac stimulation	Weak inotropic	–	–
3.	Platelets	Variable effect	–	Anti-aggregatory	Aggregation and release reaction
4.	Uterus	Contraction (*in vivo*), relaxes nongravid human uterus *in vitro*, softening of cervix	Contraction (*in vivo* and *in vitro*) softening of cervix	–	–
5.	Bronchi	Dilatation, Inhibit histamine release	Constriction	Dilatation (mild), ihibit histamine release	Constriction
6.	Stomach	↓ acid secretion ↑ mucus production	–	↓ acid secretion (week), mucosal vasodilatation	–
7.	Intestine	Contracts longitudinal and relaxes circular muscles, ↑ peristalsis, ↑ Cl^- and water secretion	Spasmogenic, ↑ fluid and electrolyte secretion (week)	Weak spasmogenic, inhibit toxin-induced fluid secretion	Weak spasmogenic

Contd.

Contd.

8.	Kidney	Natriuresis, ↓ Cl^- reabsorption, inhibit ADH action, vasodilatation, renin release	–	Natriuresis, vasodilatation, renin release	Vasoconstriction
9.	CNS	Pyrogenic, variety of effects on I.C.V. inj.			
10.	Release of NA	↑ or ↓	↑ or ↓		
11.	Afferent nerves	Sensitize to noxious stimuli → tenderness	–	Same as PGE_2	–
12.	Endocrine system	Release of ant. pituitary hormones, steroids, insulin; TSH-like action	Release of gonadotropins and prolacting, luteolysis (in animals)	–	–
13.	Metabolism	Antilipolytic, insulin like action, mobilization of bone Ca^{2+}	–	–	–

11. Buspirone acts on which receptor?

A. 5-HT 1B
B. 5-HT 1A
C. 5-HT 2A
D. 5-HT 3

Answer: Option B. 5-HT 1A

Explanation:

5-HT$_1$:	Autoreceptors: Inhibit serotonergic neural activity in brain. 5-HT$_{1A}$-Present in raphe nuclei and hippocampus; buspirone (anti anxiety) may act through these receptors. 5-HT$_{1D/1B}$-Constricts cranial blood vessels and inhibits release of inflammatory neuropeptides in them; sumatriptan (anti-migraine) acts through these receptors.
5-HT$_{2A}$:	Previously D type receptor; mot important post junctional receptor mediating direct actions of 5-HT like vascular and visceral smooth muscle contraction, platelet aggregation, neuronal activation in brain; ketanserin blocks these receptors.
5-HT$_3$:	Previously M type receptor; depolarizes neurones by gating caption channels; elicits reflex effects of 5-HT—emesis, gut peristalsis, bradycardia, transient hypotension, apnoea, pain, itch; ondansetron (anti-emetic) acts by blocking these receptors.
5-HT$_4$:	Mediate intestinal secretion, augmentation of peristalsis. Renzapride (prokinetc) is a selective 5-HT$_4$ agonist.

Buspirone

It is the first azapirone, a new class of anti-anxiety drugs, distinctly different from BZDs.

- Does not produce significant sedation or cognitive/functional impairment.
- Does not interact with BZD receptor or modify GABAergic transmission.
- Does not produce tolerance or physical dependence.
- Does not suppress BZD or barbiturate withdrawal syndrome.

- Has no muscle relaxant or anticonvulsant activity.
- Buspirone relieves mild-to-moderate generalized anxiety, but is ineffective in severe cases, in those showing panic reaction and in OCD. The therapeutic effect develops slowly; maximum benefit may be delayed up to 2 weeks.

The mechanism of anxiolytic action is dependent on **its selective partial agonistic action on 5-HT$_{1A}$ receptors**. By stimulating presynaptic 5-HT$_{1A}$ autoreceptors, it reduces the activity of dorsal raphe serotonergic neurons. After chronic treatment, adaptive reduction in cortical 5-HT$_2$ receptors may occur. Buspirone has weak dopamine D2 blocking action but no antipsychotic or extrapyramidal effects. A mild mood elevating action has been noted occasionally, which may be due to facilitation of central noradrenergic system.

Buspirone is rapidly absorbed; undergoes extensive first pass metabolism; (bioavailability <5%), one metabolite is active and excretion occurs both in urine and faeces; t½ is 2–3.5 hours.

Side effects are minor: Dizziness, nausea, headache, light-headedness, rarely excitement. It may cause rise in BP in patients on MAO inhibitors, but does not potentiate CNS depressants. Though most patients on buspirone remain alert, those operating machinery/motor vehicles should be cautioned.

12. Which of the following drug is a direct oral inhibitor of factor Xa?

A. Dabigatran B. Rivaroxaban
C. Lepirudin D. Fondaparinux

Answer: Option B. Rivaroxaban

Explanation:

ANTICOAGULANTS

I. Used in vivo

A. *Parenteral anticoagulants*
   (i) Indirect thrombin inhibitors: Heparin, Low molecular weight heparins, Fondaparinux, Danaparoid
   (ii) Direct thrombin inhibitors: Lepirudin, Bivalirudin, Argatroban

B. *Oral anticoagulants*

(i) Coumarin derivatives: Bishydroxycoumarin (dicumarol), Warfarin sod, Acenocoumarol (Nicoumalone), Ethylbiscoumacetate
(ii) Indandione derivative: Phenindione.
(iii) ***Direct factor Xa inhibitors: Rivaroxaban***
(iv) Oral direct thrombin inhibitor: Dabigatran etexilate

II. Used in vitro

- *Heparin:* Calcium complexing agents: Sodium citrate, Sodium oxalate, Sodium edetate.

Rivaroxaban

It is an orally active direct inhibitor of activated factor Xa which has become available for prophylaxis and treatment of DVT.

Its anticoagulant action develops rapidly within 3–4 hours of ingestion and lasts for ~24 hours. It is largely metabolized, but also excreted unchanged in urine; plasma t1⁄2 is 7–11 hours. Another advantage is that it requires no laboratory monitoring of PT or aPTT, and is recommended in a fixed dose of 10 mg once daily starting 6–10 hours after surgery for prophylaxis of venous thromboembolism following total knee/hip replacement. In comparative trials, its efficacy has been found similar to a regimen of LMW heparin followed by warfarin. Rivaroxaban has also been found equally effective as warfarin for preventing stroke in patients with atrial fibrillation. Side effects reported are bleeding, nausea, hypotension, tachycardia and edema.

13. Which of the following drug is a potassium channel opener?

A. Nicorandil
B. Nifedipine
C. Ranolazine
D. Tedisamil

Answer: Option A. Nicorandil

Explanation:

Nicorandil is Potassium channel opener, which causes hyperpolarization of smooth muscles and hence causes vasodilatation.

Other potassium channel openers examples: Minoxidil, Hydralazine, Diazoxide.

Nicorandil

This dual mechanism antianginal drug activates ATP sensitive K^+ channels (KATP) thereby hyperpolarizing vascular smooth muscle. The vasodilator action is partly antagonized by K^+ channel blocker glibenclamide. Like nitrates it also acts as a NO donor—relaxes blood vessels by increasing cGMP. Thus, arterial dilatation is coupled with venodilatation. Coronary flow is increased; dilatation of both epicardial conducting vessels and deeper resistance vessels has been demonstrated. No significant cardiac effects on contractility and conduction have been noted.

Beneficial effects on angina frequency and exercise tolerance comparable to nitrates and CCBs have been obtained in stable as well as vasospastic angina. Nicorandil is believed to exert cardioprotective action by simulating 'ischaemic preconditioning' as a result of activation of mitochondrial KATP channels. Ischaemic preconditioning is a phenomenon in which brief periods of ischaemia and reperfusion exert a cardioprotective effect on subsequent total vascular occlusion, and involves opening of mito. K_{ATP} channels.

Large painful aphthous ulcers in the mouth, which heal on stopping nicorandil have been reported. Nitrate like tolerance does not occur with nicorandil, but it has the potential to interact with sildenafil.

It may be useful in resistant angina when combined with other drugs. Administered I.V. during angioplasty for acute MI, it is believed to improve outcome.

Vasodilators

Venodilators (primarily ↓ preload)	**Route (for CHF)**
Glyceryl trinitrate	s.l./I.V.
Isosorbide dinitrate	s.l./Oral
Arteriolar dilators (primarily ↓ afterload)	
Pot. channel openers	
Hydralazine	Oral/I.V.
Minoxidil	I.V.
Nicorandil	–
Cal. channel blockers	–

Contd.

Contd.

Mixed ditators (↓ pre- and afterload)	
ACE inhibitors	Oral
ARBs (AT, receptor antagonists)	Oral
α_1 blocker (Prazoin)	–
PDE 3 inhibitors Amrinone, Milrinone	I.V.
Nitroprusside sod.	I.V.

14. Tolvaptan is used in which of the following condition?

A. von Willebrand disease

B. SIADH

C. Central diabetes insipidus

D. Drug resistant shock

Answer: Option B. SIADH

Explanation:

Tolvaptan

This is an orally active non-peptide vasopressin V_2 receptor antagonist introduced recently for the correction of water retention and hyponatremia occurring in **'syndrome of inappropriate ADH secretion' (SIADH)** as well as in advanced CHF. In clinical trials on CHF patients with hyponatremia, tolvaptan has afforded short-term improvement by increasing water excretion, restoring serum Na^+ and relieving dyspnea.

Tolvaptan is Vasopressin receptor antagonist:

FDA approved drug for following indication:

- The treatment of clinically significant hypervolemic and euvolemic hyponatremia [serum sodium <125 mEq/l or less marked hyponatremia that is symptomatic and has resisted correction with fluid restriction], including patients with – heart failure, cirrhosis, and *Syndrome of Inappropriate Antidiuretic Hormone.*

15. Which of the following statement is true regarding randomized clinical trial?

A. Drug efficacy on patient is determined in phase 1

B. Healthy volunteers are included for the first time in phase 2

C. Randomized clinical trial on patient is done in phase 3

D. Phase 4 is pharmacokinetics study in animals

Answer: Option C. Randomized clinical trial on patient is done in phase 3

Explanation:

Corrected options

Drug efficacy on patient is determined in phase 2

Healthy volunteers are included for the first time in phase 1

Phase 4 is postmarketing surveillance/studies.

(See Table and Figure on the next pages):

16. High plasma protein binding leads to which of the following effect?

A. Decrease in glomerular filtration of drug

B. Decrease in drug interaction

C. Increase in tubular secretion of drug

D. Increase in vascular distribution of drug

Answer: Option A. Decrease in glomerular filtration of drug

Explanation:

Plasma protein binding

The clinically significant implications of plasma protein binding are:

(i) **Highly plasma protein bound drugs** are largely restricted to the vascular compartment because protein bound drug does not cross membranes (except through large paracellular spaces, such as in capillaries). They tend to **have smaller volumes of distribution**.

(ii) The bound fraction is not available for action. However, it is in equilibrium with the free drug in plasma and dissociates

Q. No. 15

Typical characteristics of the various phases of the clinical trials required for marketing of new drugs

PHASE I **First in Human**	**PHASE II** **First in Patient**	**PHASE III** **Multi-Site Trial**	**PHASE IV** **Post-Marketing Surveillance**
10-100 participants	50-500 participants	A few hundred to a few thousand participants	Many thousands of participants
Usually healthy volunteers; occasionally patients with advanced or rare disease	Patient-subjects receiving experimental drug	Patient-subjects receiving experimental drug	Patients in treatment with approved drug
Open label	Randomized and controlled (can be placebo-controlled); may be blinded	Randomized and controlled (can be placebo-controlled) or uncontrolled; may be blinded	Open label
Safety and tolerability	Efficacy and dose ranging	Confirm efficacy in larger population	Adverse events, compliance, drug-drug interactions
Months to 1 year	1-2 years	3-5 years	No fixed duration
US $ 10 million	US $ 20 million	US $ 50-100 million	–
Success rate: 50%	Success rate: 30%	Success rate: 25-50%	–

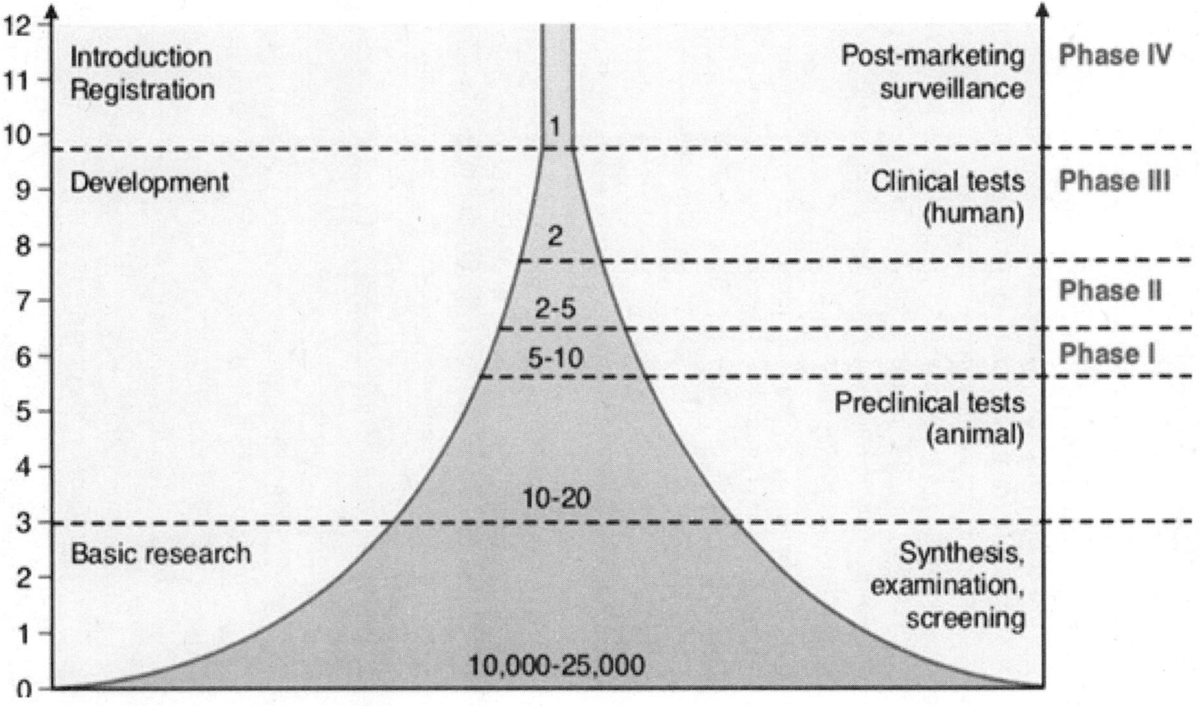
12
11
10
9
8
7
6
5
4
3
2
1
0
Introduction
Registration
Development
Basic research
1
2
2-5
5-10
10-20
10,000-25,000
Post-marketing
surveillance
Clinical tests
(human)
Preclinical tests
(animal)
Synthesis,
examination,
screening
Phase IV
Phase III
Phase II
Phase I

when the concentration of the latter is reduced due to elimination. Plasma protein binding thus tantamount to temporary storage of the drug.

(iii) **High degree of protein binding generally makes the drug long acting, because bound fraction is not available for metabolism or excretion.** Plasma protein binding in acts as a carrier mechanism and hastens drug elimination, e.g., excretion of penicillin (elimination t1⁄2 is 30 min); metabolism of lidocaine. Highly protein bound drugs are not removed by haemodialysis and need special techniques for treatment of poisoning.

(iv) The generally expressed plasma concentrations of the drug refer to bound as well as free drug. Degree of protein binding should be taken into account while relating these to concentrations of the drug that are active in vitro, e.g., MIC of an antimicrobial.

(v) One drug can bind to many sites on the albumin molecule. Conversely, more than one drug can bind to the same site. This can **give rise to displacement interactions among drugs bound to the same site(s)**. The drug bound with higher affinity will displace that bound with lower affinity. If just 1% of a drug that is 99% bound is displaced, the concentration of free form will be doubled. Some clinically important displacement interactions are:

- Aspirin displaces sulfonylureas.
- Indomethacin, phenytoin displace warfarin. Sulfonamides and vit K displace bilirubin (kernicterus in neonates).
- Aspirin displaces methotrexate.

(vi) In hypoalbuminemia, binding may be reduced and high concentrations of free drug may be attained, e.g., phenytoin and furosemide. Other diseases may also alter drug binding, e.g., phenytoin and pethidine binding is reduced in uraemia; propranolol binding is increased in pregnant women and in patients with inflammatory disease (acute phase reactant acid-glycoprotein increases).

Drugs highly bound to plasma protein	
To albumin	**To α_1-acid glycoprotein**
Barbiturates	β-blockers
Benzodiazepine	Bupivacaine
NSAIDs	Lidocaine
Valproic acid	Disopyramide
Phenytoin	Imipramine
Penicillins	Methadone
Sulfonamides	Prazosin
Tetracyclines	Quinidine
Tolbutamide	Varapamil
Warfarin	

17. Variation in sensitivity of response to different doses of a drug in different individual is obtained from:

A. Efficacy

B. Quantal dose response curve

C. Graded dose response curve

D. Potency

Answer: Option B. Quantal dose response curve

Explanation:

Quantal dose-effect curves: A response to a drug such that as the dose is increased the proportion of animals which exhibit a given response is greater. A quantal dose response is all-or-nothing: There either is or is not a response.

Quantal dose-effect curves: Animals were injected with varying doses of a drug and the responses were determined and plotted. The calculation of the therapeutic index, the ratio of the LD_{50} to the ED_{50}, is an indication of how selective a drug is in producing its desired effects relative to its toxicity. **In a quantal dose-response relationship, the percentage of the population affected increases as the dose is raised;** the relationship is quantal in that the effect is specified to be either present or absent in a given individual. This quantal dose-response phenomenon is extremely important in toxicology and is used to determine the *median lethal dose* (LD_{50}) of drugs and other chemicals.

The LD_{50} of a compound is determined experimentally, usually by administration of the chemical to mice or rats (orally or intraperitoneally) at several doses in the lethal range.

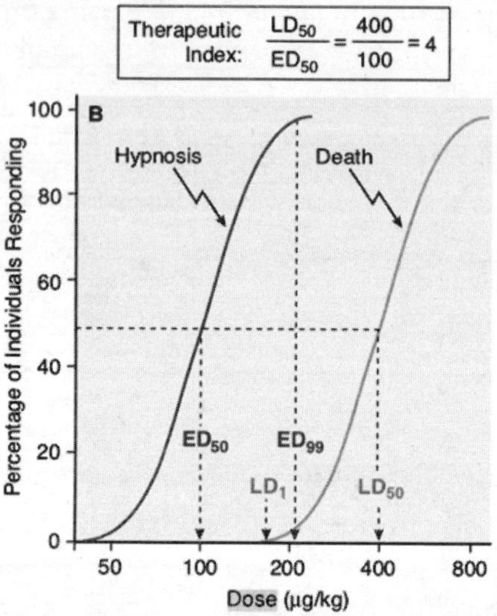

Frequency distribution curves: An experiment was performed on 100 subjects, and the effective plasma concentration that produced a quantal response was determined for each individual. The number of subjects who required each dose is plotted, giving a log-normal frequency distribution (*purple bars*). The red bars demonstrate that the normal frequency distribution, when summated, yields the cumulative frequency distribution—a sigmoidal curve that is a quantal concentration-effect curve.

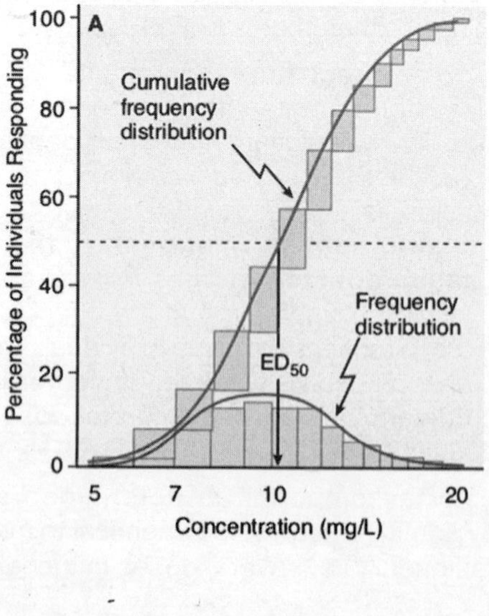

18. Drug used in a patient with scorpion bite with pulmonary edema and hypertension:

A. Prazosin
B. Furosemide
C. Mannitol
D. Clonidine

Answer: Option A. Prazosin

Explanation:

In cases of scorpion bite with cardiac arrhythmia or hypertension, prazosin (30 μg/kg orally every 6 hours for 48 hours or until clinical improvement) can be used, and in combination with immunotherapy, including in remote health centers.

Management of scorpion bite with grades

Grade	Symptoms	Treatment
I	Local pain (sometime associated with local paresthesia, erythema, ecchymosis, blisters)	Aspirin 10 mg/kg orally every 4 hours
II	Mild systemic envenoming: Idem grade I + hyperthermia + Cardiovascular and respiratory symptoms: tachycardia, arrhythmia, dyspnea, **hypertension/hypotension**, electrocardiographic abnormalities, priapism Hypersecretory syndrome (salivation, sweating, bronchorrhea, nausea, vomiting, diarrhea, urination) Digestive tract: abdominal distension, abdominal cramps Neuromuscular disorders: dysfunction of either skeletal or cranial muscles: confusion, agitation, fasciculation, dystonia, vision disorders, ptosis, aberrant eye movements Biological disorders: hyperleucocytosis, hyperglycemia, acidosis	**Prazosin** 30 μg/kg orally every 6 hours Immunotherapy: dose depending on antivenom titer Midazolam 0.05–0.2 mg/kg orally or IV (or diazepam 0.5 mg/kg IV or rectally) every 12 hours

Contd.

Contd.

III	Life-threatening envenoming: idem grade II + multivisceral failure Cardiovascular symptoms: heart failure, cardiogenic shock, pulmonary edema Diaphoresis Neuromuscular disorders: dysfunction of both skeletal and cranial muscles: convulsions, paralysis, Glasgow score ≤6 (in absence of sedation) Biological disorders: SaO_2 < 90%, increasing biomarkers of cellular necrosis, electrolytic anomalies (decrease of Na^+ and Ca^{++}, increase of K^+)	Idem + Transfer to ICU

19. Which of the following is advantage of Cis atracurium over intracurium?

A. Short duration of action
B. Better bioavailability
C. No release of histamine
D. Rapid onset of action

Answer: Option C. No release of histamine

Explanation:

Cisatracurium

This R-Cis, R-Cis enantiomer of atracurium is nearly 4 times more potent, slower in onset, but similar in duration of action. Like atracurium, it undergoes Hofmann elimination, but in contrast it is not hydrolysed by plasma cholinesterase. Most importantly, **it does not provoke histamine release.**

Side effects are fewer.

Comparative property of neuromuscular blocking drugs

Drug	Dose (mg/kg)	Onset (min)	Duration (min)	Hist. release	Gang. block	Vagal block
Long Acting						
1. d-Tubocurarine	0.2–0.4	4–6	30–60	+++	++	±
2. Pancuronium	0.04–0.1	4–6	60–120	±	±	+

Contd.

Contd.

3. Doxacurium	0.03–0.08	4–8	60–120	+	–	–
4. Pipecuronium	0.06–0.08	2–4	50–100	±	–	–
Intermediate Acting						
5. Vecuronium	0.08–0.1	2–4	30–60	±	–	±
6. Atracurium	0.3–0.6	2–4	20–40	+	–	–
7. Cisatracurium	0.15–0.2	3–6	20–40	–	–	–
8. Rocuronium	0.6–0.9	1–2	25–40	–	–	±
Short Acting						
9. Mivacurium	0.15–0.2	2–4	15–30	+	–	–
10. Succinylcholine	0.5–0.8	1–1.5	5–8	++	St.	St.

20. Which of the following carbapenem has maximum seizure activity?

A. Feropenem
B. Doripenem
C. Imipenem
D. Meropenem

Answer: Option C. Imipenem

Explanation:

Imipenem has propensity to induce seizures at higher doses and in predisposed patients. Diarrhoea, vomiting, skin rashes and other hypersensitivity reactions are the side effects.

The adverse effects of *meropenem* **are similar to imipenem, but it is less likely to cause seizures**.

Faropenem

Usual side effects are diarrhoea, abdominal pain, nausea and rashes.

Doripenem

Adverse effects are nausea, diarrhoea, superinfections and phlebitis of the injected vein. **Seizures are less likely.**

21. Mechanism of action of triazole is:

A. Inhibition of mitotic spindle
B. Inhibition of cholesterol synthesis
C. Inhibition of ergosterol synthesis
D. Affect DNA synthesis

Answer: Option C. Inhibition of ergosterol synthesis

Explanation:

The mechanism of action of triazoles.

They inhibit the fungal cytochrome P450 enzyme 'lanosterol 14- demethylase' and thus impair ergosterol synthesis leading to a cascade of membrane abnormalities in the fungus. The lower host toxicity of triazoles compared to imidazoles has correlated with their lower affinity for mammalian CYP450 enzymes and lesser propensity to inhibit mammalian sterol synthesis.

Mutation of the gene encoding for fungal 14-demethylase enzymes underlies azole resistance.

22. Which of the following is a true regarding Teduglutide?

A. It is used in DM type 1

B. It is effective orally

C. It is pancreatic enzyme

D. It is a GLP-2 analogue

Answer: Option D. It is a GLP-2 analogue

Explanation:

Teduglutide (brand names **Gattex** in the US and **Revestive** in Europe) is a 33-membered **polypeptide** and ***glucagon-like peptide-2* (GLP-2)** analog that is used for the treatment of short bowel syndrome. It works by promoting mucosal growth and possibly restoring gastric emptying and secretion. It has been granted orphan drug status.

Medical uses

Up to a certain point, the gut can adapt to partial resections that result in short bowel syndrome. Still, parenteral substitution of water, minerals and vitamins (depending on which part of the gut has been removed) is often necessary. Teduglutide may reduce or shorten the necessity of such infusions by improving the intestinal mucosa and possibly by other mechanisms.

Adverse effects

Abdominal discomfort, respiratory infections, nausea and miting, local reactions at the injection site and headache.

23. Which of the following drug inhibits granulocyte migration?

A. Infliximab
B. Colchicine
C. Aspirin
D. Montelukast

Answer: Option B. Colchicine

Explanation:

Colchicine

Colchicine is neither analgesic nor anti-inflammatory, but it specifically suppresses gouty inflammation. It does not inhibit the synthesis or promote the excretion of uric acid. Thus, it has no effect on blood uric acid levels.

Colchicine does not affect phagocytosis of urate crystals, but inhibits release of chemotactic factors and of the glycoprotein, thus suppressing the subsequent events. **By binding to fibrillar protein tubulin, it inhibits granulocyte migration into the inflamed joint and thus interrupts the vicious cycle**.

Other actions of colchicine are:

(a) Antimitotic: Causes metaphase arrest by binding to microtubules of mitotic spindle. It was tried for cancer chemotherapy but abandoned due to toxicity. It is used to produce polyploidy in plants.

(b) Increases gut motility through neural mechanisms.

Toxicity is high and dose related. Nausea, vomiting, watery or bloody diarrhea and abdominal cramps occur as dose limiting adverse effects. Accumulation of the drug in intestine and inhibition of mitosis in its rapid turnover mucosa is responsible for the toxicity. In overdose, colchicine produces kidney damage, CNS depression, intestinal bleeding; death is due to muscular paralysis and respiratory failure.Chronic therapy with colchicine is not recommended because it causes aplastic anaemia, agranulocytosis, myopathy and loss of hair.

Use

(a) Treatment of acute gout–Colchicine is fastest acting drug to control an acute attack of gout;

(b) Prophylaxis Colchicine 0.5–1 mg/day can prevent further attacks of acute gout, but NSAIDs are generally preferred.

24. Imipenem is generally used with cilastatin, reason for this combination is:

A. Cilastatin increases absorption of Imipenem

B. Cilastatin prevents hydrolysis of Imipenem in intestine

C. Cilastatin prevents hydrolysis of Imipenem in liver

D. Cilastatin prevents hydrolysis of Imipenem in kidney

Answer: Option D. Cilastatin prevents hydrolysis of Imipenem in kidney

Explanation:

Limiting feature of imipenem is its rapid hydrolysis by the enzyme dehydropeptidase I located on the brush border of renal tubular cells. An innovative solution to this problem is its **combination with cilastatin, a reversible inhibitor of dehydropeptidase I,** which has matched pharmacokinetics with imipenem (t½ of both is 1 hour) and protects it.

Imipenem-cilastatin 0.5 g I.V. 6 hourly (max 4 g/day) has proved effective in a wide range of serious hospital-acquired respiratory, urinary, abdominal, pelvic, skin and soft tissue infections including those in neutropenic, cancer and AIDS patients. For Ps. aeruginosa infections, it should be combined with gentamicin.

Meropenem is not hydrolysed by renal peptidase; does not need to be protected by cilastatin.

25. Which of the following statements is true about fixed dose combination of drugs?

A. In a patient of hepatic dysfunction, metabolism of both drugs is altered

B. Dose of any drug of the combination can be altered as per need

C. Adverse effect can be ascribed to a single drug

D. Adverse effect of one drug is neutralized by other drug

Answer: Option D. Adverse effect of one drug is neutralized by other drug

Explanation:

Fixed Dose Combinations (FDCs) of Drugs

A large number of pharmaceutical preparations contain two or more drugs in a fixed dose ratio.

Advantages

- Convenience and better patient compliance—when all the components present in the FDC are actually needed by the patient and their amounts are appropriate. It may also be cost saving compared to both/all the components administered separately.
- Certain drug combinations are synergistic, e.g., sulfamethoxazole + trimethoprim; levodopa + carbidopa/ benserazide; combination oral contraceptives, isoniazid + rifampin.
- The therapeutic effect of two components being same may add up while the side effects being different may not. For this the components of the FDC should act by different mechanisms, e.g., amlodipine + atenolol as antihypertensive.
- **The side effect of one component may be counteracted by the other, e.g. a thiazide + a potassium sparing diuretic. However, the amount of the latter may not be sufficient in all cases.**
- Combined formulation ensures that a single drug will not be administered. This is important in the treatment of tuberculosis, HIV-AIDS and falciparum malaria.

Disadvantages of FDCs:

1. The patient may not actually need all the drugs present in a combination: he is subjected to additional side effects and expense (often due to ignorance of the physician about the exact composition of the combined formulations).
2. The dose of most drugs needs to be adjusted and individualised. When a combined formulation is used, this cannot be done without altering the dose of the other component.
3. The time course of action of the components may be different: administering them at the same intervals may be inappropriate.
4. Altered renal or hepatic function of the patient may differently affect the pharmacokinetics of the components.
5. Adverse effect, when it occurs, cannot be easily ascribed to the particular drug causing it.
6. Contraindication to one component (allergy, other conditions) contraindicates the whole product.

7. Confusion of therapeutic aims and false sense of superiority of two drugs over one is fostered, specially in case of antimicrobials whose combinations should be avoided.

26. Which of the following is the drug of choice in a patient of infection with Cyclospora?

A. Vancomycin

B. Trimethoprim-sulfamethoxazole

C. Penicillin

D. Erythromycin

Answer: Option B. Trimethoprim-sulfamethoxazole

Explanation

(www.cdc.gov/parasites/cyclosporiasis/health_professionals/tx.html)

Trimethoprim-sulfamethoxazole (TMP-SMX), is the treatment of choice in a patient of infection with Cyclospora. The typical regimen for immunocompetent adults is TMP 160 mg plus SMX 800 mg (one double-strength tablet), orally, twice a day, for 7–10 days. HIV-infected patients may need longer courses of therapy.

No highly effective alternatives have been identified yet for persons who are allergic to (or are intolerant of) TMP-SMX. Approaches to consider for such persons include observation and symptomatic treatment, use of an antibiotic whose effectiveness against *Cyclospora* is based on limited data, or desensitization to TMP-SMX. The latter approach should be considered only for selected patients who require treatment, have been evaluated by an allergist, and do not have a life-threatening allergy.

Anecdotal or unpublished data suggest that the following drugs are ineffective: albendazole, trimethoprim (when used as a single agent), azithromycin, nalidixic acid, tinidazole, metronidazole, quinacrine, tetracycline, doxycycline, and diloxanide furoate. Although data from a small study among HIV-infected patients in Haiti suggested that ciprofloxacin might have modest activity against *Cyclospora*, substantial anecdotal experience among many immunocompetent persons suggests that ciprofloxacin is ineffective.

27. Which of the following is a contraindication for acetratin?

A. Severe ichthyosis

B. Pregnancy

C. Psoriasis

D. Lichen planus

Answer: Option B. Pregnancy

Explanation:

Elimination of acitretin is very slow (taking months) because of accumulation in body fat. It is highly teratogenic. Women taking acitretin must not conceive during and till 3 years after stopping it in US and 2 years in Europe. Since it affects cellular differentiation and proliferation. With the use of oral isotretinoin, malformations involving the central nervous system as well as craniofacial, cardiac and thymic structures have been reported and grouped under the term **'retinoic acid embryopathy'** which also comprises – high arched palate, anophthalmia, hip malformation, abnormalities of appendages, multiple synostosis and meningoencephalocele.

Acitretin

It is a synthetic retinoid for oral use in psoriasis, lichen planus, severe ichthyosis, etc.

It acts by binding to 'retinoic acid receptor' in epidermal cells and regulating their proliferation and maturation. Inflammation is suppressed. Because of frequent and potentially serious adverse effects, use of acitretin is restricted to recalcitrant, pustular and other forms of severe psoriasis. Combination with topical antipsoriatic drugs is advised.

Acitretin therapy has distinctive adverse effects generally typical of hypervitaminosis A. While the incidence of mucocutaneous clinical adverse effects is high, their severity does not usually necessitate withdrawal of therapy, and they are completely reversed on cessation of treatment. Adverse effects are usually dose-related, although alopecia is also dependent on the duration of therapy. Mucocutaneous reactions are most common–drying of mucous membranes of the eyes, nose and lips, and cheilitis occurs in nearly all patients. Other clinical symptoms include alopecia, desquamation of the skin, pruritus and 'sticky' skin. Changes in the lipid profile are often observed. Hypertriglyceridaemia occurs in 35% of patients treated with acitretin 50 mg/day, but increases in serum cholesterol are less frequently reported. Liver enzyme levels are also adversely affected, hepatitis has been reported and acitretin therapy may have an adverse effect on bone. Drinking alcohol should be prohibited during and till 3 months after acitretin use.

CHAPTER 5

PATHOLOGY

1. Graft from mother to son is which type of graft?

A. Iso graft
B. Xenograft
C. Allograft
D. Autograft

Answer: Option C. Allograft

Explanation:

Here is a graft from mother to son, means different individuals of same species–Allograft.

Materials and Grafts	Decription	Examples
Autogenous graft	Taken from the same organism (Autologous)	Bone grafts, transplanted teeth, Platelet rich plasma
Allogenic graft	Taken from another individual but same species (Homologous)	Banked bone (Lyophilized)
Xenograft	Taken from another species (Heterologous)	Devitalized deproteinized Bovine bone

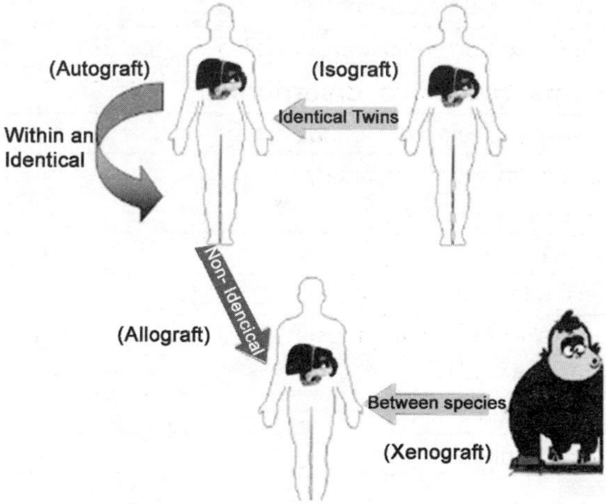

2. Achondroplasia is inherited as:

A. Autosomal recessive
B. Autosomal dominant
C. X-linked recessive
D. X-linked dominant

Answer: Option B. Autosomal dominant

Explanation:

Autosomal dominant disorders

Very **P**rideful **DOMINANT H**asti

Von Willebrand disease/**V**on Hippel-Lindau
Peudo-hypoparathyroidism
Dystrophia myotonica
Osteogenesis imperfecta/**O**sler-Weber-Rendu
Marfan syndrome
Intermittent porphyria
Neurofibromatosis
Achondroplasia/**A**dult polycystic kidney disease
Noonan syndrome
Tuberous sclerosis
Hypercholesterolemia
Huntington's disease
Hypertrophic obstructive cardiomyopathy
Hereditary spherocytosis
Hereditary non-polyposis coli
Hereditary hemorrhagic telangiectasia

Autosomal recessive disorders

Cystic fibrosis, Phenylketonuria
Galactosemia, Homocystinuria
Glycogen storage disease
Sickle cell anaemia
Thalassemias
Congenital Adrenal hyperplasia
Alkaptonuria
Friedrich ataxia
Spinal muscular atrophy

3. Wrong statement about Barret's esophagus is:

A. Predisposed by gastroesophageal reflux

B. Involves lower esophagus

C. Columnar to squamous metaplasia

D. Predisposing factor for carcinoma

Answer: Option C. Columnar to squamous metaplasia

Explanation:

Barrett esophagus is a term for intestinal metaplasia of the esophagus. It is considered the **precursor lesion for esophageal adenocarcinoma.**

Epidemiology

Barrett esophagus is thought to have a prevalence of 3-15% in patients with reflux esophagitis. Mean age at diagnosis is 55 years old. Risk factors are similar to those for **gastroesophageal reflux disease (GORD).**

Scleroderma is thought to be a risk factor, with ~37% of patients (n = 27) who underwent upper endoscopy were found to have Barrett esophagus.

Clinical Presentation

Asymptomatic. Usually discovered in a workup for GORD.

Pathology

Barrett esophagus represents progressive metaplasia of esophageal **stratified squamous cell epithelium to columnar epithelium.** Although the exact number varies, 90-100% of esophageal adenocarcinoma is thought to arise from this metaplasia.

Although patients with Barrett esophagus have a 30x risk of developing esophageal adenocarcinoma 2, the annual risk of developing adenocarcinoma depends on the degree of histological dysplasia, but may be ~1% (range 0.1-2%), and the absolute risk is low.

Radiographic Features

Because Barrett esophagus represents metaplasia, it is often occult on imaging. Early esophageal adenocarcinoma arising out of Barrett esophagus also may be difficult to see. Radiographic imaging modalities are not adequate for screening.

Fluoroscopy

Double-contrast esophagogram.

Signs of reflux esophagitis.

Long stricture in the **mid or lower esophagus.**

Large deep solitary ulcer.

Fine reticular mucosal pattern.

Thickened irregular mucosal folds.

Earliest signs of developing adenocarcinoma: Localised flattening, stiffening, or irregularity in the wall of a stricture. There is a ~70% chance of Barrett esophagus in a mid-thoracic esophageal stricture.

Treatment and Prognosis

Since Barrett esophagus is considered a premalignant lesion, confirmation with upper endoscopy and biopsy is warranted.

If Barrett esophagus is confirmed on biopsy, then aggressive therapy for gastroesophageal reflux is pursued, and perhaps endoscopic surveillance, depending on the patient's age and other risk factors.

One surveillance and biopsy protocol suggests:

Low-grade dysplasia: 6-12 months.

High-grade dysplasia: 3 months.

If there is mucosal irregularity (what would be seen on an esophagogram), then endoscopic resection has been recommended. Prophylactic resection or ablation has been used by some, particularly in younger patients.

4. Cushing ulcer occurs after:

A. Burns

B. Head injury

C. Acid ingestion

D. Food poisoning

Answer: Option B. Head injury

Explanation:

Cushing's ulcer is a gastroduodenal ulcer produced by elevated intracranial pressure caused by an intracranial tumor, head injury or other space-occupying lesion.

The ulcer, usually single and deep, may involve the esophagus, stomach and duodenum.

Increased intracranial pressure may affect different areas of the hypothalamic nuclei or brainstem leading to overstimulation of the vagus nerve or paralysis of the sympathetic system. Both of these circumstances increase secretion of gastric acid and the likelihood of ulceration of gastroduodenal mucosa. In his later years, Cushing suffered from a gastric ulcer, one that he attributed to his stressful efforts to explain this phenomenon.

GASTRODUEODENAL ULCERS

Causes

- Stress
- **Burns=Curling ulcer**
- **Cerebral disease=Cushing ulcer**
- Uremia
- Steroid therapy
- Hyperparathyroidism (25% have ulcer disease)

General Considerations

- Multiple in 2-8%.
- Coexistent duodenal ulcer disease in 5-42%.
- Duodenal to gastric ratio is 3:1.
- Multiple postbulbar duodenal ulcers should suggest Zollinger-Ellison Syndrome.

Location

- Lesser curvature aspect of body and antrum usually for benign ulcers.
- Benign ulcers also occur on posterior wall; not usually anterior wall.
- May be found in proximal half of stomach in geriatric patient.
- Almost all lesser curvature gastric ulcers <1cm are benign.
- Greater curvature benign ulcers are associated with consi-

derable mass effect which erroneously leads to conclusion of malignancy.

Imaging Findings of Benign Ulcers

- Two prerequisites for diagnosis of an ulcer:
  - Collection
  - Persistent
- Ulcer crater-collection of barium on dependent surface which usually projects beyond anticipated wall of stomach in profile (penetration).
- Hampton's line–1 mm thin straight line at neck of ulcer in profile view which represents the thin rim of undermined gastric mucosa.
- Ulcer collar–smooth, thick, lucent band at neck of ulcer in profile view representing thicker rim of edematous gastric wall.
- Ulcer mound–smooth, sharply delineated tissue mass surrounding a benign ulcer.
- Ring shadow–thin rim of contrast which represents an ulcer on the non-dependent surface of an air-contrast study.
- Thickened folds radiating directly to the base of the ulcer en face.

Imaging Findings of Malignant Ulcers

- Ulcer projects within the anticipated wall of the stomach.
- Ulcer is eccentrically located within the ulcer mound.
- Irregularly shaped ulcer crater.
- Nodular ulcer mound.
- Abrupt transition between normal and abnormal mucosa several cms away from the ulcer crater.
- Rigidity, lack of distensibility and lack of changeability.
- Associated large mass.
- Carmen meniscus sign–a relatively shallow gastric ulcerating malignancy projecting as an ulcer which is always convex inwards to the lumen and which does not project beyond the wall=Kirklin meniscus complex.

5. Partial mole has chromosome numbers:

A. 34 XX

B. 69 XXY

C. 34 XY

D. 69 XX

Answer: Option B. 69 XXY

Explanation:

Partial hydatidiform mole is a type of hydatidiform mole, which in turn falls under the spectrum of gestational trophoblastic disease.

Clinical Presentation

Clinical signs and symptoms such as abdominal pain, cramps of the lower abdomen and vaginal bleeding during pregnancy are common but non-specific. The uterus is often large for gestational age, and fetal heart beat is usually absent.

Pathology

It is characterized by its focal distribution, slower transformation, the presence of an embryo or fetus, and a triploid karyotype **(70% are 69 XXY, 27% are 69 XXX, and 3% are 69 XYY).** The extra set of chromosomes are often of paternal origin.

RADIOGRAPHIC FEATURES

Ultrasound

Described sonographic features include:

- Greatly enlarged placenta **relative to the size of the uterine cavity.**
- Cystic spaces within the placenta ("molar placenta"), which may not always be present.
- An amniotic cavity (gestational sac), either empty or containing amorphous.
- Inappropriately small fetal echoes which may be surrounded by a relatively thick rim of placental echoes with intermingling cystic spaces.
- Presence of a well-formed but growth-retarded fetus, either dead or alive with hydropic degeneration of fetal parts being frequently present.

- Some partial moles can have sonographic appearances indistinguishable from those of the common complete moles or missed abortions, although an echogenic rim around the sac, as found in missed abortion or blighted ovum, is notably absent.
- Color Doppler interrogation may show high velocity and low impedance flow.

Complete hydatidiform mole (CHM) is a type of molar pregnancy and falls at the benign end of the spectrum of gestational trophoblastic disease.

Epidemiology

CHM is the most common type of gestational trophoblastic disease.

Pathology

Complete moles are characterized by the absence of a fetus or fetal parts (i.e. no embryonic tissues). There is a non-invasive, diffuse swelling of chorionic villi.

Chromosomal composition

Approximately **90% of complete hydatidiform moles have a 46XX** diploid chromosomal pattern with **~10% having a 46XY** composition. All the chromosomes are derived from the sperm, suggesting fertilisation of a single egg that has lost its chromosomes.

Markers

Serum beta HCG levels are markedly elevated, out of proportion to the pregnancy.

RADIOGRAPHIC FEATURES

Ultrasound

- Enlarged uterus.
- Seen as an intrauterine mass with cystic spaces without fetal parts multiple cystic structures classically give a "snow storm" or "bunch of grapes" type appearance.
- Bilateral theca lutein cysts may also be seen on ultrasound.
- Color Doppler interrogation may show high velocity with a low impedance flo.

6. In case of rheumatic heart disease, fish mouth valve appearance of mitral valve is due to:

A. Thrombosis
B. Hemolytic reaction
C. Aschoff cells
D. Calcification and fibrosis

Answer: Option D. Calcification and fibrosis

Explanation:

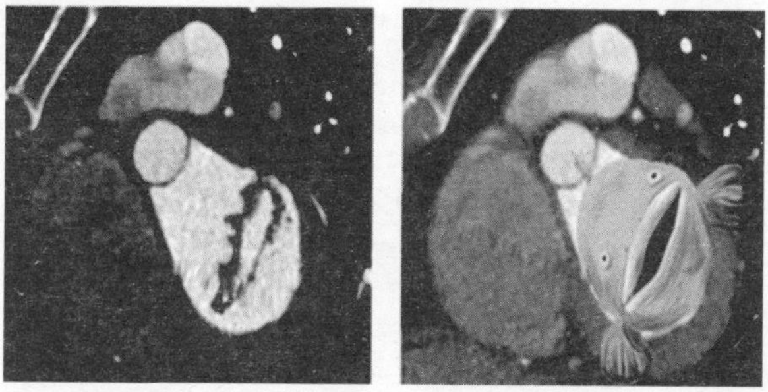

The fish mouth appearance of a cardiac valve is due to the bicuspid configuration. In the mitral valve this is the normal configuration and is demonstrated on the short axis view in echocardiography.

In CT and MR, the description 'fish mouth' has been used when the mitral valve leaflets are thickened, fibrosed and/or calcified, typically in the setting of rheumatic heart disease.

Fish Related Signs

- **Fish Hook Coeliac**: Median Arcuate Ligament Syndrome.
- **Fish Hook Ureter:** Benign prostatic hypertrophy, retrocaval ureter.
- **Fish Vertebrae:** Osteoporosis.
- **Fishtail deformity of the elbow:** Lateral trochlear ossification centers fails to develop or resorbs.

7. Which of the following gene is an apoptotic inhibitor?

A. BAD
B. BAK
C. BCL2
D. BAX

Answer: Option C. BCL2

Explanation:

Bcl-2 inhibits apoptosis by increasing the time-to-death and intrinsic cell-to-cell variations in the mitochondrial pathway of cell death.

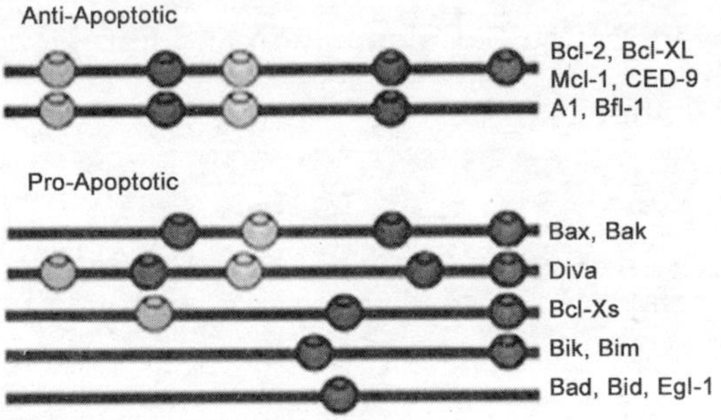

The anti-apoptotic members of this family, such as Bcl-2 and Bcl-XL, prevent apoptosis either by sequestering proforms of death-driving cysteine proteases called caspases (a complex called the apoptosome) or by preventing the release of mitochondrial apoptogenic factors such as cytochrome c and AIF (apoptosis-inducing factor) into the cytoplasm.

After entering the cytoplasm, cytochrome c and AIF directly activate caspases that cleave a set of cellular proteins to cause apoptotic changes.

In contrast, pro-apoptotic members of this family, such as Bax and Bak, trigger the release of caspases from death antagonists via heterodimerization and also by inducing the release of mitochondrial apoptogenic factors into the cytoplasm via acting on mitochondrial permeability transition pore, thereby leading to caspase activation.

Thus, the Bcl-2 family of proteins acts as a critical life-death decision point within the common pathway of apoptosis.

How to Remember:

Bcl- Banning cell lysis – means against cell lysis-apoptosis-antiapoptotic.

Bcl-2 and Bcl–XL antiapoptotic

Apoptotic genes are doing Bak-Bak

So Bak and Bax are apoptotic genes.

8. Most definitive therapy for ITP is:

A. Splenectomy

B. Antiplatelet therapy

C. Plasmapharesis

D. IV immunoglobulin

Answer: Option A. Splenectomy

Explanation:

Splenectomy is the oldest method for management of ITP and is considered to be a definitive therapy for the disease as it provides a high initial response rate (80%) and results in complete remissions in the majority of patients.

Treatment	Typical Use in ITP
Platelet transfusion	Low platelet emergency, rescue treatment
Corticosteroids	First-line treatment, rescue treatment
IVIG	First-line treatment, rescue treatment
Anti-D	Alternative to IVIG
Rituximab	Second-line treatment
Older agents	Alternative or supplementary to other ITP treatments
Other treatments	Experimental/supplementary
Splenectomy	Long-term treatment in patients with refractory/chronic disease

9. Which of the following is an intrinsic cause of hemolysis?

A. PNH

B. Leukemia

C. Autoimmune disorder

D. Medication

Answer: Option A. PNH

Explanation:

Location	Mechanism	Examples	Mode
Intrinsic	Enzyme deficiency	G6PD deficiency	Hereditary
	Hemoglobinopathies	Sickle cell anemia, thalassemia	
	Membrane abnormalities	Hereditary spherocytosis	
		PNH	
	Immune-mediated	Autoimmune; drug-induced, tx rxn	
	Traumatic	MAHA; prostheses (valves, TIPS)	
Extrinsic	Direct infections, toxins	Malaria, babesiosis; snake and spider venoms; Wilson's; hypotonic infusions	Acquired
	Entrapment	Hypersplenism	

- **Paroxysmal nocturnal hemoglobinuria (PNH)** is a disease, due to ***mutations*** in "***Phosphatidyl inositol Glycan Complementation Group A" gene (PIGA).***
- Associated with ***deficiency of glycosyl phosphatidyl inositol (GPI)*** anchor proteins along with absence of external surface membrane proteins attaching to it.
- CD55 (DAF) and CD59 (MIRL) are two such complement defense proteins.
- **CD59 deficiency:**

  Common finding in RBCs and WBCs of patients with chronic hemolysis suffering from PNH.
- **Diagnosis:**
  - ***The definite diagnosis based on demonstration of a substantial proportion of patient's RBC having increased susceptibility to complement (C), due to the deficiency on their surface of proteins (particularly CD59 and CD55).***

10. Glanzman thromboasthenia is due to defect in which receptor?

A. GpIa/Ib
B. Gp IIb/IIIa
C. Gp IIa/IIb
D. Gp Ia/IIIb

Answer: Option B. GpIIb/IIIa

Explanation:

Glanzmann's Thrombasthenia

- Autosomal recessive.
- Causes by deficiency of **glycoprotein IIb-IIIa** receptor for fibrinogen.
- Defective platelet aggregration.
- Increased bleeding time.
- Normal platelet count.

Bernard-Soulier Syndrome (BSS)

- Autosomal recessive.
- Causes by deficiency of **glycoprotein Ib-IX** receptor for von Willebrand factor.
- Defective platelet adhesion.
- Giant platelet.
- Thrombocytopenia.
- Increased bleeding time.

11. Zellweger syndrome affects which part of cell organelle?

A. Mitochondria
B. Lysosome
C. Peroxisome
D. Golgi appratus

Answer: Option C. Peroxisome

Explanation:

Peroxisome biogenesis disorders (PBDs) include the Zellweger syndrome spectrum (PBD-ZSD) and rhizomelic chondrodysplasia punctata type 1 (RCDP1).

PBD-ZSD represents a continuum of disorders including infantile Refsum disease, neonatal adrenoleukodystrophy, and Zellweger syndrome.

Collectively, PBDs are autosomal recessive developmental brain disorders that also result in skeletal and craniofacial dysmorphism, liver dysfunction, progressive sensorineural hearing loss and retinopathy.

Zellweger syndrome (ZS), also known as the cerebrohepatorenal syndrome, is a multisystem metabolic abnormality. **It is the most severe of the peroxisomal disorders.**

CNS

Ventricular enlargement.

Abnormal gyration patterns.

Pachygyria: Especially medial gyri around peri-rolandic regions.

Polymicrogyria: Laterally.

Cerebral periventricular pseudocysts.

Musculoskeletal

Scimitar-like patella calcification.

Abdominal

Hyperechoic kidneys.

Hepatomegaly.

12. The most differentiating histological factor between ulcerative colitis and Crohn's disease is:

A. Diffuse pseudopolyp B. Lymphoid aggregates

C. Crypt abscess D. Mucosal edema

Answer: Option A. Diffuse pseudopolyp

Explanation:

(*http://www.spg.pt/wp-content/uploads/2015/11/2013-ibd_biopsies_13.pdf*)

Here is the one of the most controversial question. One clue in the given options is diffuse involvement in form of pseudopolyp. Pseudopolyp formation represents severe chronic inflammation which lead to ulceration and healing leads to scar formation which look like bump-pseudopolyp. Therefore, this kind of diffuse involvement is seen only in Ulcerative colitis and not in Crohn's disease.

Crohn's disease is frequently associated with "skip lesions", discontinuous areas of active disease in the colon and small intestine with intervening segments that appear norma-

segmental affection. It forms non-caseating granuloma. In Crohn's disease–Rectum is not involved commonly.

The microscopic features that help distinguish UC and CD from one another include granulomas, architectural changes and distribution of disease. Non-cryptolytic granulomas are more useful than any other feature for discriminating between CD and UC.

Feature useful for initial diagnosis and classification of Inflammatory Bowel Disease

Feature	IBD> Infective	Infective>IBD	UC>CD	CD>UC
Architecture				
Preserved architecture		+++		+
Crypt distortion	+++		++	
Cypt atrophy	+++		++	
Diffue intersite or instrasite crypt changes (in IBD)			+++	
Non-diffue crypt changes (in IBD)				+
Irregular mucosal surface	+++		++	
Inflammation				
Basal plasmacytosis	+++			
Lymphoid aggregates	++			
Diffuse intersite or intrasite CI (in IBD)			+++	
Non-diffuse/focal CI (in IBD)				++
Inflammation upper LP		+		
Granulomas (non-cryptolytic)	++			++++
LP acute inflammation (no CI)		+		
Widespred cryptitis (in IBD)			+	
Other changes				
Mucin depletion			++	
Paneth cell metaplasia	+			
Ileal inflammation (in IBD)				++
++++, very strongly discriminant; +++, highly discriminant; ++, moderately discriminant; +, weakly discriminant; CD, Crohn's disease; CI, chronic inflammation; IBD, inflammatory bowel disease; LP, lamina propria; UC, ulcerative colitis.				

Features Favouring Ulcerative Colitis Over Crohn's Disease

Reliability/discriminant value	Feature
1. Reliable	Diffuse cypt abnormalities within and between sites
	Diffuse crypt abnormalities within a site
	Crypt atrophy
	Abnormal crypt architecture
	Villous or irregular mucosal surface
	Mucin depletion
	Absence of ileal inflammation
2. Reliable in some studies, but variably defined	Diffuse transmucosal chronic inflammation/diffuse inflammation/ heavy diffuse transmucosal lamina propria infiltrate/ transmucosal lamina proprial hypercellularity
3. Less evidence	Widespread cryptitis/'general crypt epithelial polymorphs'
	The following more prevalent distally than proximally: diffuse transmucosal inflammation; diffuse crypt changes; focal crypt changes

Features Favouring Crohn's Disease Over Ulcerative Colitis

Reliability/discriminant value	Feature
1. Reliable	Granuloma (non-cryptolytic)
	Focal or patchy lamina proprial chronic inflammation (rather than continuous/diffuse)
	Focal or segmental crypt distortion (rather than continuous/ diffuse) ileal involvement
	Absence of features of ulcerative colitis

Contd.

Contd.

2. Fairly reliable	Decreasing proximal to distal gradient of changes
3. Limited or conflicting evidence*	Disproportionate submucosal inflammation
	Focal crypt abscesses
	Focal cryptitis
4. Limited evidence from non-initial studies	Normal mucosal surface
	Segmental crypt atrophy
	Segmental mucin depletion

13. G6PD deficiency associated which pattern of inheritance?

A. Autosomal dominant B. Autosomal recessive

C. X-linked dominant D. X-linked recessive

Answer: Option D. X-linked recessive

Explanation:

X-linked recessive disorders are:

- Glucose-6-phosphate dehydrogenase deficiency.
- Red-green color blindness–most common X-linked recessive dz.
- Hemophilia A.
- Hemophilia B (Christmas Disease).
- Duchenne muscular dystrophy.
- Becker's muscular dystrophy.
- X-linked ichthyosis, X-linked agammaglobulinemia (XLA).

X-linked dominant disorders are:

- Vitamin D resistant rickets: X-linked hypophosphatemia.
- Rett syndrome (95% of cases are due to sporadic mutations).
- Alport syndrome.
- Incontinentia pigmenti.
- Giuffrè–Tsukahara syndrome.
- Goltz syndrome.
- X-linked dominant porphyria.
- Fragile X syndrome.

14. Which of the following is a positive marker of Follicular lymphoma?

A. Bcl-1 B. Bcl-2

C. Bcl-3 D. Bcl-6

Answer: Option B. Bcl-2

Explanation:

Bcl-2 and Bcl-6 are two markers linked to germinal center B cells.

The Bcl-2 gene, located at chromosome 18q21, encodes for a 25kd protein located mainly in the mitochondrial membrane.

This Bcl-2 protein is an anti-apoptosis factor that is important in normal B-cell development and differentiation.

Bcl-2 overexpression provides a survival advantage for malignant B cells and is thought to play a critical role in resistance to chemotherapy.

- Bcl-2 protein is the most frequent expression in the FL group.
- Bcl-6 is the most frequent expression in the DLBCL group.

	Mantle cell lymphoma	Chronic lymphocytic leukaemia/ lymphocytic leukaemia	Follicular lymphoma	Marginal zone lymphoma	Lymphoplasmacytic lymphoma
CD3	–	–	–	–	–
CD5	+	+	–	–	–
CD10	–	–	+	+/-	+/-
CD20	+	+	+	+	+
CD23	+	+	+/-	+/-	+/-
BCL1	–	–	–	–	–
BCL2	+	+	+	+	+
BCL6	–	–	+	–	–
MIB/ KI67	+	+	+	+	+
LEF1	–	+	–	–	–
CD 160	–	+	–	–	–
CD 200	–	+	–	–	+
SOX 11	+	–	–	–	–

Contd.

Contd.

HGAL	–	–	+	–	–
LMO2	–	–	+	–	–
Stathmin	+	–	+	–	–
GCET1	–	–	+	–	–
IRTA1	–	–	–	+	–
MNDA	+	+	–	+	+
MYD88	–	–	–	–	+

15. Which of the following causes Flask shaped ulcer?

A. Giardiasis
B. Entamoeba histolytica
C. Typhoid
D. Ancylostoma dueodenale

Answer: Option B. Entamoeba histolytica

Explanation:

Amebic invasion through the mucosa and into submucosal tissues is the hallmark of amebic colitis; lateral extension through the submucosal tissues gives rise to the classic flask-shaped ulcer of amebic colitis.

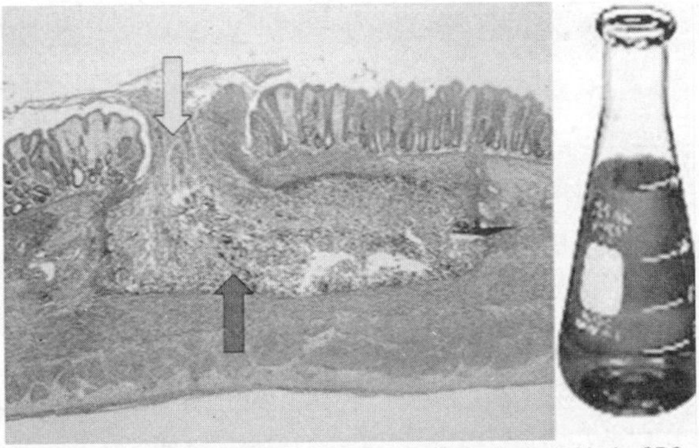

Histopathology of a typical flask-shaped ulcer of intestinal amebiasis. CDC

Classification of Amebiasis	
WHO Clinical Classification of Amebiasis infection (modified)	**Pathophysiologic Mechanisms**
Asymptomatic infection	Colonization without tissue invasion
Symptomatic infection	Invasive infection

Contd.

Contd.

Intestinal amebiasis	
A. Amebic dysentery	Fulminant ulcerative intestinal disease
B. Nondysentery gastroenteritis	Ulcerative intestinal disease
C. Ameboma	Proliferative intestinal disease
D. Complicated intestinal amebiasis	Perforation, hemorrhage, fistula
E. Post-amebic colitis	Mechanism unknown
Extraintestinal amebiasis	
A. Nonspecific hepatomegaly	Intestinal infection with no demonstrable invasion
B. Acute nonspecific infection	Amebas in liver but without abscess
C. Amebic abscess	Focal structural lesion
D. Amebic abscess, complicated	Direct extension to pleura, lung, peritoneum, or pericardium
E. Amebiasis cutis	Direct extension to skin
F. Visceral amebiasis	Metastatic infection of lung, spleen or brain

16. Multi drug resistant protein 2 is related to which of the following disorder?

A. Crigler-Najjar syndrome
B. Gilbert syndrome
C. Rotor syndrome
D. Dubin-Johnson syndrome

Answer: Option D. Dubin-Johnson syndrome

Explanation:

Dubin-Johnson syndrome results from an autosomal recessive defect in the transport protein responsible for hepatocellular excretion of bilirubin glucuronides across the canalicular membrane. Affected individuals exhibit conjugated hyperbilirubinemia. Other than having a darkly pigmented liver (from polymerized epinephrine metabolites, not bilirubin) and hepatomegaly, patients are normal.

Pathophysiology

The conjugated hyperbilirubinemia is a result of defective endogenous and exogenous transfer of anionic conjugates from hepatocytes into bile. Impaired biliary excretion of bilirubin glucuronides is due to a mutation in the canalicular multiple drug-resistance protein 2 (MRP2). A darkly pigmented liver is due to polymerized epinephrine metabolites, not bilirubin.

Dubin-Johnson syndrome is due to a defect in the multiple drug resistance protein 2 gene (ABCC2), located on chromosome 10. It is an autosomal recessive disease and is likely due to a loss of function mutation, since the mutation affects the cytoplasmic/binding domain.

Diagnosis

A hallmark of Dubin-Johnson syndrome is the unusual ratio between the byproducts of heme biosynthesis:

Unaffected subjects have a coproporphyrin III to coproporphyrin I ratio around 3–4:1.

In patients with Dubin-Johnson syndrome, this ratio is inverted, with coproporphyrin I being 3–4 times higher than coproporphyrin III. Analysis of urine porphyrins shows a normal level of coproporphyrin, but the I isomer accounts for 80% of the total (normally 25%).

Crigler-Najjar Syndrome

Type - 1 No UDP glucuronosyl transferase 1-A1 expression.

Type - 2 UGT1A1 is present at reduced but detectable levels (typically <10% of normal), because of single base pair mutations.

Gilbert's syndrome is due to a mutation in the UGT1A1 gene which results in decreased activity of the bilirubin uridine diphosphate glucuronosyltransferase enzyme.

Rotor syndrome is inherited in an autosomal recessive manner. The SLCO1B1 and SLCO1B3 genes are involved in Rotor syndrome.

17. In a patient with malignant hypertension, which type of vessel wall necrosis is seen?

A. Fibrinoid necrosis B. Fat necrosis
C. Coagulative necrosis D. Liquifactive necrosis

Answer: Option A. Fibrinoid necrosis

Explanation:

Fibrinoid necrosis

- This is seen in immune reactions in **vessels**.

- Immune complexes (antigen-antibody complexes) and fibrin are deposited in vessel walls.
- Gross: Changes too small to see grossly.
- Micro: Vessel walls are thickened and pinkish-red (called "fibrinoid" because the deposits look like fibrin deposits).

Coagulative necrosis

- See this in infarcts in any tissue (except brain).
- Due to loss of blood.
- Gross: Tissue is firm.
- Micro: Cell outlines are preserved (cells look ghostly), and everything looks red.

Liquefactive necrosis

- See this in infections and, for some unknown reason, in brain infarcts.
- Due to lots of neutrophils around releasing their toxic contents, "liquefying" the tissue.
- Gross: Tissue is liquidy and creamy yellow (pus).
- Micro: Lots of neutrophils and cell debris.

Caseous necrosis

- See this in tuberculosis.
- Due to the body trying to wall off and kill the bug with macrophages.
- Gross: White, soft, cheesy-looking ("caseous") material.
- Micro: Fragmented cells and debris surrounded by a collar of lymphocytes and macrophages (granuloma).

Fat necrosis

- See this in acute pancreatitis.
- Damaged cells release lipases, which split the triglyceride esters within fat cells.
- *Gross:* Chalky, white areas from the combination of the newly-formed free fatty acids with calcium (saponification).

- *Micro:* Shadowy outlines of dead fat cells; sometimes there is a bluish cast from the calcium deposits, which are basophilic.

Gangrenous necrosis

- See this when an entire limb loses blood supply and dies (usually the lower leg).
- This isn't really a different kind of necrosis, but people use the term clinically so it's worth knowing about.
- Gross: Skin looks black and dead; underlying tissue is in varying stages of decomposition.
- Micro: Initially there is coagulative necrosis from the loss of blood supply (this stage is called "dry gangrene"); if bacterial infection is superimposed, there is liquefactive necrosis (this stage is called "wet gangrene").

18. Which of the following type of blood group causes this type of reaction shown in image?

A. O +ve　　B. AB +ve

C. O -ve　　D. AB -ve

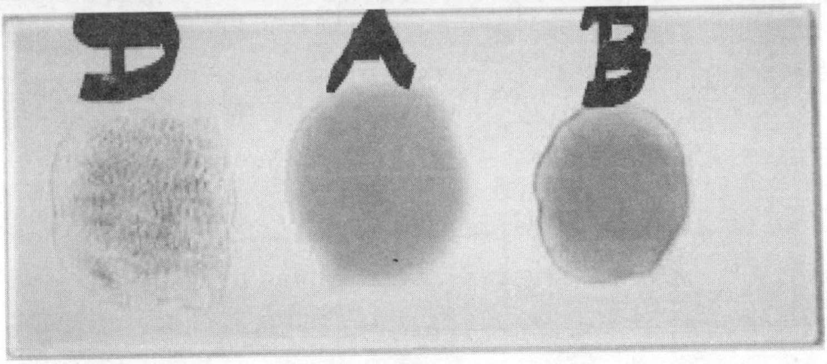

Answer: Option A. O +ve

Explanation:

Above slide showing changes of hemolysis only in anti D region, that suggest person has Rh antigen in his blood. Therefore above blood group is O positive.

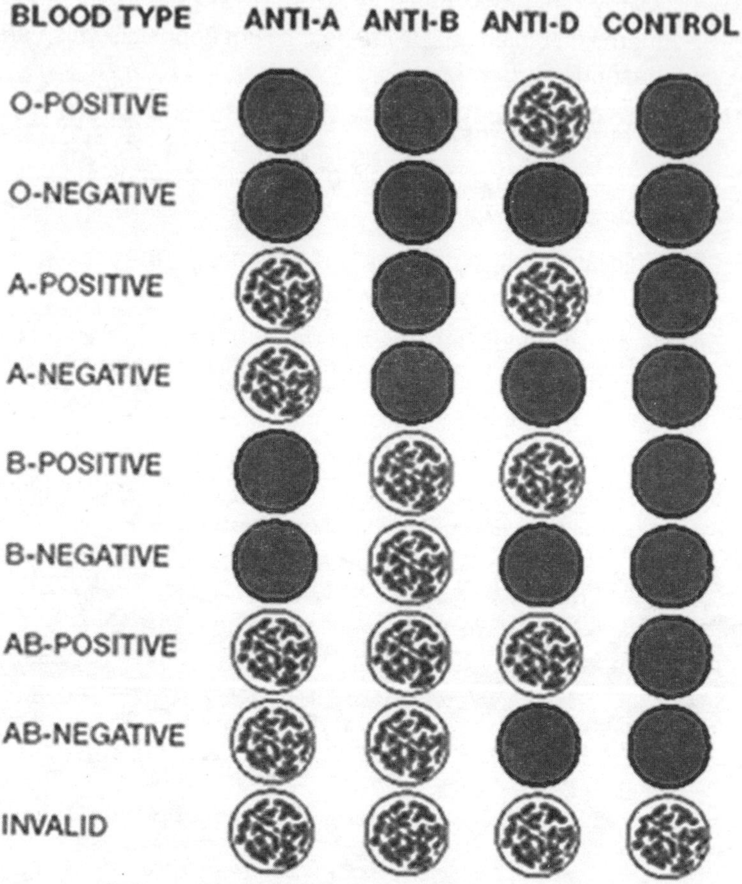

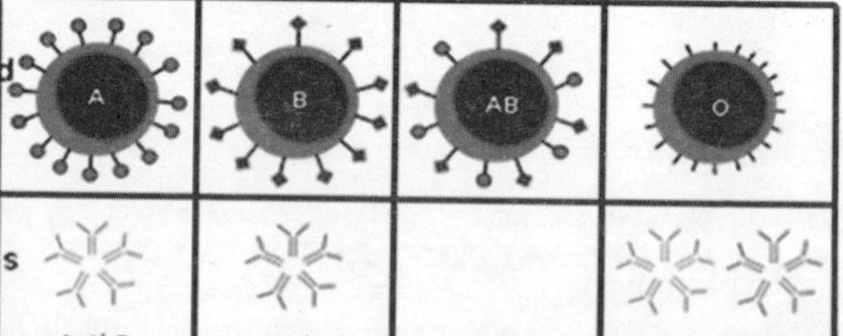

	Group A	Group B	Group AB	Group O
Red blood cell type	A	B	AB	O
Antibodies present	Anti-B	Anti-A	None	Anti-A and Anti-B
Antigens present	A antigen	B antigen	A and B antigens	None

Blood Type is Controlled by 3 Alleles

Alleles: A, B, O.

A and B are codominant, O is recessive.

Each blood group has different antigens on its surface.

Rh Factor (Rh = rhesus monkey–surface Rh antigens (and be Rh +) or no antigens (and be Rh-).

19. Which of the following is incorrect about MCH II?

A. They are not found on antigen presenting cells

B. The antigens presented by class II peptides are derived from extracellular proteins

C. Encoded by the human leukocyte antigen gene complex (HLA)

D. These cells are important in initiating immune responses

Answer: Option A. They are not found on antigen presenting cells

Explanation:

Class II MHC molecules are encoded by genes in the HLA-D region, which contains three subregions: DP, DQ and DR.

Class II molecules are heterodimers of non-covalently linked α and β subunits.

Expression of class II MHC molecules is restricted to a few cell types, mainly Antigen Presenting Cells (notably, dendritic cells), macrophages, and B cells. **They are important in initiating immune response.**

The extracellular portion of class II MHC molecules contains a cleft for the binding of antigenic peptides and a region that binds CD4. In general, class II MHC molecules bind to peptides derived from extracellular proteins synthesized outside the cell, for example, from microbes that Mare ingested and then broken down inside the cell.

This property allows CD4+ T cells to **recognize the presence of extracellular pathogens.**

They are important in Graft versus host response and Mixed leucocyte reaction.

20. Which is the advantage of CPD over ACD in a case of blood storage?

A. CPD is more acidic than ACD

B. There is less fall of 2, 3 BPG in CPD

C. There is more saturation of oxygen

D. Can be stored for prolong period

Answer: Option B. There is less fall of 2, 3 BPG in CPD

Explanation:

Citrate-phosphate-dextrose (CPD) is less acidic than ACD and maintained 2,3-diphosphoglycerate (2,3-DPG) level better than in ACD solution.

The first anticoagulant preservative was introduced by Rous and Turner in 1916.

It consisted of a citrate-glucose solution in which blood from rabbits was stored for two weeks, which prevented anaemia when transfused in another rabbit who had suffered from blood loss.

Rous Turner's solution as used for storage of human blood during the First World War (Mollison 1987).

The next important development occurred in 1943 during the Second World War when acidifieditrate dextrose (ACD) solution was introduced for clinical use by Loutit and Mollison.

In 1957 Gibson *et al.* developed an improved preservative of citrate-phosphate-dextrose (CPD), which was less acidic than ACD and maintained 2,3-diphosphoglycerate (2,3-DPG) level better than in ACD solution.

CPD eventually replaced ACD and became commonly used preservative for storage of blood/red cells in liquid form. Shelf-life of blood stored in CPD at 2-4°C was 21 days.

In 1978 citrate-phosphate-dextrose with adenine (CPDA-1) preservative was developed. The addition of adenine improved the synthesis of adenosine triphosphate (ATP) in the stored blood, Which prolonged the storage of blood/red cells at 2-4 °C to 35 days.

The average survival values of RBC between the two anti-coagulants is not significantly different at each time period.

21. Which of the following interleukin is activated by caspase 1?

A. IL-1 B. IL-6

C. IL-9 D. IL-12

Answer: Option A. IL-1

Explanation:

Several of the NLRs (NOD-like receptors) signal via a cytosolic multiprotein complex called the inflammasome, which activates

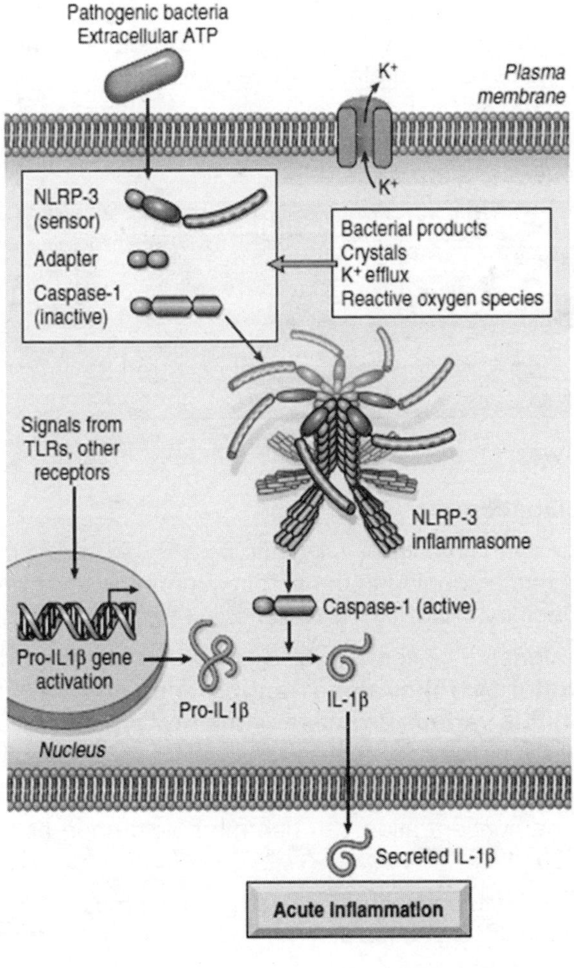

an enzyme (caspase-1) that cleaves a precursor form of the cytokine interleukin-1 (IL-1) to generate the biologically active form.

The inflammasome is a protein complex that recognizes products of dead cells and some microbes and induces the secretion of biologically active interleukin-1.

It is a complex of multiple copies of a sensor protein (a leucine-rich protein called NLRP3), an adapter, and the enzyme caspase-1, which is converted from an inactive to an active form.

The structure of the inflammasome as shown is simplified from known crystal structures. The formation of the inflammasome complex proceeds by a prion-like mechanism of propagation, in which one protein altered by activation induces conformational changes in other proteins of the same type.

The net result is the activation and assembly of a large number of identical polypeptides, forming filament-like bundles of adapters and enzymes.

22. Which is the true about alpha 1 antitrypsin?

A. It activates trypsin

B. It is inherited as X-linked disease

C. It inhibits elastase in lung

D. It is not seen in systemic circulation

Answer: Option C. It inhibits elastase in lung

Explanation:

Alpha-1-antitrypsin or α1-antitrypsin (A1AT, A1A, or AAT) is a protein belonging to the serpin superfamily. It is encoded in humans by the SERPINA1 gene.

A protease inhibitor, it is also known as **alpha1–proteinase inhibitor (A1PI) or alpha1-antiproteinase (A1AP) because it inhibits various proteases – mainly trypsin and elastase**.

As a type of enzyme inhibitor, it protects tissues from enzymes of inflammatory cells, especially neutrophil elastase, but the concentration can rise many fold upon acute inflammation.

When the blood contains inadequate amounts of A1AT or functionally defective A1AT (such as in alpha-1 antitrypsin deficiency), **neutrophil elastase** is excessively free to break down elastin, degrading the elasticity of the lungs, which results in respiratory complications, such as chronic obstructive pulmonary disease, in adults.

Normally, A1AT leaves its site of origin, the liver, and **joins the systemic circulation**; defective A1AT can fail to do so, building up in the liver, which results in cirrhosis in either adults or children.

Disorders of this protein include alpha-1 antitrypsin deficiency, an autosomal codominant hereditary disorder.

23. Vitamin A is stored in which cells?

A. Macrophage
B. Hepatocyte
C. Ito cells
D. Kupffer cells

Answer: Option C. Ito cells

Explanation:

Ito cells are pericytes in presinusoidal space. Major cells involved in liver fibrosis and cirrhosis. Vitamin A is stored in the Liver Perisinusoidal Stellate (Ito) cells as Retinyl Ester (Retinol Palmitate).

Vitamin A

Ring structure present in Vitamin A is β ionone ring Provitamin A, β carotene contain 2 β ionone ring cleaved in the intestine by a dioxygenase.

Retinoids

All compounds chemically related to retinol are called retinoids.

They are:

- Retinal: 11 cis retinal for normal vision.
- Retinoic acid: Normal morphogenesis, growth and cell differentiation.
- Retinol: Reproduction.

Vitamin A, in the strictest sense, refers to Retinol

Carotenoids

- They are provitamins of Vitamin A present in plants.

- More than 600 carotenoids in nature, and approximately 50 of them can be metabolized to vitamin A.
- β carotene is the most prevalent carotenoid in the food supply that has provitamin A activity.

Nonprovitamin A Carotenoids

- Lutein and Zeaxanthin: Protect against macular degeneration.
- Lycopene: Protect against prostate cancer.

Vitamin A Metabolism

Absorption and transport of Vitamin A

- Beta carotene from plant sources is absorbed and cleaved to two molecules of Retinal by Beta Carotene Dioxygenase. Retinal is reduced to retinol by Retinol Reductase.
- Retinol ester from animal sources is hydrolyzed in the intestinal lumen to Retinol and absorbed into the intestinal cells.
- Retinol from animal and plant sources is reesterified to retinol esters and transported in Chylomicrons to Liver. Uptake takes place in liver cells by means of apo E receptors.

Transport of Vitamin A from Liver to Target Organs Carried to target sites in the plasma as trimolecular complex bound to Retinol Binding Protein (RBP) and Transthyretin.

Vitamin A (Retinol)

1. Sources of vitamin A include cod liver oil, dairy products and egg yolk.
2. Retinol (alcohol), retinal (aldehyde), and retinoic acid are the active forms of vitamin A.
   a. β-Carotenes (i.e., provitamin A) found in dark green leafy and yellow vegetables (e.g., spinach and carrots) and retinol esters in the diet are converted into retinol, which is esterified (forming retinol esters) in the enterocytes of the small intestine.

An excess of β-carotenes in the diet turns the skin yellow, but the sclera remains white.

b. Retinol esters are packaged into chylomicrons and transported to the liver for storage.

c. Retinol is released from the liver, complexes with retinol-binding protein (RBP), and is delivered to target tissues throughout the body (except heart and skeletal muscle).

d. In the cytosol, retinol is irreversibly oxidized to retinoic acid.

e. Retinoic acid (similar to steroid hormones and vitamin D) binds to nuclear receptors, forming a complex that activates gene transcription of protein products.

24. Which of the following is the diagnosis of given histology slide (showing clonal proliferation) of patient presented with lytic lesion over skull?

A. Multiple myeloma
B. Metastasis
C. Plasmacytoma
D. Langerhans cell histiocytosis

Answer: Option D. Langerhans cell histiocytosis

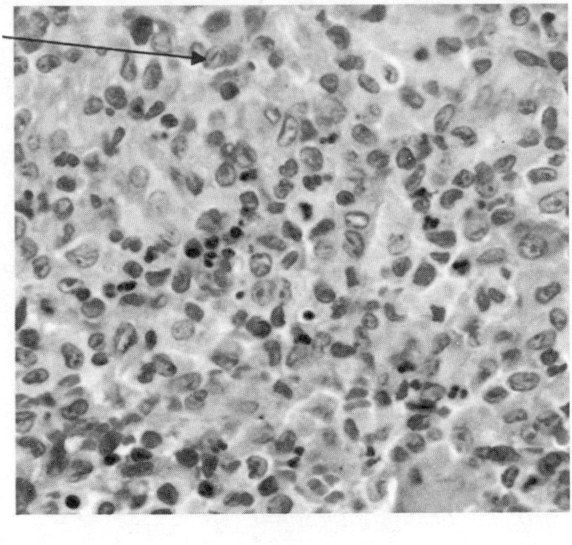

Explanation:

Here above given H and E slide shows multiple polygonal cells, eosinophilic cytoplasm, nucleus is oval shaped with longitudinal groove is seen within cytoplasm. These finding give characteristic appearance of owl eye. These are immature dendritic cells called as Langerhans cells.

Above histology features with lytic lesion at skull – diagnostic of Langerhans cell histiocytosis.

Langerhans cell histiocytosis (LCH) is a rare multi-system disease with a wide and heterogeneous clinical spectrum and variable extent of involvement.

Terminology

Langerhans cell histiocytosis was previously known as histiocytosis X. The newer term is preferred as it's more descriptive of its cellular background, and removes the ambiguity of the connotation "X".

Epidemiology

The disease is more common in the pediatric population, with a peak incidence between one and three years of age. There is also a male predilection (M:F ~ 1.5:1) .

Clinical Presentation

- *Letterer-Siwe disease*
  - Disseminated multi-organ disease.
  - Typically young children/infants less than one year old.
  - Fulminant course with poor prognosis.
- *Hand-Schüller-Christian disease*
  - Multiple lesions
    - ◊ Some authors confine the term to patients with solitary organ involvement.
    - ◊ Other authors accept multi-organ involvement (e.g., bone and spleen).
  - Confined to the one bone (usually bone).
  - Typically children.
  - Intermediate prognosis.
- *Eosinophilic granuloma (EG)*

- Lesions are confined to one organ system
  - ◊ Some authors confine the term to patients with a solitary lesion.
  - ◊ Other authors accept multiple lesions.
- 70% of cases affect bone.
- Typically children.
- Best prognosis.

Pathology

Langerhans cell histiocytosis is due to uncontrolled monoclonal proliferation of Langerhans cells (distinctive cells of monocyte-macrophage lineage) and should be considered a malignancy although its biological behavior is very variable. An immune-mediated mechanism has been postulated. This proliferation is accompanied by inflammation and granuloma formation. Electron microscopy may reveal characteristic **Birbeck granules**. Immunohistochemistry reveals expression of the following antigens:

- HLA-DR
- CD1a
- CD207 (langerin)
- S100

There is proliferation of **Langerhans cells** with an abundance of eosinophils, lymphocytes and neutrophils. These cells produce prostaglandins which result in medullary bone resorption: this is what causes the symptoms.

Location/Distribution

Patients may have one or, less commonly, many lesions. The most common locations are the skull and long bones.

- Skull: ~50%
- Pelvis: 23%
- Femur: 17%
- Ribs: 8% (most common in adults)
- Humerus: 7%
- Mandible: 7%
- Spine.

RADIOGRAPHIC FEATURES

Plain radiographs.

Skull

- Solitary or multiple punched out lytic lesions without sclerotic rim.
- Double contour or beveled edge appearance may be seen due to asymmetrical involvement of the inner and outer tables (**hole within a hole**) sign.
- **Button sequestrum** representing residual bone.
- **Geographic skull.**

Mandible

- Irregular radiolucent areas mostly involving superficial alveolar bone.
- **Floating tooth:** Loss of lamina dura.

Spine

- **Vertebra plana:** Most common cause of vertebra plana in children; more often in thoracic spine.

Long Bones

- Depends on phase of disease which is imaged.
- Permeative and aggressive appearing lesion.
- Mainly involves diaphysis or metadiaphysis and respects growth plates.
- **Endosteal scalloping, periosteal reaction** (in healing phase it can appear as solid benign periosteal reaction), cortical thinning, intracortical tunneling, and associated soft tissue mass.

Treatment and Prognosis

The prognosis can be extremely variable with eosinophilic granuloma carrying the best and Letterer-Siwe disease-carrying the worst prognosis. The prognosis is more closely related to the disease burden rather than histological features, although frankly malignant features (Langerhans cell sarcoma) do also have an impact on survival.

- Unifocal disease (eosinophilic granuloma): >95% survival.
- Two-organ involvement: 75% survival.
- Langerhans cell sarcoma: 50% survival.

MULTIPLE MYELOMA

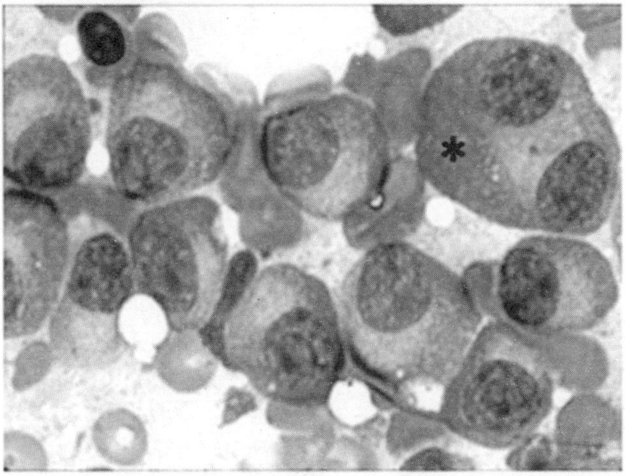

Generally on histology cells appear larger size with abundant cytoplasm and eccentric nucleus.

Variants may include:

- Bizarre cells, which are multinucleated.
- Mott cells, containing multiple clustered cytoplasmic droplets or other inclusions (sometimes confused with auer rods, commonly seen in myeloid blasts).
- Flame cells, having a fiery red cytoplasm.

25. Which of the following is a true regarding mitochondrial inheritance?

A. Mitochondrial DNA is the chromosomal DNA

B. Mitochondrial DNA is always maternally inherited

C. No children will inherit the disease from affected mother

D. Only females are affected

Answer: Option B. Mitochondrial DNA is always maternally inherited

Explanation:

- Mitochondrial DNA is the only non-chromosomal DNA in human cells.
- **Mitochondrial DNA is always maternally inherited.** Thus diseases caused by mutation in mitochondrial DNA are always inherited from mother to next generation.
- All children from affected mother will inherit the disease. But no children will inherit the disease from affected father.
- Both male and females are affected. Affected son does not transmit the disease to next generation.

Mitochondrial Inheritance

Mutations within a mitochondrial gene can lead to phenotypic defects and show a pattern of maternal genetic transmission. Since mitochondria are only present in ovum and not sperms, the inheritance is maternal. All offspring of an affected female will be affected. All affected daughters will transmit the disease. Sons will be affected but will not transmit the disease.

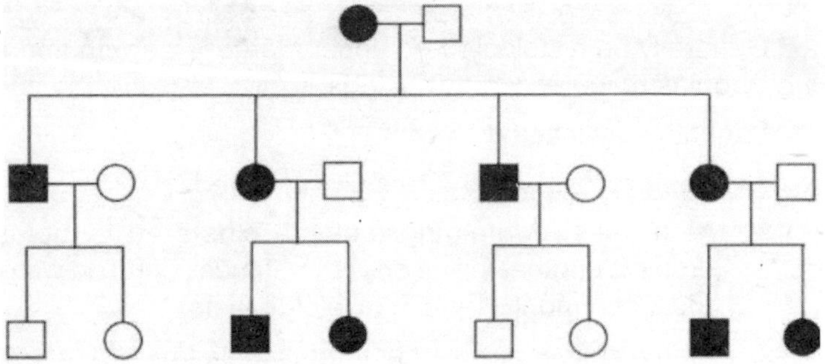

Mitochondrial Disorders

Mitochondria are mainly involved in the energy production pathway of oxidative phosphorylation (OXPHOS).

Mitochondrial disorders refer to defects in the OXPHOS pathway. Mitochondria are mainly derived from the ovum; hence, mitochondrial DNA (mtDNA) disorders are maternally inherited. Tissues such as brain, liver and kidney have high-energy requirements and are susceptible to injury.

Mitochondrial disorders can occur due to either alterations in mitochondrial DNA (mtDNA) or nuclear DNA (nDNA) mutations. The mutant mtDNA produce less energy; symptoms are apparent when energy production is less than energy requirements. Disorders that are due to nDNA mutations are autosomal recessive, autosomal dominant or X-linked. A mitochondrial disorder is often suspected with multisystem involvement such as stroke, hearing loss, muscle weakness, cardiomyopathy and/or endocrine dysfunction. The disorders due to mtDNA deletion/duplication mutations are chronic progressive external ophthalmoplegia, Kearns-Sayre Syndrome, Pearson syndrome. Disorders caused by mtDNA point mutations include (Leber hereditary optic neuropathy LHON), (maternally inherited Leigh syndrome MILS), (mitochondrial encephalopathy, lactic acidosis and stroke MELAS), (myoclonic epilepsy with ragged red fibres MERRF), (neurogenic weakness, ataxia and retinitis pigmentosa NARP), hypertrophic cardiomyopathy, mitochondrial myopathy and (non-syndromic aminoglycoside-induced sensory neural hearing loss SNHL).

Diagnosis

A markedly elevated lactate level raises the possibility of a mitochondrial disorder. An elevated lactate-to-pyruvate ratio of greater than 30 suggests an OXPHOS defect. CSF lactate and pyruvate values also are helpful in some patients. The definite method is muscle biopsy where presence of ragged red fibers as well as subsarcolemmal accumulation of mitochondria confirms mitochondropathy. Staining for succinate dehydrogenase and cytochrome C oxidase is useful.

Treatment

No specific therapy is available. Supportive treatment includes symptomatic therapy, supplementation with cofactors such as riboflavin, Co-Q, folinic acid, vitamin E, vitamin C, carnitine, high lipid, low carbohydrate diet and avoiding mitochondrial toxins such as sodium valproate and statins.

Disease	Phenotype	Most Frequent mtDNA Mutations	Homoplasmic (Usually)	Maternal
NARP, Leigh disease	Loss of central vision leading to blindness in young adult life	m.1778G>A, m.14484T>C, m.3460G>A	Heteroplasmic	Maternal
MELAS	Mitochondrial encephalomyopathy, lactic acidosis, and stroke-like episodes; may manifest only as diabetes mellitus	Point mutation in $tRNA^{leu}$	Heteroplasmic	Maternal
MERRF	Myoclonic epilepsy, ragged red fibers in muscle, ataxia, increased CSF protein, sensorineural deafness, dementia	Point mutation in $tRNA^{lys}$	Heteroplasmic	Maternal
Deafness	Progressive sensorineural deafness, one induced by aminoglycoside antibiotics	m.1555A>G mutation in 12S rRNA	Homoplasmic	Maternal
	Non-syndromic sensorineural deafness	m.7445A>G mutation in 12S rRNA	Homoplasmic	Maternal
Chronic progressive external ophthalmo-plegia (PEO)	Late-onset bilateral ptosis and ophthalmoplegia, proximal muscle weakness, and exercise intolerance	Single deletions or duplications	Heteroplasmic	Mostly sporadic, somatic mutations
Pearson syndrome	Pancreatic insufficiency, pancytopenia, lactic acidosis	Large deletion	Heteroplasmic	Sporadic, somatic mutations
Kearns-Sayre syndrome (KSS)	External ophthalmoplegia, heart block, retinal pigmentation, ataxia	The 5-kb "common deletion"	Heteroplasmic	Sporadic, somatic mutations

CHAPTER

6 MICROBIOLOGY

1. In a case of infection with polysaccharide capsule, which of the following IgG subtype will be involved?

A. IgG1 B. IgG2

C. IgG3 D. IgG4

Answer: Option B. IgG2

Explanation:

IgG1 and IgG3 subclasses are rich in antibodies against proteins such as the toxins produced by the diphtheria and tetanus bacteria, as well as antibodies against viral proteins. **IgG2 antibodies are predominantly against the polysaccharide (complex sugar) coating (capsule) of certain disease-producing bacteria (such as, Streptococcus pneumonia and Hemophilic influenza).**

The IgG in the bloodstream is 60-70% IgG1, 20-30% IgG2, 5-8% IgG3 and 1-3% IgG4. The amount of the different IgG subclasses present in the bloodstream varies with age. For example, IgG1 and IgG3 reach normal adult levels by 5-7 years of age while IgG2 and IgG4 levels rise more slowly, reaching adult levels at about 10 years of age. In young children, the ability to make IgG2 antibodies to the polysaccharide coatings of bacteria develops more slowly than the ability to make antibodies to proteins.

IgG2 or IgG3 deficiencies are the most common IgG subclass deficiencies. Since IgG1 comprises 60% of the total IgG level, deficiency of IgG1 usually drops the total IgG level below the normal range, resulting in hypogammaglobulinemia.

IgG4 is present in very low levels in children younger than 10 years of age, so IgG4 deficiencies are not usually diagnosed before age 10. IgG4 may be undetectable in the serum of many "normal" adult individuals, and therefore low IgG4 alone is insufficient evidence of an antibody deficiency disorder requiring Ig replacement.

Measurement of IgG subclasses can be recommended in the presence of known associated abnormalities, particularly if recurrent infections are also present. These circumstances include:

- IgA deficient patients with recurrent infections to determine if there is an associated IgG2 and IgG4 subclass deficiency.
- Wiskott-Aldrich and Ataxia-Telangiectasia patients at the onset of recurrent infections.
- Specific Antibody Deficiency patients with normal total immunglobulins.

2. Rubella belongs to which of the following subtype of virus?

A. Reo viridae
B. Calci viridae
C. Toga viridae
D. Flavi viridae

Answer: Option C. Toga viridae

Explanation:

(See table on the next page)

3. A 5 years old child is presented with painful, red, blister-like lesions on the tongue, gums and inside of the cheeks. A red rash, without itching but sometimes with blistering, on the palms, soles. This disease is caused by which of the following virus?

A. Echo virus
B. Entero virus
C. Coxsackie virus
D. Herpes virus

Answer: Option C. Coxsackie virus

Explanation:

Here child presented with a disease involving hand, mouth and foot which is called as hand, foot and mouth disease caused by Coxsackie virus.

(See table on the page no. 129)

Q. No. 2

	Capsid	Virion	Nucleic Acid	Virus Family	Members
DNA VIRUS					
I	Icosahedral	Naked	SS(-ve)	Parvoviridae	B-19 parvovirus
II	Icosahedral	Naked	ds circular (±)	Papovaviridae	Papilloma virus, JC, BK virus, polyomavirus
III	Icosahedral	Naked	ds (±)	Adenoviridae	Human adenovirus
IV	Icosahedral	Enveloped	ds with ss (±) circular	Hepadenoviridae	HBV
V	Icosahedral	Enveloped	ds (±)	Herpesviridae	VZ; HSV I, II; CMV; EBV
VI	Complex	Complex coats	ds (±)	Poxviridae	Variola (smallpox) Molluscum contagiosum
RNA VIRUS					
I	Icosahedral or (cubical)	Naked	SS(+)	Picornaviridae	Polio, coxsackie, entero, rhino, HAV
II	Icosahedral	Naked	SS	Astroviridae	
III	Icosahedral	Naked	SS (+)	Calciviridae	HEV, Norwalk
IV	Icosahedral	Naked	ds segmented (±)	Reoviridae	Rota, Reo, Orbivirus

Contd.

Contd.

V	Icosahedral	Enveloped	SS (+)	Togaviridae	Rubella virus
VI	Unknown or complex	Enveloped	SS (+)	Flaviviridae	HCV, HGV, yellow fever, Dengue virus
VII	Unknown or complex	Enveloped	SS (–) segmented	Arenaviridae (sandy appearance)	Lassa fever virus
VIII	Unknown or complex	Enveloped	SS (+)	Coronaviridae	
IX	Unknown or complex	Enveloped	SS diploid (+)	Retroviridae	HIV 1,2; HTLV I, II; slow virus group
X	Helical	Enveloped	SS (–) segmented	Orthomyxoviridae	Influenza A,B,C
XI	Helical		SS (–) segmented	Bunyaviridae	Hantavirus, sandfly fever virus
XII	Helical	Enveloped	SS	Bornaviridae	
XIII	Helical	Enveloped	SS (–)	Rhabdoviridae	Rabies virus, Vesicular stomatitis virus
XIV	Helical	Enveloped	SS (–)	Paramyxoviridae	Parainfluenza, RSV Mmps, rubeola New castle virus
XV	Helical	Enveloped	SS (–)	Filoviridae	Marburg virus Ebola virus

Q. No. 3

	Manifestation	Serotype of virus		
		Coxsackie virus	**Entero virus**	**Echo**
i.	Acute hemorrhagic conjunctivitis (characteristic subconjunctival hemorrhage)	A-24	Ent. 70	–
ii.	Aseptic meningitis	Most group A, all B	Ent	E
iii.	Encephalitis	A,B	Ent	E
iv.	Exanthem	A, B	Ent	E
v.	Generalized disease of newborn	B_{2-5}	–	E
vi.	Hand, foot and mouth disease	A,B (commonly by A)	Ent 71	–
vii.	Herpangina	A,B (commonly by A)	Ent 71	E
viii.	Myocarditis, pericarditis	A, B (commonly B)	–	E
ix.	Paralysis	A, B (commonly A)	Ent	E
x.	Pleurodynia (Bornholm disease)	A,B (commonly B)	–	E
xi.	Pneumonia	A,B	Ent	E
xii.	Juvenile diabetes	B-4	–	–
xiii.	Orchitis	Coxsackie	–	–
xiv.	Post viral fatigue syndrome	B	–	–

4. Which of the following culture medium is used for Legionella growth?

A. Chocolate agar
B. Thayer Martin
C. EMJH
D. BCYE

Answer: Option D. BCYE

Explanation:

Legionella

- Gram negative non-capsulated, intracellular cocobacilli.
- They are motile, aerobic, catalase and oxidase positive.

Culture

- Not grow on ordinary media.
- ***Buffered charcoal yeast extract 'BCYE'*** is selective medium used to grow legionella. It grows best at pH - 6.9 temperature 35°C and 90% humidity.
- Most common species associated with human infection is L. pneumophilia (Most common with serogroup 1).
- Other important species is L.micdadei (Pittsburgh pneumonia agent). It is partial acid fast (AFB).
- Natural habitat is aquatic bodies including lakes and streams. Shows symbiotic relations with algae, amebas, ciliated protozoa.
- Factors enhancing colonisation are warm temperature, stagnation and sediments. It can form microcolonies with in biofilms. Its eradication require disinfectants that can penetrate the biofilm.

Mode of Transmission

- Aspiration is predominant mode of transmission. Other modes include aerosolization, direct instillation in to lungs. No man to man transmission occurs. Aerosolization by A.C., nebulizer, humidifier and direct instillation into lung are other modes.

Risk Factors and Pathogenesis

- Conditions that impair mucocilliary clearance predispose to legionaires disease most commonly cigarette smoking.
- Hairy cell leukemia (not other leukemia) and immuno-compromised state are other risk factors.

- Bacteria attach host cell by type IV pili, HSP60 and major outer membrane protein. Legionella binds to CR_1 and CR_3 integrin receptor.
- Cell mediated immunity is primary mechanism of host defense (Role of neutrophil appears to be minimal).
- Humoral immunity plays no role.

Legionellosis: Legionella cause 2 clinical syndromes:

A. Pontiac fever:

- Acute febrile self-limited illness. Airbone transmission with high attack rate.
- Pneumonia does not develop. Most common symptom – malaise, fatigue and myalgia.

B. Legionnaires disease: Designation for pneumonia.

- 4th most common cause of community acquired pneumonia (Most common – S.pneumoniae 2nd most common – H.influenzae 3rd most common Chlamydia pneumoniae).
- Cause–Atypical pneumonia which is more serious than atypical pneumonia of other agents.
- Clinical features suggestive of L. pneumonia:
  - Diarrhoea
  - High fever
  - Hyponatremia
  - Proteinuria
  - Onset of symptom within 10 days after discharge from hospital suggest nosocomial logionnaires disease.
- Mostly caused by serotype 1 but serotype 6 is associated more commonly with hospital acquired and has poor prognosis.
- Relative bradycardia is useful diagnostic finding.
- Extrapulmonary legionellosis.
- Results from blood borne dissemination from lung.
- Most common extrapulmonary site is heart.
- Most cases are hospital acquired.
- Most common neurological abnormality are confusion or changed mental status.

Diagnosis

Specimen:

- Sensitivity of bronchoscopy specimens is approximately the same as that of sputum.
- Bronchoalveolar lavage fluid gives higher yield than bronchial wash specimen.

  Urinary antigen: Requires 12 weeks, so used for retrospective diagnosis or epidemiologic studies. Cheap, rapid, second in sensitivity and highly specific. Detectable within 3 days. The test is not affected by antibiotic administration.

Staining: DFA test is rapid and highly specific but less sensitive.

Culture: Requires 3-5 days to become grossly visible.

Definitive method of diagnosis:

- B'CYE media is used.

Treatment

- Azithromycin and respiratory tract quinolones (Levofloxacin, Gemifloxacin, Moxifloxacin) are DOC.
- Quinolones are preferred antibiotic in transplant recipients.

5. Infection with which of the following organism associated with conjunctival hyperemia?

A. H. Ducreyi
B. Legionella
C. Brucella
D. Leptospirosis

Answer: Option D. Leptospirosis

Explanation:

Conjunctival suffusion is an eye finding occurring early in Weil's disease, which is caused by Leptospira interrogans. Conjunctival suffusion is characterized by redness of the conjunctiva that resembles conjunctivitis, but it does not involve inflammatory exudates.

LEPTOSPIRA

- Actively motile spirochetes possessing a large number of closely wound spirals and characteristic hooked ends.
- *Culture:* Grow best under aerobic condition. For isolation EMJH media is used.
- *Pathogenesis and clinical manifestation*:

- Leptospirosis is a zoonosis with rodents being most important reservoir.
- Transmission results from ingestion or contact with urine, blood or tissue from infected animal but not from bite. Since leptospires are excreted in urine of infected rat, water is important vehicle. Human to human transmission don't occur.
- Vasculitis is responsible for most clinical manifestation.

It mainly infects:

- Liver (centritobular necrosis is found).
- Kidney (cause interstitial nephritis, tubular necrosis).

After formation of antibody, leptospires are eliminated from all sites except the eye, proximal renal tubules and brain. More than 40% of symptomatic person have mild and anticteric from of leptospirosis. Severe leptospirosis is characterized by profound jaundice, renal dysfunction, hemorrhagic diathesis called as Weil's syndrome or Icterohemorrhagic fever.

Diagnosis

1. Isolation of organism	From blood or CSF during 1st 10 days From urine after 1 week. For isolation EMJH medium is useful
2. Serology	Microscopic agglutination test (MAT) ELISA

Treatment

- Mild – Doxycycline or Ampicillin.
- Moderate/severe – Penicillin or Erythromycin.

Chemoprophylaxis: Doxycycline.

6. Which of the following organism associated with ingestion of Cysticercus cellulosae?

A. Hydatid cyst
B. Neurocysticercosis
C. Toxoplasmosis
D. Toxocara

Answer: Option B. Neurocysticercosis

Explanation:

"Neurocysticercosis is the most common parasitic disease of CNS worldwide."

NEUROCYSTICERCOSIS = CYSTICERCOSIS OF CNS

Mode of Transmission in T. solium

Ingestion of cysticercus cellulosae or bladder worm (larvae) in pork meat.

Autoinfection by finger contamination with eggs from perianal skin or feces.

Ingestion of eggs in water or vegetables which develops into larvae than into Adult worm

Autoinfection by gravid segments reaching the stomach by retrograde peristalsis from jejunum when they are digested and thousands of eggs released.

- So man is both definitive and intermediate host for T. solium but in man it is dead end infection.

Clinical Features:

- Most common manifestation is new-onset partial seizures with or without secondary generalization.

Site Symptoms

- Brain parenchyma (Most common).
- Subarachnoid or ventricular space.
- Spinal cyst.
- Seizures or focal neurological defects.
- Increased intracranial tension.
- Mimic intraspinal tumour.

Diagnosis

- By non-contrast CT.
- Most common finding on neuroimaging is parenchymal brain calcification.

Treatment

- Antiepileptic therapy + Albendazole or praziquantel.
- Site of cysticercosis.
- CNS > Subcutaneous tissue > globe of eye.

7. Which of the following test does not use labeled antibody?

A. Wasserman reaction B. ELISA

C. Hemagglutination assay D. Radioimmunoassay

Answer: Option C. Hemagglutination assay

Explanation:

All above options use antibody except hemagglutination assay.

Hemagglutination assay (HA) apply the process of hemagglutination, in which sialic acid receptors on the surface of red blood cells (RBCs) bind to the hemagglutinin glycoprotein found on the surface of influenza virus (and several other viruses) and create a network, or lattice structure, of interconnected RBC's and virus particles. The agglutinated lattice maintains the RBC's in a suspended distribution, typically viewed as a diffuse reddish solution. The formation of the lattice depends on the concentrations of the virus and RBC's, and when the relative virus concentration is too low, the RBC's are not constrained by the lattice and settle to the bottom of the well. Hemagglutination is observed in the presence of staphylococci, vibrios, and other bacterial species, similar to the mechanism viruses use to cause agglutination of erythrocytes. The RBC's used in HA assays are typically from chickens, turkeys, horses, guinea pigs, or humans depending on the selectivity of the targeted virus or bacterium and the associated surface receptors on the RBC.

Hemagglutination inhibition assay is closely related to the HA assay, but includes anti-viral antibodies as "inhibitors" to interfere with the virus-RBC interaction.

Following are Antigen Antibody Reactions

1. **Precipitation Reaction**

   When soluble antigen combines with its antibody in presence of electrolytes, it forms insoluble precipitates/ floccules.

   - This reaction show "zone phenomenon" (also in agglutination) either in the form of prozone (antibody excess) or postzone (antigen excess).
   - It occur in zone of equivalence due to lattice formation (also in agglutination).

- It is very sensitive in antigen detection (but relatively less sensitive for antibody detection).

  It is of following types:
- Ring test
- Slide test
- Tube test
- Immunodiffusion (ppt in gel) – E.g., Elek test for toxigenicity in diphtheria (double diffusion).
- Electroimmune diffusion – E.g., Rocket electrophoresis for quantitative estimation of antigen.

  Simplest type–E.g., Ascoli's thermoprecipitin test and streptococcal lancefield grouping.
  - VDRL test of syphilis.
  - Kahn test of syphilis.

2. **Agglutination Reaction**

   It is more sensitive than precipitation for antibody detection. Occur in presence of electrolytes.
   - Incomplete or monovalent antibodies (usually Ab are bivalent) do not cause agglutination, though they combine with the antigen. They also act as blocking Ab since they inhibits agglutination by complete Ab. Agglutination is of following types:
   - Slide agglutination–used for blood grouping and cross matching.
   - Tube agglutination–E.g., Widal test, Brucellosis, Weil-Felix reaction, Paul Bunnel test, cold agglutination and Streptococcus MG test.
   - Antiglobulin (Coombs) test–used for detecting in complete Ab of brucellosis; anti-RhAb.
   - Passive agglutination test–used to detect Ab by adsorbing soluble Agon carrier particles so precipitation reaction converts into agglutination test which are more convenient and more sensitive. E.g., Rose waller test, test detecting RA factor by using amboceptor.
   - Latex agglutination test (latex fixation test)–for detection of ASO, CRP, RA factor, HCG; Streptozyme test.
   - Reversed passive agglutination – Estimation of antigen by adsorbing antibody to carrier particles.

3. **Complement Fixation Test (CFT)**

- Antigen may be soluble or particulate.
- Source of complement is guinea pig serum, E.g. (i) ***Wassermann reaction***; coagulating complement adsorption test using horse complement; immuno adherence of V.cholera and T. pallidum. (ii) Immobilization test of T. pallidum. (iii) Cytolytic or cytocidal test. (iv) Neutralisation Test includes virus neutralisation test (plaque inhibition test), Toxin neutralisation (Schick, anti-streptolysin O) test. (v) ***Radioimmunoassay (RIA).*** vi. ***Enzyme Immunoassay (EIA).***
- Most common labels used are radio-isotopes and enzymes.
- It measures analytes upto picogram (10^{-12}g) quantities.
- Used for quantitation of hormones, drugs, tumour markers, IgE and viral antigen.
- Measures enzyme labelled antigen, hapten or antibody.
- It may be homogenous or heterogenous.
- Major type of heterogenous EIA is ***ELISA*** which involves the use of immunosorbent – an absorbing material specific for one of components of reaction, the antigen or antibody. E.g., ELISA for detection of Rotavirus in feces or HIV antibody in serum.

8. Which of the following test does not use in immediate evaluation of UTI screening?

A. Blood test

B. Nitrite test

C. Bed side culture

D. Leukocyte esterase test

Answer: Option C. Bed side culture

Explanation:

Urine may be assessed both at the bedside (dipstick) and **in the laboratory (**microscopy, **culture,** sensitivity and urinary electrolytes).

Bedside analysis

- Urine Colour
- Urine Transparency
- Urine Odour
- Dipstick Urine Analysis

Parameters
Nitrite test
Leukocyte esterase test
Blood test
Nitrite and/or leukocyte esterase
Leukocyte esterase and/or blood
Nitrite and/or blood
Nitrite and/or blood and/or leukocyte esterase

Leucocytes (White cell count (WCC))

- Determines the presence of whole or lysed white cells in the urine (pyuria) by detecting leucocyte esterase activity.
- A positive leucocyte esterase test correlates well with pyuria. However, the diagnosis may be missed in up to 20% of cases if a negative urinalysis dipstick is used to exclude UTI.
  - **False positive:** Contaminated specimen, trichomonas vaginalis, drugs or foods that colour the urine red.
  - **False negative:** Intercurrent or recent antibiotic therapy (especially gentamicin, tetracycline and cephalosporins), glycosuria, proteinuria, high specific gravity. Low bacteria count UTI (especially in women).

Nitrites

- Nitrates in the urine are converted to nitrites in the presence of Gram-negative bacteria such as E.coli and Klebsiella.
- A positive nitrite test is a surrogate marker of bacteruria.
- Positive test strongly suggests infection but negative test does not exclude it (PPV 95% and NPV 25-70%).
  - **False negative:** Drugs or foods that colour the urine red. Certain bacteria such as S. saprophyticus, acinetobacter and most enterococci.

Blood

- Dipstick urinalysis is able to detect haemolysed and nonhaemolysed blood in the urine.
- The pseudoperoxidase reaction of erythrocytes, free haemoglobin or myoglobin catalyses chromogen oxidation on the dipstick to produce a colour change.
- A positive result may be indicative of haematuria from trauma, infection, inflammation, infarction, calculi, neoplasia, clotting disorders or chronic infection (see haematuria chapter).
- Haemaglobinuria may be associated with intravascular haemolysis, burns, sudden cold, eclampsia, sickle cell crisis, multiple myeloma, alkaloids (mushrooms) and transfusion reactions.
- **Dip stick analysis can also be used for ketones, glucose, bilirubin, urobilinogen.**

9. Which of the following is false regarding needle stick injury?

A. Non-dominant hand is generally involved

B. Injured site should be washed in running tap water

C. Highest rate of transmission

D. All sharp injury do not require reporting

Answer: Option C. Highest rate of transmission

Explanation:

Needle stick injury has lowest rate of transmission (<1%) and highest rate of transmission occurs through sexual intercourse.

Transmission route	%
Sexual intercourse	**70-80**
Mother-to-child-transmission	5-10
Blood transfusion	3-5
Injecting drug use	5-10
Health care–e.g.: needle stick injury	<0.01

MODES OF TRANSMISSION

A. Sexual transmission

- The most common mode of transmission worldwide is heterosexual transmission.
- Chance of infection from male to female is twice as from female to male.
- Anal intercourse has higher risk of transmission.

B. Transmission by blood and blood products:

- Transmission of whole blood. Packed red cells, platelets, leucocytes and plasma are all capable of transmitting HIV infection.
- Hyperimmunoglobulin, hepatitis B immunoglobulin, plasma derived hepatitis B vaccine and Rh immunoglobulin have not been associated with transmission of HIV infection.
- Risk of getting HIV infection from transfusion of a unit of infected blood is > 95%.

C. Maternal fetal transmission – Risk is 30%

- Occurs most commonly in perinatal period.
- Cesarean section decrease risk of transmission.
- Risk of infection is high if the mother is newly infected or if she has already developed AIDS.
- Vitamin A deficiency increase risk of transmission.
- Exclusive breastfeeding carries lower risk of transmission than mixed feeding.
- Presence of mastitis, low maternal CD4+ T cells counts and maternal vitamin A deficiency increase risk of transmission.

D. Transmission by other body fluids

- HIV can be isolated in low titres from saliva, but saliva cannot transmit HIV infection due to presence of endogenous antiviral factors of which most important is secretory leucocyte protease inhibitor (SLPI).

NEEDLE STICK INJURY

Protocol

1. ***Immediate***
    - *For Injury:* Wash with soap and running water.
    - *For Non-intact Skin Exposure:* Wash with soap and water.
    - *For Mucosal Exposure:* Wash thoroughly.
2. ***Reporting***
    - ***All sharps injury and mucosal exposure MUST be reported*** to the immediate supervisor, and to the Casualty Medical Officer to evaluate the injury. Details of the needle stick injury should be filled by the supervisor and handed over to the HIC nurse for further follow-up.
3. ***Management***
    - Management is on a case to case basis.
4. ***Follow-Up***
    - Follow-up and statistics of needle stick injury are done by the HIC nurse on a weekly basis. This information is presented at the HICC meeting and preventive actions to avoid needle stick injuries, if any, are recorded.

POST-HIV EXPOSURE MANAGEMENT/PROPHYLAXIS (PEP)

Occupational exposure

Occupational exposure refers to exposure to potential blood-borne infections (HIV, HBV and HCV) that occurs during performance of job duties.

"Exposure" which may place an HCP at risk of blood-borne infection is defined as:

- A percutaneous injury (e.g., needle stick or cut with a sharp instrument).
- Contact with the mucous membranes of the eye or mouth.
- Contact with non-intact skin (particularly when the exposed skin is chapped, abraded, or afflicted with dermatitis), or
- Contact with intact skin when the duration of contact is prolonged (e.g., several minutes or more) with blood or other potentially infectious body fluids.

As needle is held in dominant hand (right in most cases), left hand is used to fix the lump. NSI (Needle Stick Injury) was **the most common in non-dominant hand,** i.e., left in 52.4% (33 out of 57) and right in 22.2% (14 out of 57). Both hands were injured in 14.3% (9 out of 57).

10. Hyper Ig E syndrome is associated with:

A. Joint infection

B. Meningitis

C. Non-silent pulmonary infection

D. Recurrent cold abscess

Answer: Option D. Recurrent cold abscess

The most characteristic features of hyper IgE syndrome are recurrent Staphylococcal cold abscesses and recurrent relatively silent pulmonary infection.

Hyperimmunoglobulin E (hyper IgE) syndrome (HIES), also known as **Job syndrome**, consists of a heterogeneous group of complex hereditary combined B- and T-cell immune deficiency diseases characterized by recurrent *Staph aureus* chest infections, characteristic coarse facial appearance and dental problems with eczema-like pruritic dermatitis.

Terminology

There are two types of HIES:

- Autosomal dominant (**STAT3 deficiency**)
  - More common.
  - Caused by a mutation in STAT3 gene.
- Autosomal recessive
  - Etiology unknown.

This article is concerned with the more common autosomal dominant HIES.

Clinical Presentation

First sign of disease is pustules and eczematoid rashes in the face and scalp. Skeletal manifestations include scoliosis, minimal trauma fractures due to osteoporosis, and hyperextensibility of the joints. Failure of exfoliation of primary teeth. After delayed shedding of primary teeth or extraction, the normal secondary teeth will emerge. Facial changes such as facial asymmetry, broad nose, and deep-set eyes with a prominent forehead, facial skin thickening with prominent pores occur during adolescence.

Radiographic Features

Recurrent chest infections in childhood with Staph aureus usually are less symptomatic than in immunologically normal children hence in most cases, delayed treatment results in severe damage to the lung parenchyma. Besides, even after adequate treatment of the acute infection, healing process in these patients causes severe parenchymal injury, bronchiectasis, scarring, and large pneumatocele formation. After initial injuries, lungs become susceptible to the secondary indolent infections with *Pseudomonas* and *Aspergillus* infections which are difficult to treat and they usually worsen the parenchymal and bronchial damage.

11. Dose of diphtheria antitoxin is:

A. 10-100 IU

B. 100-1000 IU

C. 20,000-1,00,000 IU

D. 1,00,000- 2,00,000 IU

Answer: Option C. 20,000-1,00,000 IU

Diphtheria antitoxin (Antidiphtheritic serum ADS). It is obtained from horse and is used therapeutically in clinical diphtheria without waiting for bacteriological report, because each hour's delay increases the dose requirement and decreases beneficial effects: damage already caused by the toxin is not reversed. The antitoxin neutralizes the exotoxin released at the site of infection and that circulating in blood but not that fixed to tissues.

Dose: 20,000–40,000 IU I.M. or I.V. for pharyngeal/laryngeal disease of upto 48 hours duration. Higher dose (upto 100,000 IU may be needed).

Diphtheria Antitoxin 10,000 IU in 10 ml amp.

Appropriate antimicrobials should also be given. Unprotected child contacts should be given ADS (1000 IU) along with diphtheria toxoid for prophylaxis.

12. A 28 years old male working as IT profession visited China and ate crayfish. Thereafter he developed cough, fever and malaise. Which of the following organism is associated with these symptoms?

A. Fasciola buski

B. Schistosoma hematobium

C. Fasciola hepatica

D. Paragonimus westermani

Answer: Option D. Paragonimus westermani

Here this person has history of ingestion of cray fish, which is an intermediate host in transmission of paragonimus westermani organism.

- Trematodes (also known as flukes).
- Man is definitive and snails are intermediate host usually.
- They are classified as:

(See table on page 21)

13. A 36 years old, veterinarian person has developed black eschar over hand region. Based on these features which of the following is a cause of these features?

A. HSV   B. C. diphtheria

C. Bacillus anthrax   D. CMV

Answer: Option C. Bacillus anthrax

Explanation:

Here above case patient is 36 years old and he is working as veterinarian (so, must be contact with animal) presenting with black eschar over hand region. So this is a case of cutaneous anthrax caused by shaving brushes of animal hair, which can lead to black eschar.

(See table on Page No.146)

Q. No. 12

Flukes	Habitat	Intermediate Host	Mode of Transmission
A. Blood flukes			
i. Schistosoma (Bilharzia) hematobium	Vesical and pelvic vein plexuses	Snail which is infected by miracidium	Water borne disease Man is infected by bathing in contaminated water when carcaria penetrates unbroken skin
ii. S. mansoni	Inferior mesentric vein (Intestinal bilharziasis) or Schistosomal dysentery		
iii. S. japonicum or oriental schistosomiasis	Superior mesentric vein (katayama disease)		
B. Live flukes			
i. Clonorchis sinensis (=Chinese liver flukes)	Biliary tract (associate with cholangiocarcinoma)	1st intermediate host: snail 2nd intermediate host: fish	Fish containing metacercariae are eaten raw or inadequately processed
ii. Fasciola hepatica (=sheep liver fluke)	Biliary tract	Primary host: man/sheep Intermediate host: snails	Ingestion of watercress or other water vegetation containing metacercaria
C. Intestinal flukes			
i. Fasciolopsis buski (Giant intestinal fluke)	Duodenum or jejunum	Molluscum Snails	Ingestion of roots of lotus, bulb of water chestnut and other acquatic vegetations
ii. Heterophytes	Small intestine	Molluscum Snails	Ingestion of fishes since cercriae encyst on fishes
iii. Metagonimus yokogawai	Small intestine	1st intermediate host: fresh water snail 2nd intermediate host: fish	Ingestion of raw fish

Contd.

Contd.

iv. Gastrodiscoides hominis (only fluke inhabiting human large intestine)	Large intestine	Molluscum	Ingestion of water plants
D. Lung fluke			
Paragonimus Westermani = Oriental lung fluke	Cystic space of lung	1st intermediate host: snail; 2nd intermediate host: fresh water cray fish or crab fish	Inadequately cooked crabs, cray fish

Q. No. 13

Cutaneous anthrax (Hide porter's disease) (=Malignant pustule)	Gastrointestinal anthrax (Wool sorter's disease)	Pulmonary anthrax (= Inhalation anthrax)
• Most common type of anthrax • Usual sites–arms, hand, face, neck • Characterized by presence of malignant pustule • Central necrotic painless lesion covered by black eschar surrounded by satellite lesions • Generally resolved spontaneously but 10-20% patients develop fatal septicemia • Also caused by shaving brushes of animal hair or occasionally by insect bite	• Earliest symptom are typically viral like prodrome with fever, malaise, abdominal or chest symptoms • 100% fatal though with prompt treatment, survival is possible • Characteristic X-ray mediastinal widening, hemorrhagic pleural effusion	• Rare form • High mortality rate • Primary lesion is most often located on tonsil

14. Which of the following method used as disc-diffusion antibiotic susceptibility test?

A. Muller – Hinton agar method

B. Chocolate agar method

C. Thayer Martin media method

D. Kirby-Bauer method

Answer: Option D. Kirby-Bauer test

Explanation:

The disk-diffusion test, or agar diffusion test, or Kirby-Bauer test (disc-diffusion antibiotic susceptibility test, disc-diffusion antibiotic sensitivity test, KB test), is a test of the antibiotic sensitivity of bacteria. It uses **antibiotic discs** to test the extent to which bacteria are affected by those antibiotics. In this test, wafers containing antibiotics are placed on an agar plate where bacteria have been placed, and the plate is left to incubate. If an antibiotic stops the bacteria from growing or kills the bacteria, there will be an area around the wafer where the bacteria have not grown enough to be visible. This is called a zone of inhibition.

The size of this zone depends on many factors, one being how effective the antibiotic is at stopping the growth of the bacterium. Another factor that will influence the size of a zone is the diffusion of the antibiotic within the agar medium and varies based on the molecular configuration of the antibiotic. Once the zone diameter is measured it must be compared to a database of zone standards to determine if the bacterium being studied is susceptible, moderately susceptible or resistant to the antibiotic in question.

A pure bacterial culture is suspended in buffer, standardized to turbidity and swabbed uniformly across a culture plate. A filter-paper disk, impregnated with the compound to be tested, is then placed on the surface of the agar. The compound diffuses from the filter paper into the agar. The concentration of the compound will be highest next to the disk, and will decrease as distance from the disk increases. If the compound is effective against bacteria at a certain concentration, no colonies will grow where the concentration in the agar is greater than or equal to the effective concentration. This is the zone of inhibition. This along with the rate of antibiotic diffusion are used to estimate the bacteria's susceptibility to that particular antibiotic. In general, larger zones correlate with smaller minimum inhibitory concentration (MIC) of antibiotic for that bacteria. Inhibition produced by the test is compared with that produced by known concentration of a reference compound. This information can be used to choose appropriate antibiotics to combat a particular infection.

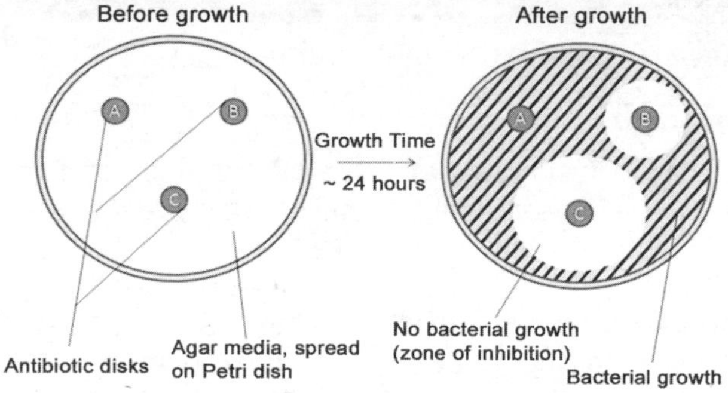

The disk-diffusion agar method tests the effectiveness of antibiotics on a specific microorganism. An agar plate is first spread with bacteria, then paper disks of antibiotics are added. The bacteria is allowed to grow on the agar media, and then observed. The amount of space around every antibiotic plate indicates the lethality of that antibiotic on the bacteria in question. Highly effective antibiotics (disk C) will produce a wide ring of no bacterial growth, while an ineffective antibiotic (disk A) will show no change in the surrounding bacterial concentration at all. The effectiveness of intermediate antibiotics (disk B) can be measured using their zone of inhibition. This method is used to determine the best antibiotic to use against a new or drug-resistant pathogen.

15. A 30 years old patient presented with abdominal pain and rectal prolapse. Infection with which of the following organism causes these symptoms?

A. Trichuris trichura

B. Enterobius vermicularis

C. Strongyloides stercoralis

D. Tape worm

Answer: Option A. Trichuris trichura

Explanation:

Heavy infections with trichuris trichura, especially in small children, can cause gastrointestinal problems such as abdominal pain, diarrhea, rectal prolapse.

- **Trichuris – Trichura = Whipworm**

Life cycle in one host only (monoxenous).

Adult worm lives in caecum and appendix (Large intestine).

Mode of infection : Feco-oral when mature embryonated eggs containing infective rhabditiform larva are swallowed in food or water.

Life cycle

The unembryonated eggs are passed with the stool. In the soil, the eggs develop into a 2-cell stage, an advanced cleavage stage, and then they embryonate; eggs become infective in 15 to 30 days. After ingestion (soil-contaminated hands or food), the eggs hatch in the small intestin, and release larvae that mature and establish themselves as adults in the colon. The adult worms (approximately 4 cm in length) live in the cecum and ascending colon. The adult worms are fixed in that location, with the anterior portions threaded into the mucosa. The females begin to oviposit 60 to 70 days after infection. Female worms in the cecum shed between 3,000 and 20,000 eggs per day. The life span of the adults is about 1 year.

Clinical Presentation

Most frequently asymptomatic. Heavy infections, especially in small children, can cause gastrointestinal problems (abdominal pain, diarrhea, rectal prolapse) and possibly growth retardation.

Laboratory Diagnosis

Microscopic identification of whipworm eggs in feces is evidence of infection. Because eggs may be difficult to find in light infections, a concentration procedure is recommended. Because the severity of symptoms depend on the worm burden, quantification of the latter (e.g. with the Kato-Katz technique) can prove useful.Examination of the rectal mucosa by proctoscopy (or directly in case of prolapses) can occasionally demonstrate adult worms.

Treatment

Whipworm is effectively treated with albendazole, mebendazole or ivermectin.

CHAPTER

7 FORENSIC MEDICINE

1. Which of the following poison permits gastric lavage?

A. Sulfuric acid
B. Carbolic acid
C. Nitric acid
D. Hydrochloric acid

Answer: Option B. Carbolic acid

Explanation:

The only absolute contraindication for gastric lavage is corrosive poisoning except for carbolic acid which permits gastric lavage. Rest of sulfuric acid, nitric acid and hydrochloric acid do not permit gastric lavage.

GASTRIC LAVAGE

It is useful any time wihin 3 hours after ingestion of a poison. It is done using a stomach tube (Ewald's or Boa's, tube) or ordinary soft, non-collapsible rubber tube of one cm diameter and one-and-half metre length, with a glass funnel attached at one end, and a mark about 50 cm from the other end, which should be rounded with lateral openings to avoid any injury when it is being passed. At about the midpart of the tube there is a suction bulb, used to pump out the stomach contents.

Stomach contents can be aspirated by a 20 ml syringe. Preserve this for chemical analysis. If there is any bleeding, abandon the procedure. Gastric lavage may be done with water; 1:5000 potassium permanganate; five per cent sodium bicarbonate; four percent tannic acid; one percent sodium or potassium iodide; one to three percent calcium lactate; saturated lime water or starch solution, or 0.9% saline. Next, use about half litre of suitable solution and repeat till clear and odourless fluid comes out. This indicates that there is no further interaction between the antidote and poison. At this stage, the stomach is not completely emptied but a small quantity of the fluid containing the antidote or activated charcoal suspension (one gm/kg body weight, or/and a cathartic) is left behind in the stomach, so that it may neutralise whatever small quantity of the poison is left behind. Ryle's tube or a number 10 to 12 French catheter can be used for infants and children, and about 25 cm is necessary to reach the stomach. After a recent heavy meal, the bulky contents are first removed by emetics. Stomach wash is better than emesis because of the discomfort caused to the patient in vomiting.

In poisoning with salicylates, phenothiazines, tricyclic antidepressants, antihistamines, lavage can be done up to 12 to 18 hours after ingestion of the poison.

Contraindications

The only absolute contraindication is corrosive poisoning (except carbolic acid), owing to the danger of perforation. In the following conditions stomach wash can be done by taking proper precautions. (1) **Convulsant poisons,** as it may lead to convulsions. Lavage should be done after controlling the convulsions. (2) **Comatose patients,** because of the risk of aspiration of fluid into the air-passages. The airway should be sealed by cuffed endotracheal tube (8 to 9 mm) and lavage done. (3) **Volatile poisons,** which may be inhaled. (4) Upper alimentary disease, e.g., oesophageal varices. (5) In patients with marked hypothermia, and haemorrhagic diathesis.

Complications: (1) Laryngeal spasm. (2) Aspiration pneumonitis. (3) Perforation of stomach. (4) Sinus bradycardia.

2. **Which of the following is not true regarding identical twin?**
   A. They have same fingerprint
   B. Identical twin share one placenta
   C. Identical twin has same DNA
   D. Identical twins grow differently based on environment

Answer: Option A. They have same fingerprint

Explanation:

Fingerprint pattern is different in identical twins.

Identical twins is monozygotic twins, so they share one placenta. Identical twins are created when a single zygote splits into two in this way **share the same DNA. Environmental factors can influence a person's physical appearance,** for example, and epigenetic factors create differences as twins age. The epigenome describes chemical changes within DNA as an organism ages. These factors explain why identical twins can be different, whether in appearance, temperament, or personality.

The majority of twins are dizygotic, produced when two separate eggs are fertilized by two different sperm. One way to find out if a pair of twins of the same gender is identical or fraternal (different-sex twins are always fraternal), is through DNA testing. DNA from non-identical (fraternal or dizygotic) twins will generally be about 50 percent to 75 percent similar.

Each person's **retina** has an unique pattern which is not changed from birth until death. The pattern is different even in identical twins. As such, it appears to be the most precise and reliable biometric.

3. Rigor mortis occurs first in which organ?

A. Shoulder B. Eyelid

C. Facial muscles D. Myocardium

Answer: Option D. Myocardium > B Eyelid

Explanation:

Here there is a controversy regarding answer between myocardium and eyelid because different textbook gives different answer.

1. **The Essentials of Forensic Medicine and Toxicology (33rd edition)–*Dr. K.S. Narayan Reddy***

It first appears in involuntary muscles; the myocardium becomes rigid in an hour.

Eyelid muscle is the levator palpebrae superioris, composed of both skeletal and smooth muscle fibers therefore it has voluntary and involuntary both types of fibers.

Rigor mortis (death stiffening; cadaveric rigidity) is a state of stiffening of muscles, sometimes with slight shortening of the fibres. Individual cell death takes place in this stage.

The Order of Appearance of Rigor:

All muscles of the body, both voluntary and involuntary are affected. It does not start in all muscles simultaneously (Nysten's rule).

It first appears in involuntary muscles; the myocardium becomes rigid in an hour. It begins in the eyelids, neck and lower jaw and passes upwards to the muscles of the face, and downwards to the muscles of the chest, upper limbs, abdomen and lower limbs and lastly in the fingers and toes. The lactic acid enters blood stream and reconverted to glycogen in the liver. In individual limbs, it usually progresses from above downwards. Such a sequence is not constant, symmetrical or regular. In individual limbs, it disappears in the same order in which it has appeared. Rigor mortis always sets in, increases and decreases gradually.

2. **Concise Textbook of Forensic Medicine and Toxicology (3rd edition)–*R.K. Sharma***

The rigor mortis follows a definite course. **It starts first in muscles of eyelids,** muscles of the back of neck and lower jaw, front of neck, face, chest and upper extremities and then progresses to muscles of the abdomen and lower extremities.

3. **Simpson's Forensic Medicine (12th edition)**

Rigor develops uniformly throughout the body but **it is first detectable in the smaller muscle groups such as those around the eyes** and mouth, the jaw and the fingers. It appears to 'spread' down the body from the head to the legs as larger and larger muscle groups are rendered stiff.

4. **Textbook of Forensic Medicine and Toxicology (5th edition)–*Krishan Vij***

In 1811, the French Physician and Chemist PH Nysten published the first scientific description of rigor mortis. He stated, "Cadaveric rigidity affects successively the masticatory mus- cles, those of the face and neck, those of the trunk and arms, and finally those of the lower limbs". It is often added that resolution occurs in the same order. Even today, almost the same holds good, and it is considered to **appear first in the muscles of the eyelids by 1–2 hours** of death and then progresses on to muscles of face, neck, lower jaw, muscles of the chest, upper limbs, abdomen and lower limbs. The proximodistal progression is only apparent one.

Rigor mortis involves the involuntary muscles also, where it makes its existence earlier than the voluntary muscles. It may be due either to their small mass or more speedy loss of irritability. **It appears in the heart usually within an hour of death** and may stay for 10–12 hours. Left ventricles contracted by rigor may not be deemed hypertrophied.

4. Which section of IPC defines punishment for perjury?

A. IPC 151
B. IPC 191
C. IPC 193
D. IPC 153

Answer: Option C. IPC 193

193. Punishment For False Evidence.

Whoever intentionally gives false evidence in any stage of a judicial proceeding, or fabricates false evidence for the purpose of being used in any stage of a judicial proceeding, shall be punished with imprisonment of either description for a term which may extend to seven years, and shall also be liable to fine; and whoever intentionally gives or fabricates false evidence in any other case, shall be punished with imprisonment of either description for a term which may extend to three years, and shall also be liable to fine.

196. Using Evidence Known To Be False.

Whoever corruptly uses or attempts to use as true or genuine evidence any evidence which he knows to be false or fabricated, shall be punished in the same manner as if he gave or fabricated false evidence.

199. False Statement Made In Declaration Which Is By Law Receivable As Evidence.

195. Prosecution For Contempt Of Lawful Authority Of Public Servants, For Offences Against Public Justice And For Offences Relating To Documents Given In Evidence.

Offence of **perjury** has been defined in **Section 191** of the **Indian Penal Code**.

Few Other IPC Useful for Exam

31 IPC Testamentary capacity

44 Injury

45 IEA witness

53(1) CPC accused can be examined and evidence can be collected without his consent and by use of force

53(2) CPC whenever a female is to be examined the examination should be made only by or under the supervision of a female RMP 61 to 69 Summons

Sec 84 Act of a person of unsound mind/McNaughtens Rule

Sec 85 Act of a person who is intoxicated against will

90 IPC if age of the subject is under 12 years written consent of parent or guardian is taken

114 IPC if a female says she didn't consent for sex, the court shall presume that she didn't consent

Sec 191 and Sec 193 definition and Punishment of perjury (Punishment up to 7 years)

Sec 197 Issuing or signing false certificate

Sec 228 identity of rape victim should not be disclosed

Sec 294 IPC punishment for exhibitionism upto 3 months or fine

Sec 299 Culpable Homicide

Sec 300 Murder

Sec 302 Punishment of murder/infanticide*

Sec 304 Culpable Homicide not amounting to murder

Sec 304 A Causing death by negligence* (punishment upto 2 years/fine)

Sec 304 B Dowry death

Sec 312 to Sec 316 Abandonment of Child under 12 years

Sec 317 Concealment of birth

Sec 318 Hurt

Sec 319 Grievous Hurt

Sec 320 Assault

Sec 327 CrPC inquest into a rape case in camera

Sec 351 Assault to Outrage the Modesty of Women

Sec 354 Rape

Sec 375 Definition Punishment

Sec 376 Punishment for rape

[Section 228A Disclosure of identity of the victim of certain offences etc like Sec 376]

Criminal Procedure Code

Sec 377 Unnatural sexual offense

Sec 497 Adultery

Sec 498 Battered wife

Sec 174 Police Inquest

Sec 176 Magistrate's Inquest

Indian Evidence Act

Sec 32 Dying Declaration

5. Which of the following is not used for preservation of visceral specimen?

A. Saturated sodium chloride
B. Rectified spirit
C. Potassium fluoride
D. Formalin

Answer: Option D. Formalin

Explanation:

The viscera **should not be preserved in formaldehyde/ formalin** because extraction of poison, especially non-volatile organic compounds become difficult.

Preservatives

(1) Saturated **sodium chloride** solution, except in poisoning from corrosive acids, alkalis, corrosive sublimate and aconite.

(2) **Rectified spirit,** except in cases of suspected poisoning by (a) alcohol, kerosene, (b) chloroform, ether, (c) chloral hydrate, (d) formic acid, (e) formaldehyde, acetic acid, (f) phenol, (g) phosphorus, and (h) paraldehyde, because the organic acids and paraldehyde are soluble in alcohol and the phosphorescence of phosphorus is diminished by alcohol.

(3) Ten mg/ml of sodium or **potassium fluoride** (prevents glycolysis, inhibits enzyme enolase and inhibits bacteial growth) and 3 mg potassium oxalate (anti-coagulant) should be used for preserving blood. Fluoride should also be added to urine, CSF, and vitreous humour if alcohol estimation is required, and also to samples for analysis for cocaine, cyanide and Co. In poisoning by oxalic acid,

ethylene glycol, fluoride and CO, 30 mg sodium citrate should be added for 10 ml of blood as preservative. **One ml of concentrated hydrochloric acid or 100 mg of thymol or 100 mg of sodium fluoride can be used for 10 ml urine as a preservative. Toluene is better.**

Preservative is not necessary if (1) viscera can be analysed within 24 hours, (2) if sample can be kept in a refrigerator or ice box, (3) bone, hair, nails, (4) lung for detecting inhaled poisons.

6. Which of the following is not true about battered baby syndrome?

A. Direct manual violence is the most common method of injury

B. Lesions are not related to age

C. Lesions are at different stage healing

D. Delayed reporting of injuries may lead to suspicion for this

Answer: Option B. Lesions are not related to age

Explanation:

Battered Baby Syndrome or Caffey's Syndrome

It is also known commonly as 'battered baby or, child abuse syndrome'. They usually have multiple injuries of various durations. It suggests that the child has been beaten many a times over a certain period of time. They may have multiple rib injuries, multiple bruises over various parts of the body. Usually, parents deny any injury happening to child accidentally. These children usually come from problem families having multiple problems like parental maladjustment, foster parents, alcoholism or poverty in family. Sexual abuse of the child may also be seen in such cases.

A battered child is one who has received repetitive physical injuries as a result of non-accidental violence, produced by a parent or guardian. In addition to physical injury, there may be non-accidental deprivation of nutrition, care and affection.

Features:

1. **Age:** Usually less than three years old, though it may occur at any age.
2. **Sex:** Slightly more in males (55 to 63%).

3. **Position in family:** One child of a family, commonly the eldest or the youngest and often unwanted, such as the result of pregnancy before marriage, failure of contraception or an illegitimate child.
4. **Socio-economic factors:** Parents tend to be young between 20 to 30 years, and belong to lower social class and lower education. The family is usually isolated. There is often a history of family disharmony, long-standing emotional problems or financial problems. Many of the fathers have criminal records, or unemployed or socially unstable. Many mothers have multiple social and psychiatric problems with a chaotic and violent home background. The mother is of lower I.Q., often pregnant or in the premenstrual period at the time of battering. Unhappy childhood experiences are common in both parents and many battering parents were "battered children" themselves. Most of the parents suffer guilt-amnesia.
5. **History:** There is obvious difference between the nature of the injuries and the explanation given by the parents, which may change on several times of repetition, each time the child is taken to a different doctor.
6. **Treatment:** There is always delay between the injury and medical attention.
7. **Precipitating factors:** Violence is precipitated by actions of the child itself, e.g., crying, refusal to be quiet, persistent soiling of napkins, etc.

Injuries: Direct manual violence is the most common method of injury.

Surface Injuries: Soft tissue injuries are very common and may be seen almost anywhere on the child's body.

Visceral Injuries: Subdural haemorrhage is found in about 40% of fatal cases.

Skeletal Injuries: Skull fractures are common in occipito-parietal area. The fractures are multiple, depressed and wide.

Eye: Retinal separation, lens displacement, retinal haemorrhages, vitreous haemorrhages, subconjunctival haemorrhages.

Burns: Stubbing of cigarette ends upon the skin produce small circular, pitted burns which are pink or red when fresh.

Diagnosis: The diagnosis depends upon (1) nature of injuries, (2) time taken to seek medical advice, and (3) recurrent injuries. Differential diagnosis has to be made from scurvy, congenital syphilis, osteomyelitis, leukaemia, rickets, juvenile osteoporosis with stress fractures, paralytic disease with fractures, infantile cortical hyperostoses and osteogenesis imperfecta. Radiological manifestations of trauma and especially the metaphyseal lesions are specific to the battered baby syndrome.

Head injury is the most common cause of death followed by rupture of an abdominal organ.

The patterns of injury are fairly constant and mainly comprise bruises and fractures. The classic feature is repetition of injuries.

Major suspecting points may include:

1. Delayed reporting of injuries.
2. Injuries not corresponding to those that would be anticipated from the explanation given.
3. Injuries may be of recent origin and/or different ages, and
4. Sudden death in case of fatality.

Six patterns of child abuse are recognized: 1. Physical abuse 2. Nutritional deprivation 3. Sexual abuse 4. Intentional drugging 5. Neglect of medical care/safety and 6. Emotional abuse.

7. Which of the following firearm injury has blackening, tattooing and burns?

A. Close shot injury
B. Contact shot injury
C. Distant shot injury
D. Near shot injury

Answer: Option A. Close shot injury

Explanation:

Type of firearm injury	Features
Contact (in touch with skin)	Largest size, stellate shape, blast effect, edge eversion seen, Blackening, tattooing,singeing, abrasion collar and grease collar missing.
Close shot 2.5–7.5 cm from skin	Bullet size entry wound, circular, blast effects absent, no edge eversion. Blackening, tattooing, singeing, abrasion collar and grease collar seen.

Contd.

Contd.

Near shot 30–60 cm	Entry wound smaller than bullet size, circular in shape. No blast effects seen. Blackening and singeing almost absent. Tattooing, abrasion collar and grease collar seen.
Distant shot More than 60 cm	Entry wound smaller and circular. No blast effects seen. No blackening, tattooing, abrasion collar or grease collar seen.

1. **Contact Wounds:** The following subtypes can be seen:
   (a) *Firm contact with skin with bone beneath:* Such situation is seen when the firearm is held in close contact with the head. In this case the gases and projectile enter the skull through scalp but after resistance from the skull bone. Some amount of gases or parts of bullet may be reverted backward causing eversion of margins. In such cases the entry wound is seen as cruciate or star-shaped with everted, rugged margins. Since the discharge of the firearm enters skull completely, the underlying bone is fractured in multiple pieces with margins drawn inwards. The effect of flame and soot particles is seen around the entrance wound.
   (b) *Firm contact with skin with no bone underneath:* In such cases, the discharge enters completely into the soft tissue along with the bullet as there is no firm resistance. In both of the above cases, carbon monoxide present in the discharge enters tissues and combines with haemoglobin to impart pinkish colour to whole of the track. All along the track laceration of muscles, nerves and vessels is seen. Soot particles can also be seen along the track. The bullet may finally hit the bone or enter the cavity or may come out of body through exit wound. The muzzle imprint can be seen in some cases when the weapon is held against the head forcefully.
2. **Close-shot wounds:** There is no definite distance of close range wounds but the distance is sufficient to produce

flame and soot particles effect. The burning and singeing of hair around the wound is seen, if no clothings are present. Soot particles can be seen around the wound. It is more common with black gun powder than nitrocellulose. Unburnt powder particles of the propellent may produce tattooing of the skin.

The presence of carboxyhaemoglobin can be demonstrated in diminishing concentration all along the track. The abrasion and contusion collar may be seen, but observed less easily due to effect of flame and smoke.

3. **Near shot wounds:** In short range wounds, the effect of flame may not be present but tattooing due to powder deposition may be seen. In medium range wounds, the tattooing is not seen. The entrance wound is clearly observed. It is usually oval, margins are inverted and are smaller than the diameter of the bullet. The direction is inward and backward. The **abrasion collar** around the wound is seen as the margins are abraded. Sometimes, a **contusion collar** is also seen around the wound. The 'grease or dirt collar' may also be seen around the margins of the wound due to deposition of bullet lubrication or gun oil from the barrel of the gun.
4. **Distant shot wounds:** Since in these cases, the body is away from the useful range of the firearm, the bullet does not have momentum to enter the body. In such cases, laceration of the skin may be seen.

8. Which of the following method involves showing images and words associated with the case thereby the investigator wants to know if the subject has memories about the case thereby finding out the criminal?

A. Polygraph
B. Narco analysis
C. Brain mapping
D. Hypnosis

Answer: Option C. Brain mapping

Explanation:

Brain mapping or Brain fingerprinting is based on the principle that by showing images and words associated with the case, the investigator wants to know if the subject has memories about the case.

Brain Mapping or Brain Fingerprinting: In late 1980s in USA, Institute of Medicine of the National Academy of Science started evaluating the importance of integrating neuroscientific information by MRI, EEG, positron emission tomography (PET) and other non-invasive scanning techniques to map anatomy, psychology, perfusion, function and phenotypes of human brain. The brain mapping was started for study of memory, learning, aging and drug effects especially in schizophrenics, autistics and depressed people. This led to the establishment of the human brain project and later international consortium on brain mapping evolved.

Now this technique is used in crime detection also. It is based on the principle that by showing images and words associated with the case, the investigator wants to know if the subject has memories about the case. When a subject is shown an image or words associated with the case, a wave known as P300 is generated (the name is so given because the wave is generated 300 millisecond after the images or words are shown). This P300 wave can be documented. This test is non-invasive. This test was patented in 2001 by Lawrence Farwell, USA. The subject is made to sit on a chair and a band containing six to seven neurosensors is attached. First the control experiments are done. Then the subject is shown images, words or incidents related to the case, and his responses are recorded. If a person has seen these images, P300 wave is generated. The test usually takes 5-6 hours. Permission from the court is not needed. The results are not admissible in court of law but can provide leads to the investigative agencies to solve the case. This test has been done in many cases in recent past like in Telgi case.

Other Methods of Criminal Detection

1. ***Polygraph or Lie Detector Test:*** This method was invented by Dr. John Larson, USA in 1921. It is based on the fact that there are changes in the body which occur when a person lies and these changes can be effectively documented. In this process, the subject is made to lie on a bed and a lot of sensors are attached to his body. These sensors measure changes in breathing, blood pressure, pulse, respiratory rate and sweating. During this process, the subject is asked some standard questions (also called control questions) which are correct and then his responses are recorded on a polygraph. Then actual

questions are asked which are mixed with fillers and the person's response to these questions is documented. It has been generally found that if a person is lying, his blood pressure and heart rate increase along with high perspiration. The person's response to some fillers is also documented. Since all these responses are recorded on a polygraph, it is also called 'polygraph test'. Usually the subject's examination lasts about 2 hours. This test is quite important in cases of non-habituated criminals but it fails in highly determined and highly motivated criminals as they can speak lie very easily. No permission is needed from the court to conduct this study. The findings of this test are not admissible in the court of law but can provide leads to the investigating agencies.

2. ***Narco-analysis or Truth Serum Test:*** In 1930s, a number of psychiatrists started analysing patients after giving drugs to them. This induced a state of sleep in them which decreased the effectiveness of the patients in controlling their conscious stage. The term narco-analysis was coined as the drugs were narcotics or sleep inducers.

   This test is performed under the supervision of an anaesthetist and clinical psychologist. The fitness of the subject is evaluated by anaesthetist—whether drug can be administered to him or not. His physical examination is documented. Sodium pantothenol or sodium amytal, which is commonly used in hospital practice to induce anaesthesia, is administered in low doses. This drug causes sedation just like alcohol and the person becomes talkative and less inhibited. His ability to hide truth decreases. Now a set of questions are asked to him in a controlled manner. His responses are recorded via sound recorder. Most of the time, the subject is able to reveal the truth as his guilt complex decreases. This test can be performed only with the permission of the court and the subject himself as nobody can be forced to give evidence against himself. The report of this test is not admissible in the court of law but it can provide leads to the investigating team to reach the truth. The test is controversial but has been performed in many cases in recent past.

3. ***Hypnosis:*** Hypnosis is a trance stage induced by suggestion. In this, the subject is given commands to relax,

and slowly by giving suggestions, he is taken to a deep sleep stage, where his unconscious mind can be probed. During the entire stage, the subject remains conscious. This test can be done only with the active help of the subject. This test is quite useful in investigation of cases where information is sought from persons who witnessed the crime instead of committing it. It may help them giving details about the persons who committed the crime. The report of this test is also not admissible in court of law but can provide leads to the investigators about the persons who committed the crime.

4. ***Writing Analysis or Graphology:*** 'Graphology' or 'handwriting analysis' is done to know the genuineness of documents and to create psychological profile of the person concerned. It is also used in various industries to know about an employee's character. The report of this is admissible in court of law in many cases of forged documents.

5. ***Voice Stress Test:*** It is based on the principle that when a subject is lying, there are changes in his voice patterns which can be documented objectively. No consent of the individual is required but its report is not admissible in court of law.

CHAPTER 8

PREVENTIVE AND SOCIAL MEDICINE

1. Which of the following range is included in 1 Standard deviation in either side of curve?

A. 34% B. 68%

C. 46% D. 56%

Answer: Option B. 68%

Explanation:

68% range is included in 1 Standard deviation in either side of curve.

Poisson Distribution

- Is a 'discrete probability distribution' that expresses the 'probability of a number of events occurring in a fixed period of time' (if these events occur with a known average rate and independently of the time since the last event).
- It can also be used for the number of events in other specified intervals such as distance, area or volume. Is generally used to model the number of events occurring within a given time interval. Is a discrete distribution which takes on the values X = 0, 1, 2, 3.

Normal Distribution

- Is also known as 'Gaussian distribution' or 'Standard distribution'.
- Type of distribution: Is the distribution of values of a quantitative variable such that they are symmetric with respect to a middle value with same mean, median and mode, and then the frequencies taper off rapidly and symmetrically on both sides – 'bell shaped distribution'.

Is based on mean (m) and standard deviation (s)

- Mean, Median and Mode coincide (Mean = Median = Mode)
- Has Mean (m) = 0 and SD (m) = 1
- SD = √Variance

In Normal distribution, SD (s) = 1, thus Variance = 1

- Mean ± 1SD (μ ± 1σ) covers 68% values
- Mean ± 2SD (μ ± 2σ) covers 95% values
- Mean ± 3SD (μ ± 3σ) covers 99% values
- Actual parameters in a Normal (Gaussian) distribution:
  - Mean ± 1 SD (m ± 1m) limits include 68.27% values
  - Mean ± 2 SD (m ± 2s) limits include 95.45% values
  - Mean ± 1.96 SD (m ± 1.96s) limits include 95% values
  - Mean ± 3 SD (m ± 3m) limits include 99.73% values
  - Mean ± 2.58 SD (m ± 2.58s) limits include 99% values.

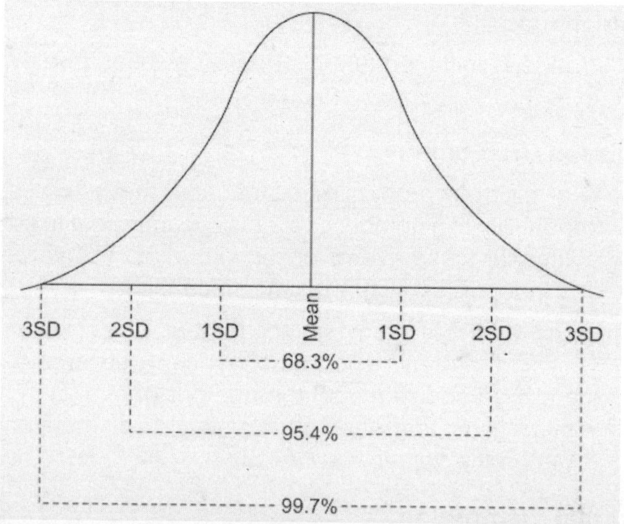

2. Cross product ratio is included in which of the following study?

A. Cross-sectional study
B. Cohort study
C. Case control study
D. Ecological study

Answer: Option C. Case control study

Explanation:

In a Case Control Study, we calculate 'an estimate of Relative Risk', known as 'Odds Ratio' (Cross Product Ratio). Case Control Study cannot provide with incidences, so Relative Risk cannot be calculated.

Odds Ratio (OR):

Ratio of odds that cases were exposed to a risk factor to the odds that the controls were exposed.

- Is used to *'measure strength of association in a case control study'*.
- Is also known as *'Cross product ratio'* or *'Relative odds'*.
- Is an *'estimate of Relative risk (RR)'*, which is used to measure strength of association in a cohort study.
- *'RR is more accurate than OR'* as a measure of strength of association.
- *OR calculation*: *CORRECT TABLE CONSTRUCTION in a case control study* requires that table will have disease at the top (row) and history of exposure/risk factor on the left (column).

	Disease Present (cases)	**Disease Absent (controls)**
Exposure present	**a**	**b**
Exposure absent	**c**	**d**

Odds Ratio (Cross Product Ratio) = ad/bc

- *Odds ratio is a good estimate of RR when the derivation of Odds ratio is based on 3 assumptions*:
  1. The disease being investigated must be relatively rare.
  2. The cases must be representative of those with the disease.
  3. The controls must be representative of those without the disease.
- *Interpretation of Odds ratio is just like relative risk*: OR can be >1, = 1 or < 1.

Odds Ratio:

INTERPRETATION EXAMPLE

Risk /Exposure Disease

OR > *1* So many times odds that cases were exposed to a risk factor is *more* to the odds that the controls were exposed **(Positive Association)** OCPs Thromboembolism.

OR = *1* Odds that cases were exposed to a risk factor is same as the odds that the controls were exposed **(No Association)** Smoking HIV/AIDS.

OR < *1* So many times odds that cases were exposed to a risk factor *is less than* the odds that the controls were exposed **(Negative Association)** Regular physical activity – CHD.

	Relative Risk (RR)	**Odds Ratio (OR)**
Synonyms	Risk ratio	Cross product ratio
Estimates strength of association	In a cohort study	Association in a case control study
Measure of strength of association	More accurate	Less accurate
Calculation	Exposed/non-exposed	ad/bc

3. Which of the following is defined as paradoxical carrier?

A. Person who shed infectious agent during incubation period of disease

B. A person who harbors the microorganism bud had never suffered from any disease by it

C. A person who acquires the microorganism due to his contact with the patient

D. Infection is transmitted from one carrier to another carrier

Answer: Option D. Infection is transmitted from one carrier to another carrier

Explanation:

Paradoxical carrier: A person is a paradoxical carrier when he acquires the microorganism from another carrier.

Contact carrier: A person can become a contact carrier when he acquires the microorganism due to his contact with the patient.

CARRIERS

- **Carriers:** Infected person or animal that harbours a specific agent in the absence of discernible clinical disease and serves as a potential source of infection for others.
  - Carriers are less infectious than cases but are more dangerous epidemiologically.
- **Carriers by Type:**
  - ***Incubatory Carriers:*** Shed infectious agent during incubation period of disease, e.g. Measles, Mumps, Polio, Pertussis, Influenza, Diphtheria, Hepatitis-B.
  - ***Convalescent Carriers:*** These are the persons who had been infected by that microorganism and are recovering from that infection. Even though they have no more symptoms of the disease, they continue to shed the microorganism into the environment, e.g., Typhoid, Bacillary Dysentery, Amoebic Dysentery, Cholera, Diphtheria and Pertussis (Clinical recovery does not coincide with bacteriological recovery).
  - ***Healthy carriers:*** These are the persons who harbor the microorganism bud had never suffered from any disease by it, e.g., Poliomyelitis, Cholera, Meningococcal Meningitis, Diphtheria and Salmonellosis.
- **Carriers by Duration:**
  - ***Temporary Carriers:*** Shed infectious agent for short periods of time, less than 6 months, e.g., Incubatory carriers, Convalescent carriers, Healthy carriers.
  - ***Chronic Carriers:*** Excretes infectious agents for indefinite periods, beyond 6 months, e.g., Typhoid, Hepatitis-B, Dysentery, Meningococcal Meningitis, Malaria, Gonorrhoea, etc.
- **Carriers by Portal of Exit:**
  - Urinary carriers, e.g., typhoid
  - Intestinal carriers, e.g., typhoid, cholera, amoebiasis
  - Nasal carriers, e.g., Diphtheria, staphylococcal food poisoning
  - Respiratory carriers
  - Nasopharyngeal carriers, e.g., Meningococcus

4. Which of the following is not included in malarial parasite measures?

A. Annual blood examination rate

B. Annual parasite index

C. Infant parasite rate

D. Annual falciparum incidence (AFI)

Answer: Option B. Annual parasite index

Its annual parasite incidence not annual parasite index which is included in malarial parasite measures.

Malariometric Measures in Eradication Era

- ***Annual parasitic incidence (API):*** Sophisticated measure of malaria incidence in a community

$$API = \frac{\text{Confirmed cases during one year}}{\text{Population under surveillance}} \times 1000$$

- ***Annual blood examination rate (ABER):*** Index of operational efficiency

$$ABER = \frac{\text{Number of slides examined}}{\text{Population}} \times 100$$

- ***Annual falciparum incidence (AFI)***

- ***Slide positivity rate (SPR)***

$$SPR = \frac{\text{No. of blood smears + ve for parasite}}{\text{No. of blood smears examined}} \times 100$$

- ***Slide falciparum rate (SFR).***

Malariometric Measures in Pre-eradication Era

- ***Spleen rate:*** Percentage children 2–10 years age showing enlargement of spleen.
  - Index used for measuring endemicity of malaria in a community.
- **Average enlarged spleen.**
- ***Parasite rate:*** Percentage children 2–10 years age showing parasites in blood films.

- **Parasite density index.**
- ***Infant parasite rate:*** Percentage infants showing parasites in blood films.
  - Is 'most sensitive index of recent malaria transmission' in a locality.
  - If IFR is zero for 3 consecutive years, it is regarded as absence of malaria transmission (even though anopheline may remain).
- ***Proportional case rate:*** Is no. of clinical malaria cases diagnosed per 100 patients attending hospitals and dispensaries.

5. Which of the following is defined as probability that person with a positive screening test truly have a disease?

A. Sensitivity

B. Negative predictive value

C. Positive productive value

D. Specificity

Answer: Option C. Positive productive value

Explanation:

Positive productive value is defined as probability that person with a positive screening test truly have a disease.

PPV is also known as 'post-test probability of a disease' or 'precision rate'.

Positive predictive value (PPV): Ability of a screening test to identify correctly all those who have the disease, out of all those who test positive on a screening test.

$$PPV = a \times 100/a + b \text{ or } \frac{TP \times 100}{TP + FP}$$

- *PPV of a screening test depends on:*
  - Sensitivity
  - Specificity
  - Prevalence of disease in the population.
- PPV of a screening test is directly proportional to prevalence of disease in the population.

$$PPV = \frac{\text{Sensitivity} \times \text{Prevalence}}{[\text{Sensitivity x Prevalence}] + [(1 - \text{Specificity})(1 - \text{Prevalence})]} \times 100$$

- *Actual Baye's Theorem:* Gives relationship between post-test probability of a disease in a population (PTP = PPV) and

  Sensitivity, Specificity and Post-test probability of a disease in a population (pTP = Prevalence)
  - Post-test probability of a disease in a population (pTP) IS SAME AS PPV.
  - Pre-test probability of a disease in a population (pTP) IS SAME AS Prevalence.
- **PPV of a screening test is directly proportional to prevalence of disease in the population**
  - **PPV α Prevalence of disease.**
  - **As the prevalence of a disease increases in a population, PPV increases for the screening test.**

6. Which of the following vaccine is changed every year?

A. Rabies
B. Influenza
C. Measles
D. Rubella

Answer: Option B. Influenza

Explanation:

Influenza vaccine has to be changed every year because of following reasons:

1. The body's immune response from **vaccination** declines over time, so an annual **vaccine** is needed for optimal protection.
2. Because **flu** viruses are constantly **changing**, the formulation of the **flu vaccine** is reviewed **each year** and updated as needed to keep up with **changing flu** viruses.

Influenza viruses are constantly changing. They can change in two different ways:

One way the change is called "antigenic drift". These are small changes in the genes of influenza viruses that happen continually over time as the virus replicates. These small genetic changes usually produce viruses that are pretty closely related to one another, which can be illustrated by their location close together on a phylogenetic tree. Viruses that are closely related to each other usually share the same antigenic properties and an immune system exposed to a similar virus will usually recognize it and respond. (This is sometimes called cross-protection.) But these small genetic changes can accumulate over time and result in viruses that are antigenically different (further away on the phylogenetic tree). When this happens, the body's immune system may not recognize those viruses.

This process works as follows: A person infected with a particular flu virus develops antibody against that virus. As antigenic changes accumulate, the antibodies created against the older viruses no longer recognize the "newer" virus, and the person can get sick again. Genetic changes that result in a virus with different antigenic properties is the main reason why people can get the flu more than one time. This is also why the flu vaccine composition must be reviewed each year, and updated as needed to keep up with evolving viruses.

The other type of change is called "antigenic shift". Antigenic shift is an abrupt, major change in the influenza A viruses, resulting in new hemagglutinin and/or new hemagglutinin and neuraminidase proteins in influenza viruses that infect humans. Shift results in a new influenza A subtype or a virus with a hemagglutinin or a hemagglutinin and neuraminidase combination that has emerged from an animal population that is so different from the same subtype in humans that most people do not have immunity to the new (e.g., novel) virus. Such a "shift" occurred in the spring of 2009, when an H1N1 virus with a new combination of genes emerged to infect people and quickly spread, causing a pandemic. When shift happens, most people have little or no protection against the new virus.

While influenza viruses are changing by antigenic drift all the time, antigenic shift happens only occasionally. Type A viruses undergo both kinds of changes; influenza type B viruses change only by the more gradual process of antigenic drift.

7. Which of the following is not included in Concurrent list of Indian Constitution?

A. Vital statistic

B. Drugs and poisons control

C. Promotion of research through research centers

D. Adulteration of food prevention

Answer: Option C. Promotion of research through research centers

Explanation:

Concurrent List under Union Ministry of Health and Family Welfare includes:

(These are responsibility of both Union and State governments).

[Mnemonic: WE (V) CLAPPED]

- **V**ital statistics
- **C**ommunicable diseases spread prevention
- **L**abour welfare
- **A**dulteration of food prevention
- **P**opulation control and family planning
- **P**orts other than major
- **E**conomic and social planning
- **D**rugs and poisons control

8. Which of the following test is used to determine differences between the means of 2 groups?

A. Z test

B. Student's t-test

C. ANOVA test

D. Chi-square test

Answer: Option B. Student's t-test

Explanation:

Student's t-test checks difference between the means of 2 groups.

ANOVA checks difference between the means of 3 or more groups.

Parametric Tests

- *Paired Student's t-test:* Comparing means (+ SD) in paired data (in same group of individuals before and after an intervention).
- *Unpaired Student's t-test:* Comparing means (+ SD) in two different groups of individuals
  - Z-test: Is a variant of student's t-test which is used when sample size is > 30.

Student's t-test: Comparison of two means

Theory

Among the most commonly used statistical **significance tests** applied to small data sets (populations samples) is the series of Student's tests. One of these tests is used for the comparison of two means, which is commonly applied to many cases. Typical examples are:

Example 1: Comparison of analytical results obtained with the same method on samples A and B, in order to confirm whether both samples contain the same percentage of the measured analyte or not.

Example 2: Comparison of analytical results obtained with two different methods A and B on the same sample, in order to confirm whether both methods provide similar analytical results or not.

General aspects of significance tests

The outcome of these tests is the **acceptance** or **rejection** of the **null hypothesis (H_0)**. The null hypothesis generally states that: "Any differences, discrepancies, or suspiciously outlying results are purely **due to random** and **not systematic errors**". The **alternative hypothesis (H_a)** states exactly the opposite.

The null hypothesis for the aforementioned examples is:

The means are the same, i.e., in **Example 1**: both samples contain the same percentage of the analyte; in **Example 2**: both methods provide the same analytical results. The differences observed (if any) are purely due to random errors.

The alternative hypothesis is:

The means are significantly different, i.e. in **Example 1**: each sample contains a different percentage of the analyte; in

Example 2: The methods provide different analytical results (so at least one method yields systematic analytical errors).

An erroneous rejection of H_0 (even though it is true) constitutes a **Type 1 error**, whereas an erroneous acceptance of H_0 (even though it is false) constitutes a **Type 2 error**.

All significance tests provide results within a predefined **confidence level %** (CL%). Confidence levels commonly used are 90%, 95% and 99%, with most usual (at least in the field of chemical analysis) the 95%.

A CL 95% means that: In case of rejecting $\mathbf{H_o}$, we are **95% or more** certain that we did the right thing. In other words, we risk a probability of **no more** than (100-95)/100 = 0.05 for a **Type 1 error**.

We can decrease or increase the confidence level of a significance test, but one has to consider the following pitfalls:

(a) By decreasing CL say to 90% (making thus the rejection of H_0 easier) the probability of **Type 1 error** obviously increases.

(b) By increasing CL say to 99% (making thus the rejection of H_0 harder) the probability of **Type 2 error** increases.

A CL 95% is generally considered as a fair compromise between these two different risks.

Student's t-test for the comparison of two means

This test assumes:

(a) A normal (gaussian) distribution for the populations of the random errors.

(b) There is no significant difference between the standard deviations of both population samples.

The ***t*-test** is any statistical hypothesis test in which the test statistic follows a Student's t-distribution under the null hypothesis.

A *t*-test is most commonly applied when the test statistic would follow a normal distribution if the value of a scaling term in the test statistic were known. When the scaling term is unknown and is replaced by an estimate based on the data, the test statistics (under certain conditions) follow a Student's *t* distribution.

The *t*-test can be used, for example, to determine if two sets of data are significantly different from each other.

Uses

Among the most frequently used *t*-tests are:

- A one-sample location test of whether the mean of a population has a value specified in a null hypothesis.
- A two-sample location test of the null hypothesis such that the means of two populations are equal. All such tests are usually called Student's t-test's, though strictly speaking that name should only be used if the variances of the two populations are also assumed to be equal; the form of the test used when this assumption is dropped is sometimes called Welch's t-test. These tests are often referred to as "unpaired" or "independent samples" *t*-tests, as they are typically applied when the statistical units underlying the two samples being compared are non-overlapping.

9. Which of the following is the best management in a patient of breast carcinoma?

A. Radiotherapy

B. Chemotherapy

C. Early diagnosis and treatment

D. Surgery

Answer: Option C. Early diagnosis and treatment

Explanation:

Breast Cancer Nanagement

A. Primary prevention

There is limited knowledge of etiology of breast cancer in current scenario.

However aim should be reduction or elimination of risk factors, such as fatty diet, reduced physical activity.

B. Secondary prevention

Secondary prevention includes early diagnosis of breast cancer by screening method, which in turn influence treatment and mortality.

Another important component of secondary prevention is follow up–which will helpful to find out early recurrence as early as possible, detect cancer in opposite breast at early stage.

Current treatment modalities have not yet shown in major improvement in survival rates.

So for breast cancer, best management is early diagnosis and treatment.

10. Which of the following is false regarding confounding factor?

A. It is a risk factor itself

B. There is independent association with risk factor and disease

C. It is associated with both exposure and outcome

D. It has an independent effect in causation of outcome

Answer: Option B. There is independent association with risk factor and disease

Explanation:

Confounding: Any factor associated with both exposure and outcome, and has an independent effect in causation of outcome is a confounder– It is found unequally distributed between the study and control groups.

- Is associated with both exposure and outcome.
- Has an independent effect in causation of outcome (thus is a risk factor itself).

Methods Used to Control Confounding

Method	Utility to control confounding
Randomization	*Most ideal method*
Restriction	Limiting study to people who have particular characteristics
Matching	Mostly useful in case control studies
Stratification	Useful for larger studies
Statistical modeling	When many confounding variables exist simultaneously

11. Which of the following test is used to determine differences between 2 or more proportions?

A. Z test
B. T test
C. T test
D. Chi-square test

Answer: Option D. Chi-square test

Explanation:

Chi-square test is used to determine differences between 2 or more proportions or percentages of categorical outcomes (not mean values).

Chi-square test: Comparing percentage, proportions and fractions in two or more different group of individuals.

- **Chi-Square Test (C^2 Test)**

  Is a 'non-parametric test' of significance.

  Is used to 'test significance of association between 2 or more qualitative characteristics'.

  Is used to compare proportions in 2 or more groups.

  Is used for non-Normal (non-Gaussian) distributions.

  Applications of Chi-square test:

  - Test of proportions
  - Test of association
  - Test of goodness of fit

  Essential requirements for calculation of Chi-square test:

  - Random sample
  - Qualitative data
  - Lowest expected frequency not < 5.
  - Fischer's test: Is a variant of Chi-square test when sample size is < 30.

- Advantages of Chi-square test over 'Standard error of difference between two proportions' test as a test of proportions has:

  Can be used to compare values of 2 binomial samples even if they are less than size of 30.

  1. Apply correction factor – yates correction.
  2. Expected value must not be < 5 in any cell.

3. Can be used to compare frequencies of 2 multinomial samples.

- Chi-square test as a test of association between 2 events in binomial of multinomial samples is its 'most important application'.

  Chi-square test tells about the presence or absence of association between 2 events/characteristics but 'do not tell about strength of association'. If strength of association (Relative Risk or Odds Ratio) found in a study is close to value of 1: Chi-square test can be used to find whether or not RR/OR is really statistically significantly different from value of 1.

- If in any cell frequency is < 5: Fischer's exact test is used.

  McNemar's Chi-square test: is a non-parametric test used to test significance of association between 2 sampled paired test.

  Chi-square test is applied when you have two categorical variables from a single population. It is used to determine whether there is a significant association between the two variables.

  For example, in an election survey, voters might be classified by gender (male or female) and voting preference (Democrat, Republican, or Independent). We could use a Chi-square test for independence to determine whether gender is related to voting preference. The sample problem at the end of the lesson considers this example.

  The test procedure described in this lesson is appropriate when the following conditions are met:

  - The sampling method is simple random sampling.
  - The variables under study are each categorical.
  - If sample data are displayed in a contingency table, the expected frequency count for each cell of the table is at least 5.

12. Below image is showing death certificate, which of the following is an underlying cause in this death certificate?

A. Cardiac arrest B. Diabetes mellitus

C. Carcinoma breast D. Metastasis

Answer: Option C. Carcinoma breast

CAUSE OF DEATH		Time interval between onset and death
I		
Immediate cause	(a) Cardiac arrest	
State the disease, injury or complication Which caused death, not the mode of dying such as heart failure, asthenia etc.	(due to or as a consequences of)	
Antecedent cause	(b) Diabetes Mellitus	
Morbid conditions, if any, giving rise to the above cause, stating underlying conditions last	(c) Carcinoma breast (due to or as a consequences of)	
II Metastasis		
Other significant conditions contributing to the death but not related to the disease or conditions causing it (due to or as a consequences of)		

Explanation:

A full explanation of the cause of death includes four items:

- The immediate cause of death, here is the **cardiac arrest.**
- The antecedent cause, which triggered the immediate cause, here is **diabetes mellitus.**
- **The main antecedent or underlying causes, which triggered the chain of events leading to death, here is carcinoma of breast.**
- Any other diseases and disorders the person had at the time of death, even though they did not directly cause the death, here is **metastasis.**

13. Which of the following organism show bird-arthropode-human life cycle?

A. Toxocariasis
B. Neurocysticercosis
C. Hyadatid cyst
D. Japanese encephalitis

Answer: Option D. Japanese encephalitis

Explanation:

Japanese encephalitis show bird-arthropode-human life cycle.

Pond herons, cattle egrets, poultry and ducks–mosquitoes– Man (dead end host).

Japanese Encephalitis (JE)

- *Causative agent:* Group B arbovirus (Flavivirus).
- *Host factors:*
  - *Pigs are 'Amplifier Hosts':* Pigs themselves do not manifest overt symptoms but circulate the virus.
  - *Cattle and buffaloes are 'Mosquito attractants':* Infected but not the natural hosts of JE virus.
  - Horses are only domestic animals which show signs of encephalitis due to JE virus.
  - *Birds are also involved in Natural History:* Pond herons, cattle egrets, poultry and ducks.
  - *Man is an 'Incidental Dead end Host':* Man to Man transmission is not seen.
- 85% cases occur in Children < 15 years of age.
- *Vectors of JE:* Culicine mosquitoes and some Anophelines Culex tritaeniorhynchus (most important vector), Culex vishnuii and Culex gelidus.
- *IP of JE in man:* 5 – 15 days (9 – 12 days in mosquitoes).
- *Case fatality rate:* 20 – 40% (may reach upto 58%).
- *Epidemiology in India:*
  - JE has been reported by 26 states and UT's in India.
  - Gorakhpur District of UP contribute the largest no. of cases.
  - 85% of cases of JE are reported in age below 15 years but JE Is Infrequent In Infancy.
  - Not all humans bitten by mosquitoes develop the disease: Ratio of JE overt disease to inapparent infection varies from 1:300 to 1:1000.
  - Endemicity of JE in India: 1-2 cases per village.

JE Vaccines

Vaccine	Strain
Mouse brain derived, purified and inactivated	Nakayama Strain, Beijing Strain
Cell culture derived inactivated vaccine	Beijing P3 Strain
Cell culture derived live attenuated vaccine	SA 14-14-2 Strain (in India)

- *Mouse brain derived inactivated vaccine:*
  - 2 primary doses 4 weeks apart, booster after 1 year and subsequently at 3 yearly intervals until the age of 10-15 years.
  - *Dose:* 0.5 ml for children aged < 3 years (1 ml for age > 3 years).
  - *Route:* Subcutaneous.
  - Vaccine is most useful in interepidemic period.
  - *Pre-exposure prophylaxis*: 3 Primary doses on day 0, 7, 28 (or 2 primary doses 4 weeks apart).
  - Booster after 1 year and then every 3 years.

14. What is the requirement of land for 10,000 populations per year for disposal of refuse according to trench method where the depth of trench is 6 feet (2 meter)?

A. Three acre
B. Ten acre
C. One acre
D. Five acre

Answer: Option C. One acre

Explanation:

Where compacted refuse is placed in the fill to a depth of 2 m (6 ft.). It is estimated that **one acre** of land per year will be required for 10, 000 population. (*Park, 23rd edition, page 763*)

The Trench Method

Trench composting, or trenching, is a way of composting by burying food scraps directly in the garden. This method of composting is good for composting materials that attract rodents such as meat, dairy, breads, and processed foods. It is also a safe and effective way of composting pet waste. Trenching is a great a way of depositing nutrients into soil at the exact place where plants need it – at their root zones.

A long trench is dug out–2 to 3 m (6-10 ft.) deep and 4 to 12 m, (12-36 ft.) wide, depending upon local conditions.The refuse is compacted and covered with excavated earth.

Trench composting offers some advantages:

- It virtually eliminates all smell and rodent problems if materials are buried at least 45 cm (18") deep and well covered with garden soil.
- The anaerobic process will retain more nutrients than hot composting which loses much of its nitrogen in the decomposition process.
- It requires no investment in containers or materials.

15. Which of the following graph gives best representation of incidence of disease over period of time?

A. Pictogram
B. Sector diagram
C. Line diagram
D. Bar diagram

Answer: Option C. Line diagram

Explanation:

Line Chart/Graph diagram best represents trend of an event or incidence of disease over a period of time.

Quantitative data	Qualitative data
Frequency polygon	Bar diagram
Histogram	Pictogram/Picture diagram
Frequency curve	Map diagram/Spot map
Scatter/Dot diagram	Pie/Sector diagram
Cumulative frequency diagram (Ogive)	
Line chart/graph	

Histogram

- Is graphical presentation for 'continuous quantitative data'.

- Continuous groups are marked on x-axis (abscissa) while frequencies are marked on y-axis (ordinate).

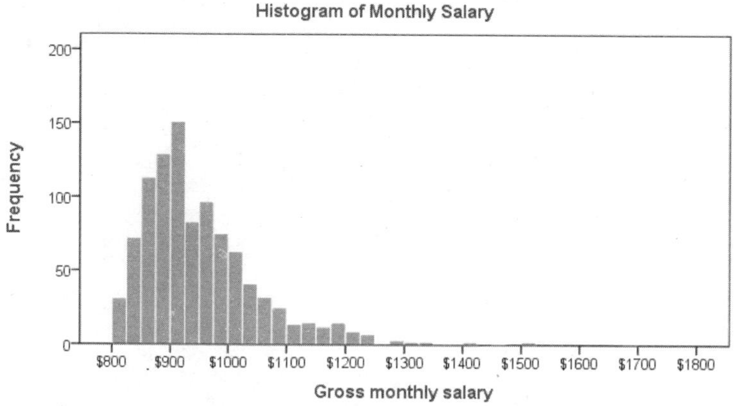

Frequency Polygon

- Is an area diagram of frequency distribution developed over a histogram.
- Made by joining mid-points of class intervals at the heights of frequencies

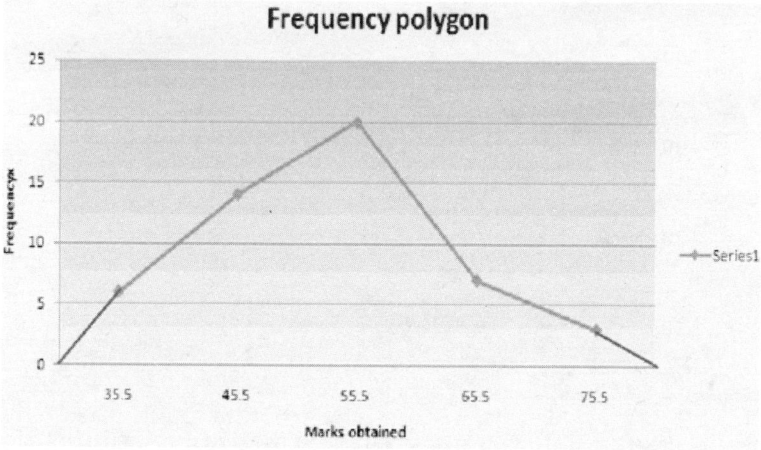

Frequency Curve

- When no. of observations is large and group-interval is reduced: Frequency polygon loses its angulations to become a curve.

FREQUENCY CURVE

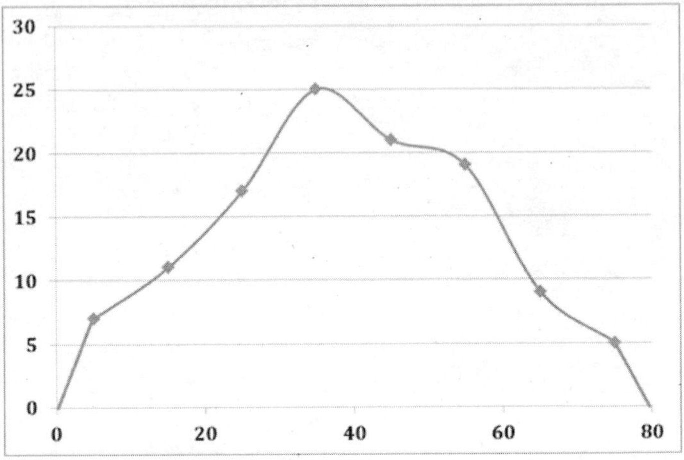

Line Chart/Graph

Is a frequency polygon presenting variations by line – It shows the trend of an event over a period of time.

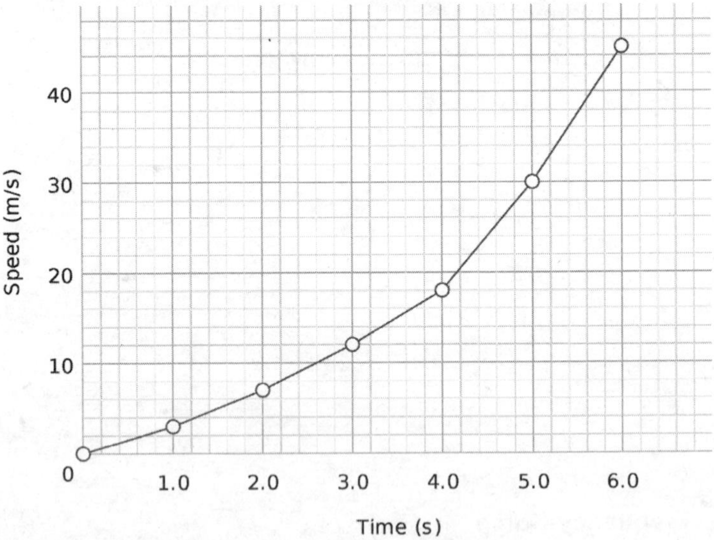

Cumulative Frequency Diagram (Ogive)

- Is graph of cumulative relative frequency distribution.

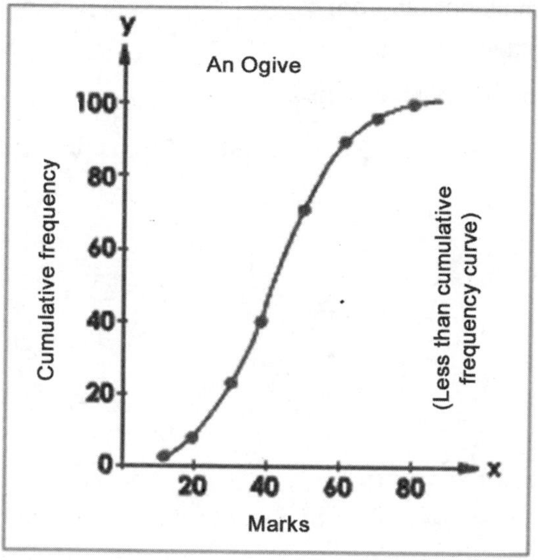

Scatter/Dot Diagram

Also known as 'Correlation diagram'– Is used to depict 'correlation (relationship) between 2 quantitative variables'– Vertical axis in scatter diagram: should be the dependent or the outcome variable – In a scatter diagram, 2 imaginary lines are drawn along the distribution of dots/scatter.

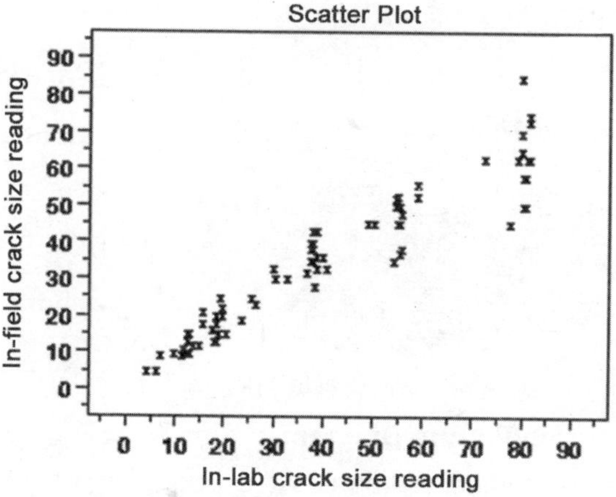

Bar Diagram

- Is for visual comparison of magnitude of different frequencies in discrete data – Is 'the most versatile of all statistical diagrams'– Bar diagram is of 3 types:

- Simple bar diagram
- Multiple bar diagram
- Proportional bar diagram.

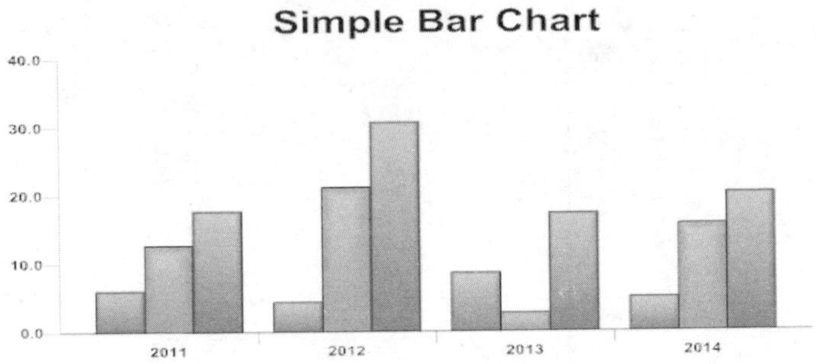

Pie/Sector Diagram

- Is for 'presentation of discrete data of qualitative characteristics'.
- All pie categories are mutually exclusive, with a total of 100% (360°).

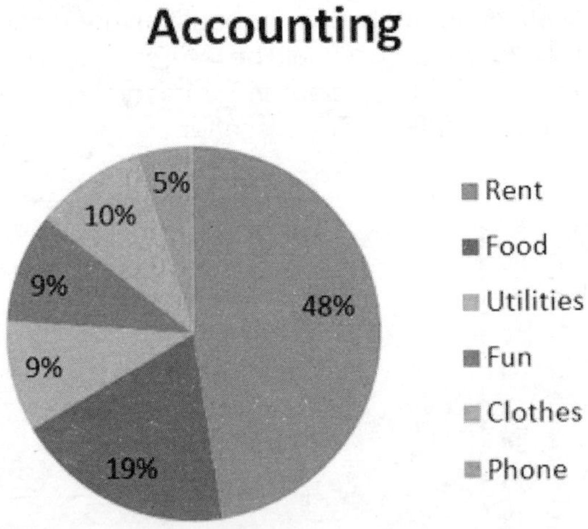

Pie (Sector) diagram

Pictogram/Picture Diagram

- Is a method to impress the frequency of occurrence of events to common man.

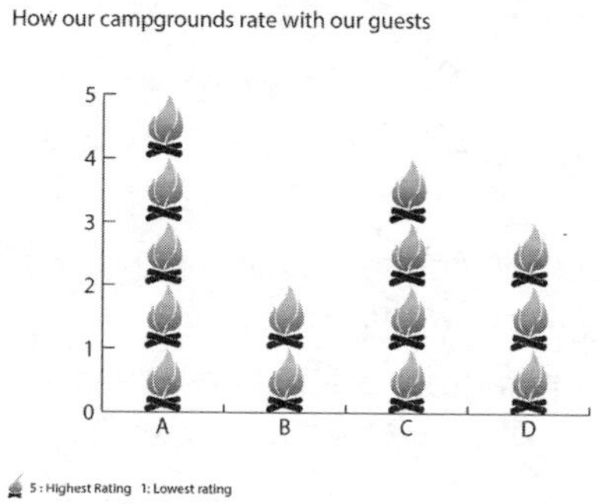

Map Diagram/Spot Map

- Is prepared to show geographical distribution of frequencies of characteristic.
- Each spot (dot) marks one frequency.

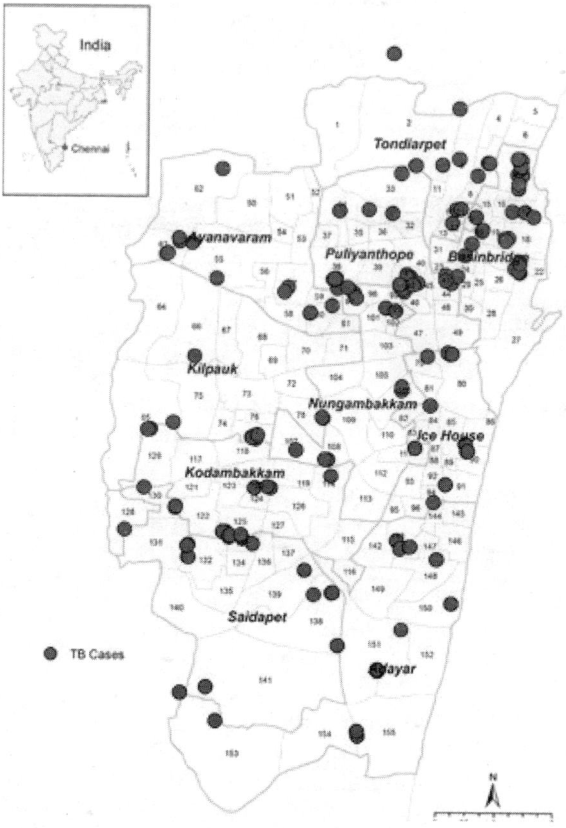

Scatter Diagram

Also known as '*Correlation diagram*' or '*Dot diagram*'

- Is used to depict '*correlation (relationship) between 2 quantitative variables*'.
- Vertical axis in scatter diagram: should be the dependent or the outcome variable.
- In a scatter diagram, 2 imaginary lines are drawn along the distribution of dots/scatter.

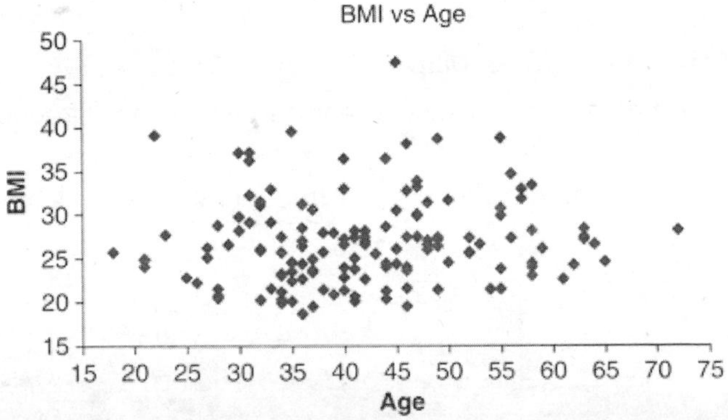

16. Which of the following diagram is shown in below image?

A. Scatter diagram
B. Component bar diagram
C. Pie diagram
D. Pictogram

Answer: Option B. Component bar diagram

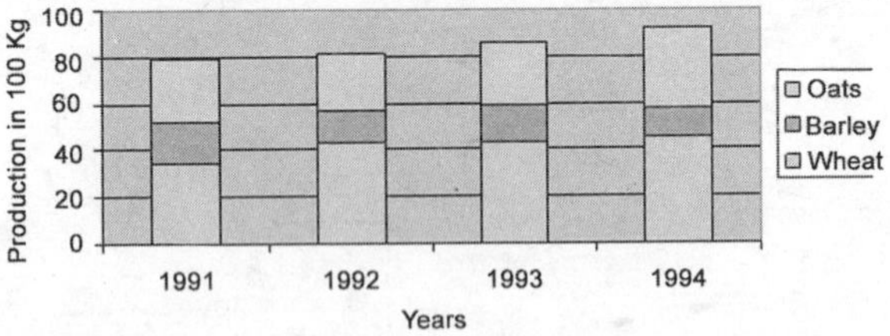

Explanation:

Above bar diagram shows the various components (quantity) in hundred kgs of wheat, barley and oats produced in a certain form during the years 1991 to 1994. Therefore, above diagram is the component bar diagram.

Component bar diagram

A sub-divided or component bar chart is used to represent data in which the total magnitude is divided into different or components.

In this diagram, first we make simple bars for each class taking the total magnitude in that class and then divide these simple bars into parts in the ratio of various components. This type of diagram shows the variation in different components within each class as well as between different classes. A sub-divided bar diagram is also known as a component bar chart or stacked chart.

17. Peripheral most unit in RCH planning is:

A. State
B. Sub centre
C. District
D. PHC

Answer: Option B. Sub centre

Explanation:

Sub Centre – A sub centre is the most peripheral contact point between the Primary Health Care system and Community. It is manned by one Multi Purpose Worker Male and one MPW Female or ANM. A sub centre to cover a population of 5,000 in plain areas and for 3000 population in hilly and tribal areas. Under RCH program, Kit A, B are kept at sub centre level.

- **RMNCH+A (Reproductive, Maternal, Newborn, Child and Adolescent Health) Strategy**

PLUS indicates:

- Inclusion of adolescence as a distinct 'life stage'.
- Linking of maternal and child health to reproductive health and other components.
- Linking of community and facility-based care as well as referrals.

Goals for RMNCH+A strategy (As per 12th Five-year plan)

- Reduction of IMR to 25 per 1,000 live births by 2017.
- Reduction in MMR to 100 per 100,000 live births by 2017.
- Reduction in TFR to 2.1 by 2017.
- *4Ds:* Defects, Deficiencies, Diseases and Disability in children (0–18 years).
- *5 × 5 Matrix of RMNCH+A: Minimum Essential Commodities.*

Reproductive health	Maternal health	Newborn health	Child health	Adolescent health
FP commodities: Tubal rings, CuT 380A, IUCD 375	Injection Oxytocin	Injection Vitamin K	ORS	Tablet Albendazole
OCPs, Mala N, Condoms	Tablet Misoprostol	Mucus extractor	Zinc dispersible tablets	Tablet Dicyclomine
Emergency contraceptive pills (LNG 1.5 mg)	Inj. Magnesium sulphate	Vaccines: BCG, OPV, Hep B	Salbutamol syrup/ nebulising solution	
Pregnancy testing kits – Nischay			Vaccines: DPT, OPV, Measles, Hep-B, JE, Pentavalent vaccine	
Tablet Mifepristone			Syrup Vitamin A	

Components of Reproductive and Child Health Programme

- Community Needs Assessment Approach (CNAA)
- Integrated packages of services for mother and child
- MTP services at PHC and safe abortion
- Control and prevention of RTI/ STI
  - Adolescent health
  - Services in urban slums
  - Improving quality of services
  - Unmet needs and sub-centre action plans
  - Communication strategy
  - Gender sensitiveness
  - Greater involvement of Panchayati Raj Institutions (PRIs), NGOs and community.

18. Which of the following is true about community needs assessment approach?

A. It is top to bottom manner

B. It is target free manual

C. It alters population goals

D. Its aim is to increase quantity of services

Answer: Option B. It is target free manual

Explanation:

Community needs assessment approach uses target free manual without altering population goals with main emphasis is to increase quality of service.

- Previously, the achievements of family welfare programs were assessed in terms of targets provided by the central planning authorities.
- There were many demerits to this approach. They were:
  - The actual needs of the local community was not taken into consideration.
  - The emphasis was on the quantity of the services rather than quality.

  - Because of the existence of pre allotted targets and cash benefits, contraceptive methods were provided without first assessing whether the recipients were good candidates for the same (for example, Intrauterine Contraceptive Devices were introduced without first checking for presence of any reproductive tract infections) – This resulted in low acceptance and high discontinuity rate.
  - The health workers were tempted to falsify the reports so as to gain benefits.
- Because of these defects, the targets were replaced by community needs assessment approach.
- In this approach, at the beginning of the year, the Axillary Nurse Midwife (ANM) will consult the different families in her allotted area for assessing their needs for that year.
- Based on the needs assessment, the workload for that year is calculated.
- The sum total of the workload for the different ANM's will become the workload for a PHC.
- The requirements of the district can be calculated by combining the workload of the different PHC's.
- Thus instead of a top to bottom manner, the planning is based on the community needs and hence is more successful. **So it is bottom to top manner.**

19. Which of the following is the probability of genetic disease in consanguineous marriage?

A. 5% B. 10%

C. 15% D. 20%

Answer: Option A. 5%

The birth defects frequency in consanguineous marriage is estimated to be around 2–3% points more than the background rate among newborns in the general population (around 2–3%). So it's around 4 to 6%.

The main impact of consanguineous marriage is an elevation in the rate for homozygotes in recessive disorders. On average, first cousins have an extra risk of 1.7–2.8% of having a child with an autosomal recessive disorder. Rates of consanguinity are highly variable between and within countries, but the prevalence is highest in North Africa, the Middle East, South Asia and among migrant communities in North America, Europe and Australia.

The reproductive health criteria related to consanguinity show that in first cousin marriages as opposed to non-consanguineous marriages, fertility rate is slightly higher, abortion rate is not different, stillbirths and infant mortality rates are slightly higher. Furthermore, consanguineous unions lead to increased expression of autosomal recessive disorders. The offspring of consanguineous unions may be at increased risk for recessive disorders because of the expression of autosomal recessive gene mutations inherited from a common ancestor. The closer the biological relationship between parents, the greater is the probability that their offspring will inherit identical copies of one or more detrimental recessive genes. For example, first cousins are predicted to share 12.5% (1/8) of their genes. Thus, on average, their progeny will be homozygous at 6.25% (1/16) of gene loci.

In general, consanguinity does not increase the risk for autosomal dominant conditions in offspring when one of the parents is affected, nor for X-linked recessive conditions if neither parent is affected.

Most of the literature studying the association of Down syndrome with parental consanguinity concluded that no such association existed.

- **Genetic Risk:** First cousin marriages compared to non-consanguineous marriages
  - Fertility rate slightly higher
  - Miscarriage rate not different
  - Still births and infant mortality rates slightly higher
  - Congenital anomalies 2-3% higher than background population risk (2-3%)
  - Increased likelihood of autosomal recessive conditions
  - Increased risk for almost all multifactorial birth defects including congenital heart defects, clefting, club feet, etc
  - Complex diseases–really not known–could be significant if high susceptibility gene present in family.

20. Following is the cycle of disease. Which of the following statement truly represents in below given options?

Health–sub clinical disease—clinical disease → Died / → Recovers

A. Types of disease

B. Natural course of disease

C. Intervention in disease

D. Spectrum of disease

Answer: Option B. Natural course of disease

Explanation:

The natural history of a disease is defined as the "natural course of a disease from the time immediately prior to its inception, progressing, through its presymptomatic phase and different clinical stages to the point where it has ended and the patient is either cured, chronically disabled or dead without external intervention." By "natural course" they mean here that no external intervention is applied that might change this pathway from health to disease to expression: possible interventions include preventative health measures (designed to stop or delay disease initiation), and treatment for symptoms (designed to change or delay the expression of a disease).

The **natural history of disease** is the course a disease takes in individual people from its pathological onset ("inception") until its eventual resolution through complete recovery or death. The inception of a disease is not a firmly defined concept. The natural history of a disease is sometimes said to start at the moment of exposure to causal agents. Knowledge of the natural history of disease ranks alongside causal understanding in importance for disease prevention and control. Natural history of disease is one of the major elements of descriptive epidemiology.

Natural History and Spectrum of Disease

Natural history of disease refers to the progression of a disease process in an individual over time, in the absence of treatment. For example, untreated infection with HIV causes a spectrum of clinical problems beginning at the time of seroconversion (primary HIV) and terminating with AIDS and usually death. It is now recognized that it may take 10 years or more for AIDS to develop after seroconversion. Many, if not most, diseases have a characteristic natural history, although the timeframe and specific manifestations of disease may vary from individual to individual and are influenced by preventive and therapeutic measures.

The process begins with the appropriate exposure to or accumulation of factors sufficient for the disease process to begin in a susceptible host. For an infectious disease, the exposure is a microorganism. For cancer, the exposure may be a factor that initiates the process, such as asbestos fibers or components in tobacco smoke (for lung cancer), or one that promotes the process, such as estrogen (for endometrial cancer).

After the disease process has been triggered, pathological changes then occur without the individual being aware of them. This stage of subclinical disease, extending from the time of exposure to onset of disease symptoms, is usually called the **incubation period** for infectious diseases, and the **latency period** for chronic diseases. During this stage, disease is said to be asymptomatic (no symptoms) or inapparent. This period may be as brief as seconds for hypersensitivity and toxic reactions to as long as decades for certain chronic diseases. Even for a single disease, the characteristic incubation period has a range. For example, the typical incubation period for hepatitis A is as long as 7 weeks. The latency period for leukemia to become evident among survivors of the atomic bomb blast in Hiroshima ranged from 2 to 12 years, peaking at 6–7 years.

21. Which of the following arthropod is shown given below image?

A. Ixodid tick

B. Pediculus humanus capitis

C. Sarcoptes scabiei

D. Phthirus pubis

Answer: Option C. Sarcoptes scabiei

Explanation:

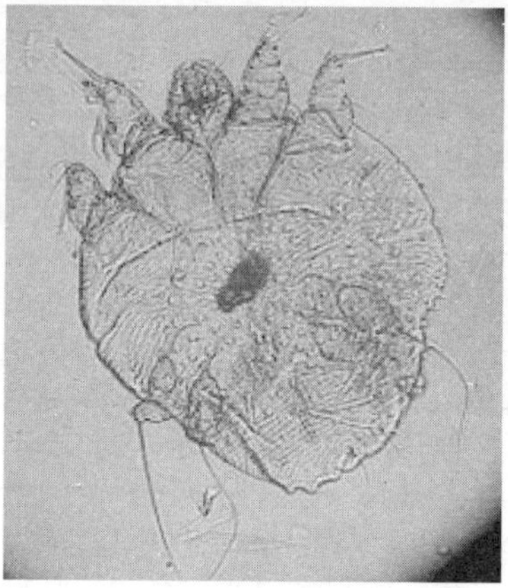

Here above given image is of adult sarcoptes scabiei mite which can be recognized by their oval, ventrally flattened and dorsally convex tortoise-like bodies and multiple cuticular spines with four pairs of legs (two pairs in front and two pairs behind). No demarcation into cephalothorax or abdomen occurs, and the mite's surface has folds covered with short bristles. The front legs end in long, tubular processes known as suckers, and the hind legs end in long bristles.

Sarcoptes scabiei or the **itch mite** is a parasitic mite (an arthropod) that burrows into skin and causes scabies.

The scabies mite *Sarcoptes scabiei* var. *hominis* goes through four stages in its lifecycle: egg, larva, nymph and adult.

Upon infesting a human host, the adult female burrows into the *stratum corneum* (outermost layer of skin), where she deposits two or three eggs per day.

The action of the mites moving within the skin and on the skin itself produces an intense itch that may resemble an allergic reaction in appearance. A delayed Type IV hypersensitivity reaction to the mites, their eggs, or scybala (packets of feces) occurs approximately 30 days after infestation. The presence of the eggs produces a massive allergic response that, in turn, produces more itching. Individuals who already are sensitized from a prior infestation can develop symptoms within hours.

Sarcoptes is a genus of skin parasites, and part of the larger family of mites collectively known as "scab mites". They are also related to the scab mite *Psoroptes*, also a mite that infests the skin of domestic animals. Sarcoptic mange affects domestic animals and similar infestations in domestic fowls causes the disease known as "scaly leg". The effects of *S. scabiei* are the most well-known, causing "scabies", or "the itch". The adult female mite, having been fertilized, burrows into the skin (usually at the hands or wrists, but other parts of the body may also be affected), and lays its eggs.

The burrowing is carried out using the mouth parts and special cutting surfaces on the front legs. While these are being used, the mite anchors itself with suckers on its feet. Eggs are laid in small numbers as the mite burrows, and, as these hatch, six-legged larvae climb out on to the skin and search for hair follicles, where they feed and moult (discard old cuticles to grow). In the hair follicles, the larvae show the first nymphal stages, with eight legs.

In the nymphal stages, the creature feeds and moults, and if male, gives rise to the adult. In the case of females, another moult occurs before adulthood. The female has more moults than a male, so takes longer—17 days compared to 9 to 11 days for a male—to reach adulthood. The female is about twice the size of the male.

Although the life-cycle is only about two weeks, individual patients are seldom found to have more than about a dozen mites on them. Even so, this number can cause agonising itching, especially at night, and severe damage to the skin often comes as a result of scratching, in particular by the introduction of infective bacteria, which may lead to impetigo or eczema.

The eggs are laid by the female at a rate of about two to three eggs a day for about two months. About 2% of the British population is thought to be infected with these mites, which take about 25 minutes to an hour to burrow into the skin.

The best conditions in which to harbor *S. scabiei* is in areas with frequent skin-to-skin contact, such as the hands and wrists, as the mites are transmitted by skin contact with carriers, and they very easily spread. Infestations of *S. scabiei* are commonly found in pigs. They significantly depress growth and feeding rate, but usually die out in around five days in typical farm conditions. However, once in a herd, the mites are very difficult to eliminate without great measures taken.

22. Which of the following is true about triage?

A. It is based on first come first serve

B. Red colour is given priority for transport

C. Highest priority is given for moribund patient

D. It classify the patient based on severity of injury

Answer: Option D. It classify the patient based on severity of injury

Explanation:

Triage is a method of rapidly classifying the injured persons 'on the basis of severity of their injuries and likelihood of their survival'.

Triage

- *Triage:* Consists of rapidly classifying the injured *'on the basis of severity of their injuries and likelihood of their survival'* with prompt medical intervention.
  - First come first serve is NOT followed in emergencies.
  - Triage yields best results when carried out at the site of disaster.
- *Triage sieve:* Quick survey to separate the dead and the walking from the injured.
- *Triage sort:* Remaining casualties are assessed and allocated to categories.
- *Triage system:* Most commonly uses FOUR color code system:
  - *Red (Highest Priority)*: Immediate resuscitation or limb/life saving surgery in next 6 hours.
  - *Yellow (High Priority)*: Possible resuscitation or limb/life saving surgery in next 24 hours.
  - *Green (Low Priority)*: Minor illness/AMBULATORY patients.
  - *Black (Least Priority)*: Dead and moribund patients.

	Red indicates high priority treatment or transfer, e.g., Massive Hemorrhage, Tension Pneumothorax.
	Yellow signals medium priority, e.g., Isolated Simple Femur fracture.
	Green is used for ambulatory patients, e.g., Isolated Abrasions, contusions, sprains.
	Black for dead or those with minimal chance of survival, e.g., Massive Head Injuries, 95% coverage with third degree burns.

- *Tagging:* Is the procedure where identification, age, place of origin, triage category, diagnosis and initial treatment are tagged on to every victim of disaster through a Colour Coding.

Types of Triage

- *Triage is of two types:*
  - *Simple triage*: Simple triage is used in a scene of mass casualty, in order to sort patients into those who need critical attention and immediate transport to the hospital and those with less serious injuries.
    - ◊ This step is required before transportation becomes available.
    - ◊ The categorization of patients based on the severity of their injuries can be aided with the use of printed triage tags or colored flagging.
  - *Rapid triage*: S.T.A.R.T. (*Simple Triage and Rapid Treatment*) is a simple triage system that can be performed by lightly-trained lay and emergency personnel in emergencies.
    - o It is not intended to supersede or instruct medical personnel or techniques.
    - o It may serve as an instructive example.
    - o It has been field-proven in mass casualty incidents such as train wrecks and bus accidents.
- *Reverse Triage*: In addition to the standard practices of triage as mentioned above, there are conditions where sometimes the less wounded are treated in preference to the more severely wounded. This may arise in:

- A situation such as war where the military setting may require soldiers be returned to combat as quickly as possible.
- Disaster situations where medical resources are limited in order to conserve resources for those likely to survive but requiring advanced medical care.

23. Which of the following drug is used for prophylaxis of diphtheria?

A. Linezolid B. Ciprofloxacin

C. Erythromycin D. Cefixime

Answer: Option C. Erythromycin

Explanation:

Erythromycin is used for prophylaxis of diphtheria.

Disease	Chemoprophylactic drug
Pertussis	Azithromycin
Cholera	Tetracycline/ Furazolidone
Bacterial conjunctivitis	Erythromycin ointment
Diphtheria	**Erythromycin and 1st dose of vaccine**
Meningococcal meningitis	Ciprofloxacin > Rifampicin
Plague	Tetracycline
Tuberculosis	Isoniazide alone or with rifampicin
Influenza A OR B	Amantadine/Oseltamivir
Malaria < 6 weeks > 6 weeks	 Doxycycline Mefloquine
Toxoplasmosis	Cotrimoxazole
Rheumatic fever	Benzathin penicillin

Diphtheria

- *Causative agent:* Corynebacterium diphtheriae, a gram positive non-motile organism.
- Diphtheria is an endemic disease in India.
- *Source of infection:* Case or carrier.

- *Carriers are more important as source of infection:* 95% of total disease transmission.
- Nasal carriers are more dangerous than throat carriers.
- *Incidence of carriers in a community:* 0.5-1%.
- Immunization does not prevent carrier state.

- *Incubation Period:* 2-6 days.
- *Mode of transmission:* Droplet infection (main mode), directly from cutaneous lesions and fomites.
- *Period of Infectivity:* 14-28 days from onset of disease; longer for carriers.
  - A case/carrier may be considered non-communicable when atleast 2 cultures from nose and throat, 24 hours apart, are negative.

Management of Diphtheria Contacts

- ***Immunisation:***
  - If primary immunization or booster was received in previous 2 years: No further action.
  - If primary immunization or booster was received more than 2 years ago: 1 booster dose.
  - If unimmunized contact: Active immunization + 1000-2000 units Antitoxin + Prophylactic penicillin/ erythromycin.
- ***Examination:***
  - Physical examination: Daily for 1 week after exposure.
  - Throat swabbing: Weekly for several weeks.

CHAPTER

9 EAR, NOSE AND THROAT

1. Which of the following is the diagnosis based on the given below image of 9 years old child?

A. Inverted papilloma B. Laryngeal chondroma

C. Laryngeal hemangioma D. Laryngeal papilloma

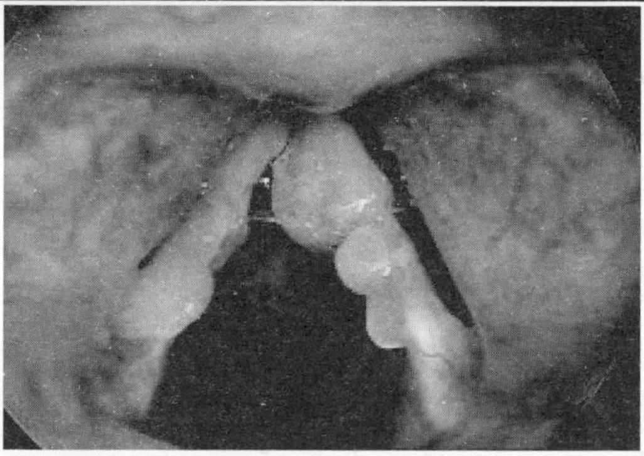

Answer: Option D. Laryngeal papilloma

Explanation:

Here, above given image (of 9 years old child) is showing multiple intraluminary polypoidal papillary projection arising from vocal cord on both sides. So the diagnosis here is laryngeal papilloma.

SQUAMOUS PAPILLOMAS OF LARYNX

Most common benign tumour of larynx and *most common site vocal cord.*

They can be divided into (a) juvenile and (b) adult-onset types.

(a) **Juvenile papillomas:** They are viral in origin caused by human papilloma virus subtype 6 and 11 and less commonly by subtypes 16 and 18 and multiple, often involving infants and young children who present with hoarseness and stridor. They are mostly seen on the true and false cords and the epiglottis, but they may involve other sites in the larynx and trachea. Clinically, they appear as glistening white irregular growths, pedunculated or sessile, friable and bleeding easily. They are known for recurrence after removal and therefore multiple laryngoscopies may be required. They tend to disappear spontaneously after puberty. They have been treated by endoscopic removal with cup forceps, cryotherapy and micro electrocautery. These days, CO laser is preferred because of the precision in removal and less bleeding. Interferon therapy is being tried to prevent recurrence and has been found successful.

(b) **Adult-onset papilloma:** Usually, it is single, smaller in size, less aggressive and does not recur after surgical removal. It is common in males (2:1) in the age group of 30-50 and usually arises from the anterior half of vocal cord or anterior commissure. Treatment is the same as for juvenile type.

Infantile hemangioma involves the subglottic area and presents with stridor in first 6 months of life.

2. Which of the following is the diagnosis based on the given below image?

A. Brandt-Daroff exercises
B. Epley maneuver
C. Lempert maneuver
D. Semont maneuver

Answer: Option C. Lempert maneuver

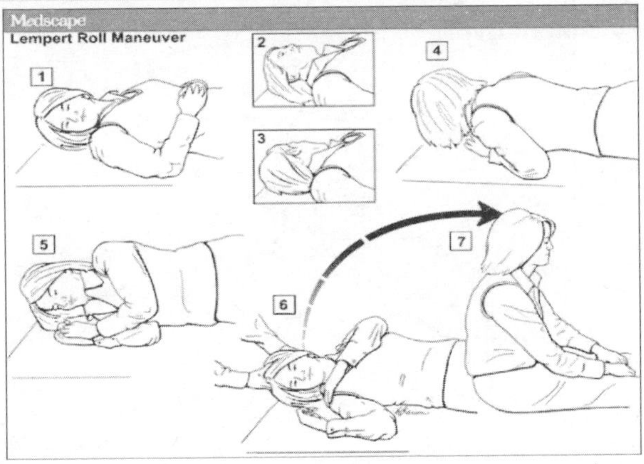

Explanation:

The patient is in straight supine position (1) The head is turned to the right side (2) with observation of nystagmus and then turned back to face up. Then the head is turned to the left side (3). Then head is turned to the prone (4). Then the head is turned to the right side (5). From Step 5, the patient positions his or her body to the back (6) in preparation for the rapid and simultaneous movement from the supine face up to the sitting position (7). So, this is Lempert maneuver.

Lempert Maneuver

Lempert described a maneuver (Barbecue Maneuver or Roll Maneuver), which is the most commonly employed maneuver for the treatment of lateral canal BPPV. This maneuver involves rolling the patient 360 degrees in a series of steps to effect particle repositioning.

The patient is in supine position; the patient's head is turned 90 degrees slowly toward the unaffected side. The head is held in this position, and the body is turned to lateral decubitus. Then, the head is turned to the facedown position and the body is moved to the ventral decubitus. Later the patient's head is turned 90 degrees, and the body is placed on lateral decubitus.

Gradually, the patient resumes the supine position. Each step is maintained for 15 seconds for slow migration of the particles, in response to gravity. To complete the maneuver, the patient is brought into the upright sitting position with head bowed down at 30 degrees.

Epley's Maneuver

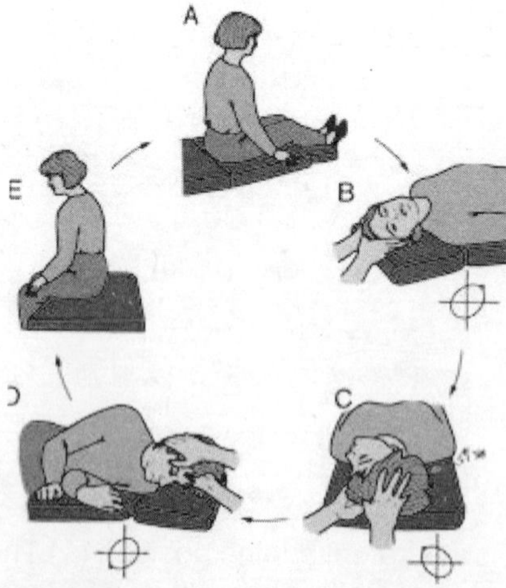

The principle of this maneuver is to reposition the otoconial debris from the posterior semicircular canal back into the utricle. The doctor stands behind the patient and the assistant on the side. The patient is made to sit on the table so that when he is made to lie down, his head is beyond the edge of the table as is done in Dix-Hallpike maneuver. His face is turned 45° to the affected side.

The maneuver consists of five positions:

Position 1. With the head turned 45°, the patient is made to lie down in head-hanging position (Dix-Hallpike maneuver). It will cause vertigo and nystagmus. Wait till vertigo and nystagmus subside.

Position 2. Head is now turned so that affected ear is up.

Position 3. The whole body and head are now rotated away from the affected ear to a lateral recumbent position in a face-down position.

Position 4. Patient is now brought to a sitting position with head still turned to the unaffected side by 45°.

Position 5. The head is now turned forward and chin brought down 20°.

There should be a pause at each position till there is no nystagmus or there is slowing of nystagmus, before changing to the next position. After maneuver is complete, patient should maintain an upright posture for 48 hours. Eighty percent of the patients will be cured by a single maneuver. If the patient remains symptomatic, the maneuver can be repeated. A bone vibrator placed on the mastoid bone helps to loosen the debris.

Semont Maneuver (Liberatory Maneuver)

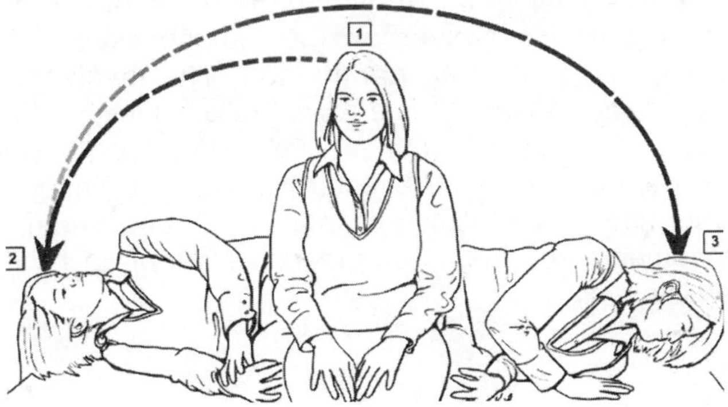

The maneuver described by Semont is indicated for the treatment of posterior canal cupulolithiasis. If the posterior canal is affected, the patient is seated in the upright position; then the patient's head is turned 45 degrees toward the unaffected side, and then is rapidly moved to the side-lying position. Nystagmus and vertigo may be observed. This position is held for 1 to 3 minutes. The patient is rapidly moved to the opposite side-lying position without pausing in the sitting position and without changing the head position relative to the shoulder. Gradually the patient resumes the upright sitting position. If the superior semicircular canal is affected, the movement is performed in the direction opposite to the procedure for posterior semicircular canal. Figure demonstrates the Semont Maneuver for treatment of right-sided posterior semicircular canal cupulolithiasis.

Brandt-Daroff Exercises

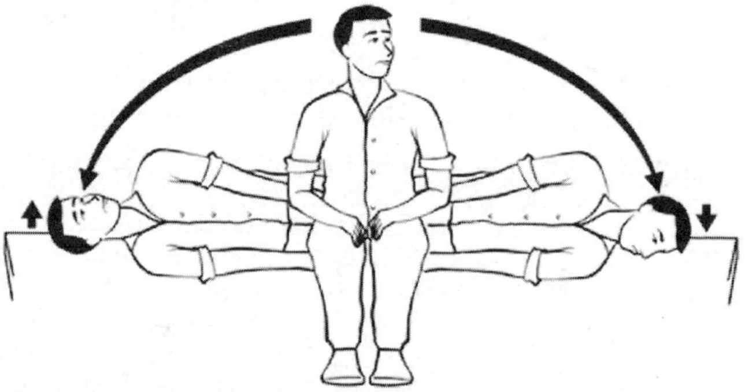

The Brandt-Daroff exercises were developed for home self-administration, as an additional therapy for patients who have been symptomatic, even after Epley or Semont maneuver. Some authors indicate them one week before the therapeutic maneuver, aiming to improve the patient's tolerability. The Brandt-Daroff exercises are positioning exercises that, theoretically, promote habituation. The involvement of more than one semicircular canal is not unusual. In these cases, the repositioning maneuver will be applied in steps. The treatment of each affected semicircular canal will be performed, in protocols according to the observed ocular movements and the correct identification of each affected semicircular canal.

Hallpike Maneuver (Positional Test) – Diagnostic Test for Benign Paroxysmal Positional Vertigo

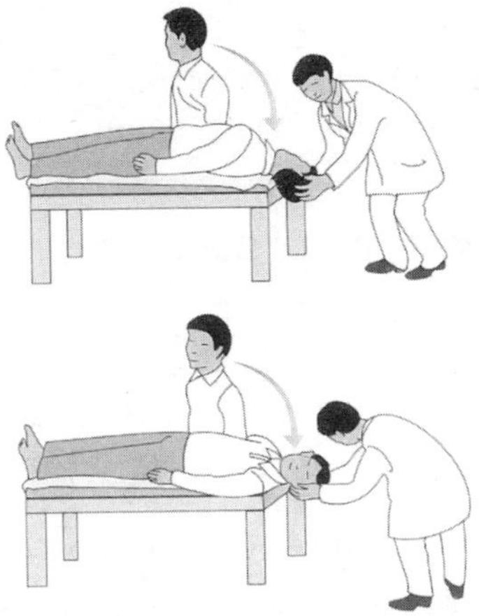

This test is particularly useful when patient complains of vertigo in certain head positions. It also helps to differentiate a peripheral from a central lesion.

Method: Patient sits on a couch. Examiner holds the patient's head, turns it 45° to the right and then places the patient in a supine position so that his head hangs 30° below the horizontal. Patient's eyes are observed for nystagmus. The test is repeated with head turned to left and then again in straight head-hanging position. Four parameters of nystagmus are observed: *latency, duration, direction* and *fatiguability.* In benign paroxysmal positional vertigo, nystagmus appears after a latent period of 2—20 seconds, lasts for less than a minute and is always in one direction, i.e., towards the ear that is undermost. On repetition of the test, nystagmus may still be elicited but lasts for a shorter period. On subsequent repetitions it disappears altogether, i.e., nystagmus is fatiguable. Patient also complains of vertigo when the head is in critical position.

3. A 26 years old male patient has developed Pott's puffy tumor. Which of the following statement is best defining this condition?

A. Maxillary carcinoma

B. Maxillary sinusitis

C. Sub periosteal frontal sinus osteomyelitis

D. Mastoid abscess

Answer: Option C. Sub periosteal frontal sinus osteomyelitis

Explanation:

Puffy swelling under the periosteum of frontal bone is called as Pott's puffy tumor which occurs due to subperiosteal osteomyelitis of frontal sinus.

Osteomyelitis of Frontal Bone

Organism causing:

- Staphylococcus
- Streptococcus
- Anaerobes

Osteomyelitis of the frontal bone is most common as:

- It is a diploic bone and the lesion is essentially thrombophlebitis of diploic bone. It follows infection of frontal sinus.
- It is more often seen in adults, as frontal sinus is not developed in infants and children.
- Osteomyelitis of frontal bone results from acute infection of frontal sinus either directly or through the venous spread. It can also follow trauma or surgery of frontal sinus in the presence of acute infection.
- Pus may form externally under the periosteum as soft doughy swelling (Pott's puffy tumour), or internally as an extradural abscess.
- Treatment consists of large doses of antibiotics for 4-6 weeks, drainage of abscess through frontonasal duct and trephining of frontal sinus through its floor. Sometimes, it requires removal of sequestra and necrotic bone by raising a scalp flap through a coronal incision.

4. A 30 years old female presented with chronic ear discharge. Which of the following is the diagnosis, based on the given below image?

A. Primary acquired cholesteatoma

B. Congenital cholesteatoma

C. Keratosis obturans

D. Secondary acquired cholesteatoma

Answer: Option D. Secondary acquired cholesteatoma

Explanation:

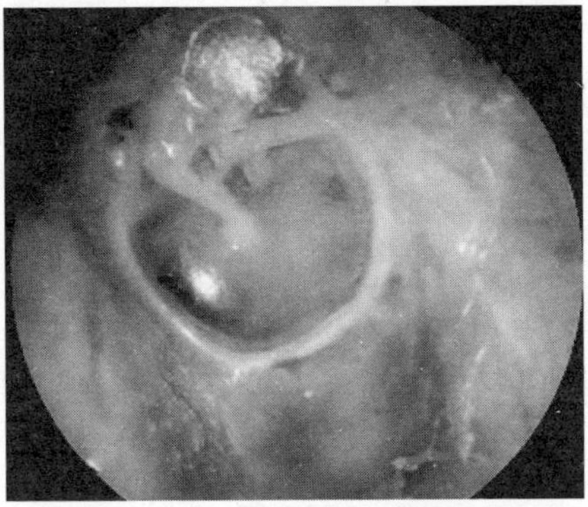

Here above image is showing **perforation of tympanic membrane** (not seen in congenital and primary acquired cholesteatoma) with cholesteatoma formation at middle ear, ill defined margin of head of malleus and adjacent peripheral area. These features are seen in secondary acquired cholesteatoma.

Keratosis obturans is Collection of a pearly white mass, seen in external ear or deep meatus (not seen in our case).

1. **Congenital cholesteatoma:** It arises from the embryonic epidermal cell rests in the middle ear cleft or temporal bone.
   - Squamous epithelium trapped within the temporal bone during embryogenesis.
   - Typically develop in the **anterior mesotympanum**
   - Usually identified in early childhood.
   - Unlike other cholesteatomas, the congenital type is usually **identified behind an intact, normal-appearing tympanic membrane.** The child often has no history of recurrent suppurative ear disease, previous otologic surgery, or tympanic membrane perforation.

   Congenital cholesteatoma occurs at three important sites: middle ear, petrous apex and the cerebellopontine angle, and produces symptomatology depending on its location.

   A middle ear congenital cholesteatoma presents as a white mass behind an intact tympanic membrane and causes conductive hearing loss. It may sometimes be discovered on routine examination of children or at the time of myringotomy.

It may also spontaneously rupture through the tympanic membrane and present with a discharging ear indistinguishable from a case of chronic supportive otitis media (CSOM).

2. **Primary acquired cholesteatoma:** It is called primary as there is no history of previous otitis media or a preexisting perforation.
   - Develops as a result of medial retraction of the tympanic membrane.
   - Medial retraction of the tympanic membrane continues beyond the heads of the ossicles and into the posterior epitympanum.
   - A variant of primary acquired cholesteatoma occurs when posterior quadrant of the tympanic membrane retract into the posterior middle ear which usually produce **facial nerve lesion** and **destruction of the ossicles**.

   Theories on its genesis are:

   (a) *Invagination of pars flaccida:* Persistent negative pressure in the attic causes a retraction pocket which accumulates keratin debris. When infected, the keratin mass expands towards the middle ear. Thus, attic perforation is in fact the proximal end of an expanding invaginated sac.

   (b) *Basal cell hyperplasia:* There is proliferation of the basal layer of pars flaccida induced by subclinical childhood infections. Expanding cholesteatoma then breaks through pars flaccida forming an attic perforation.

   (c) *Squamous metaplasia:* Normal pavement epithelium of attic undergoes metaplasia, keratinising squamous epithelium due to subclinical infections. Such a change has also been demonstrated in cases of otitis media with effusion.

3. **Secondary acquired cholesteatoma**

   In these cases, there is already a pre-existing perforation in pars tensa. This is often associated with posterosuperior marginal perforation or sometimes large central perforation.
   - Usually caused by injury to the tympanic membrane (surgery, perforation, infection, otitis media).

- Deep retraction pockets can also trap desquamated epithelium which can then lead to secondary acquired cholesteatoma.

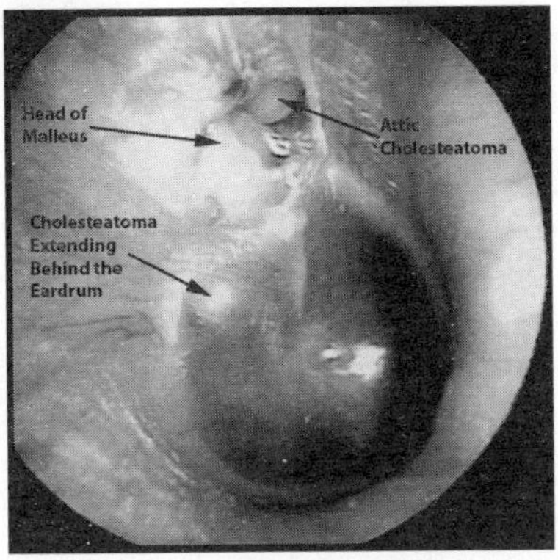

Theories on its genesis include:

(a) *Migration of squamous epithelium:* Keratinising squamous epithelium of external auditory canal or outer surface of tympanic membrane migrates through the perforation into the middle ear. Perforations, involving tympanic annulus as in acute necrotising otitis media, are more likely to allow in-growth of squamous epithelium.

(b) *Metaplasia:* Middle ear mucosa undergoes metaplasia due to repeated infections of middle ear through the pre-existing perforation.

4. **Keratosis obturans:** Collection of a pearly white mass of desquamated epithelial cells in the deep meatus is called keratosis obturans. This, by its pressure effect, causes absorption of bone leading to widening of the meatus so much so that facial nerve may be exposed and paralysed.

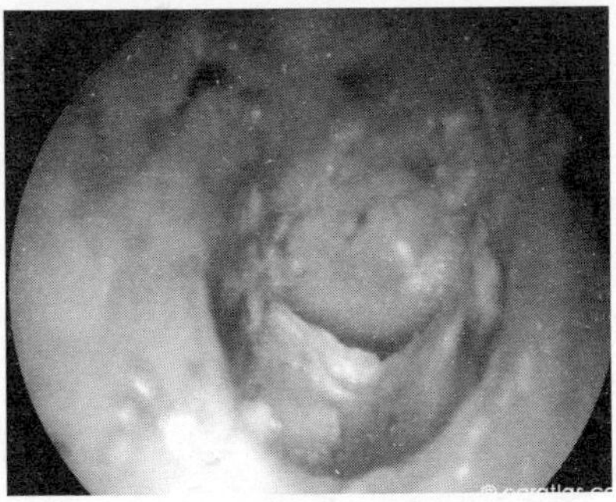

Aetiology: It is commonly seen between 5 and 20 years and may affect one or both ears. It may sometimes be associated with bronchiectasis and chronic sinusitis. Normally, epithelium from surface of tympanic membrane migrates onto the posterior meatal wall. Failure of this migration or obstruction to migration caused by wax may lead to accumulation of the epithelial plug in the deep meatus.

Clinical features: Presenting symptoms may be pain in the ear, hearing loss, tinnitus and sometimes ear discharge.

On examination, ear canal may be full of pearly white mass of keratin material disposed in several layers. Removal of this mass may show widening of bony meatus with ulceration and even granuloma formation.

Treatment: Keratotic mass is removed either by syringing or instrumentation, similar to the techniques employed for impacted wax. Secondary otitis externa may be present and should be treated. Patient should be periodically checked and any reaccumulations removed. Recurrence can be checked to some extent by the use of keratolytic agent such as 2% salicylic acid in alcohol.

5. A 6 years old child presented with complaints of throat pain, fever and cough. His throat examination image is given below. Which of the following is the diagnosis?

A. Vincent's angina

B. Aphthous ulcers

C. Membranous tonsillitis

D. Tonsillar Diphtheria

Answer: Option D. Tonsillar Diphtheria

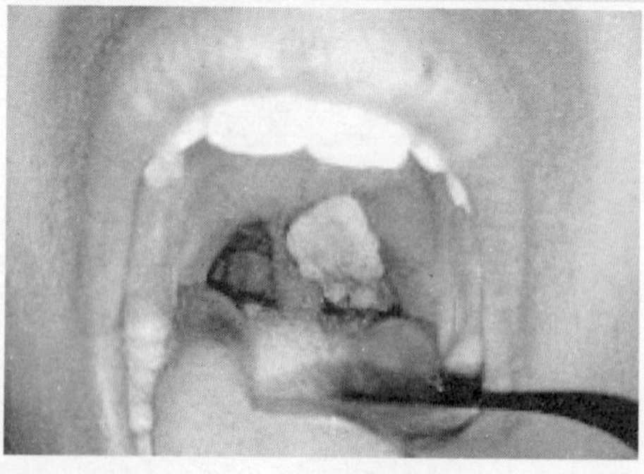

Explanation:

Here 6 years old child presented with complains of throat pain, fever and cough–suggest throat infection. And his throat image shows presence of greyish white membrane over tonsil on left side with reddish area on removal part. These features are seen in infection with diphtheria.

Aetiology

It is an acute specific infection caused by the Gram-positive bacillus, *Corynebacterium diphtheriae.* It spreads by droplet infection. Incubation period is 2—6 days. Some persons are "carriers" of this disease, i.e. they harbour organisms in their throat but have no symptoms.

Clinical Features

Children are affected more often though no age group is immune. Oropharynx is commonly involved and the larynx and nasal cavity may also be affected.

General symptoms: Onset is insidious with low-grade fever (100–101°F), sore throat and malaise but patient is very toxaemic with tachycardia and thready pulse.

Membrane: Greyish white membrane is seen on the tonsil, pharynx and soft palate. It is adherent and its removal leaves a bleeding surface. Similar membrane is seen over the larynx and trachea.

In the oropharynx, a greyish white membrane forms over the tonsils and spreads to the soft palate and posterior pharyngeal wall. It is quite tenacious and causes bleeding when removed. Cervical lymph nodes, particularly the jugulodigastric become enlarged and tender, sometimes presenting a "bull-neck" appearance. Patient is ill and toxaemic but fever seldom rises above 38°C.

Complications

Exotoxin produced by C. *diphtheriae* is toxic to the heart and nerves. It causes *myocarditis, cardiac arrhythmias* and *acute circulatory failure.*

Neurological complications usually appear a few weeks after infection and include *paralysis of soft palate, diaphragm* and *ocular muscles.*

In the larynx, diphtheritic membrane may cause airway obstruction.

Treatment of diphtheria is started on clinical suspicion without waiting for the culture report. Aim is to neutralise the free exotoxin still circulating in the blood and to kill the organisms producing this exotoxin. Dose of antitoxin is based on the site involved and the duration and severity of disease. It is 20,000 to 40,000 units for diphtheria in less than 48 hours, or when the membrane is confined to the tonsils only; and 80,000 to 120,000 units, if disease has lasted longer than 48 hours, or the membrane is more extensive. Antitoxin is given by I.V. infusion in saline in about 60 minutes. Sensitivity to horse serum should be tested by conjunctival or intracutaneous test with diluted antitoxin, and adrenaline should be at hand for any immediate hypersensitivity. In the presence of hypersensitivity reaction, desensitization should be done.

Antibiotics used are benzyl penicillin 600 mg 6 hourly for 7 days. Erythromycin is used in penicillin-sensitive individuals (500 mg 6 hourly orally).

Differential Diagnosis of Membrane Over Tonsil

1. ***Membranous tonsillitis:*** It occurs due to pyogenic organisms. An exudative membrane forms over the medial surface of the tonsils, along with the features of acute tonsillitis.
2. ***Diphtheria:*** Unlike acute tonsillitis which is abrupt in onset, diphtheria is slower in onset with less local discomfort, the membrane in diphtheria extends beyond the tonsils, on to the soft palate and is dirty grey in color. It is adherent and its removal leaves a bleeding surface. Urine may show albumin. Smear and culture of throat swab will reveal *Corynebacterium diphtheriae.*
3. ***Vincent's angina:*** It is insidious in onset with less fever and less discomfort in throat. Membrane, which usually forms over one tonsil, can be easily removed revealing an irregular ulcer on the tonsil. Throat swab will show both the organisms typical of disease, namely fusiform bacilli and spirochaetes.
4. ***Infectious mononucleosis:*** This often affects young adults. Both tonsils are very much enlarged, congested and covered with membrane. Local discomfort is marked.

Lymph nodes are enlarged in the posterior triangle of neck along with splenomegaly. Attention to disease is attracted because of failure of the antibiotic treatment. Blood smear may show more than 50% lymphocytes, of which about 10% are atypical. White cell count may be normal in the first week but rises in the second week. Paul-Bunnell test (mono test) will show high titer of heterophil antibody.

5. ***Agranulocytosis:*** It presents with ulcerative necrotic lesions not only on the tonsils but elsewhere in the oropharynx. Patient is severely ill. In acute fulminant form, total leucocytic count is decreased to < 2000/cu mm or even as low as 50/cu mm and polymorph neutrophils may be reduced to 5% or less. In chronic or recurrent form, total count is reduced to 2000/cu mm with less marked granulocytopenia.
6. ***Leukaemia:*** In children, 75% of leukaemias are acute lymphoblastic and 25%> acute myelogenous or chronic, while in adults 20% of acute leukaemias are lymphocytic and 80% non-lymphocytic.

   Peripheral blood shows TLC > 100,000/cu mm. It may be normal or less than normal. Anaemia is always present and may be progressive. Blasts cells are seen on examination of the bone marrow.
7. ***Aphthous ulcers:*** They may involve any part of oral cavity or oropharynx. Sometimes, it is solitary and may involve the tonsil and pillars. It may be small or quite large and alarming. It is very painful.
8. ***Malignancy tonsil.***
9. ***Traumatic ulcer:*** Any injury to oropharynx heals by formation of a membrane. Trauma to the tonsil area may occur accidentally when hit with a tooth brush, a pencil held in mouth or fingering in the throat. Membrane appears within 24 hours.
10. ***Candidal infection of tonsil.***

6. Which of the following condition causes inspiratory stridor?

A. Glottic stenosis B. Pharyngeal stenosis

C. Subglottis stenosis D. Supraglottic stenosis

Answer: Option D. Supraglottic stenosis

Explanation:

Stridor is noisy respiration produced by turbulent airflow through the narrowed air passages. It may be heard during inspiration, expiration or both.

- ***Inspiratory stridor is often produced in obstructive lesions of supraglottis*** or pharynx, e.g., laryngomalacia or retropharyngeal abscess.

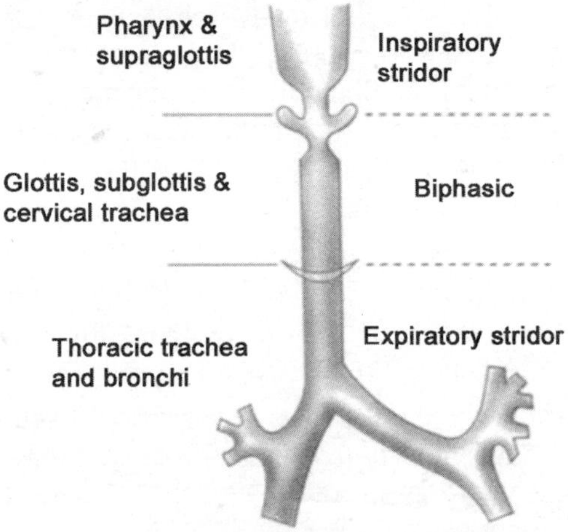

- ***Expiratory stridor*** is produced in lesions of thoracic trachea, primary and secondary bronchi, e.g., bronchial foreign body, tracheal stenosis. *Biphasic stridor* is seen in lesions of glottis, subglottis and cervical trachea, e.g., laryngeal papillomas, vocal cord paralysis and subglottis stenosis.

Common Causes of Stridor

(a) *Nose:* Choanal atresia in newborn.

(b) *Tongue:* Macroglossia due to cretinism, haemangioma or lymphangioma, dermoid at base of tongue, lingual thyroid.

(c) *Mandible:* Micrognathia, Pierre-Robin syndrome. In these cases, stridor is due to falling back of tongue.

(d) *Pharynx:* Congenital dermoid, adenotonsillar hypertrophy, retropharyngeal abscess, tumours.

(e) *Larynx:*

1. *Congenital:* Laryngeal web, laryngomalacia, cysts, vocal cord paralysis, subglottic stenosis.
2. *Inflammatory:* Epiglottitis, laryngotracheitis, diphtheria, tuberculosis.
3. *Neoplastic:* Haemangioma and juvenile multiple papillomas, carcinoma in adults.
4. *Traumatic:* Injuries of larynx, foreign bodies, oedema following endoscopy, or prolonged intubation.
5. *Neurogenic:* Laryngeal paralysis due to acquired lesions.
6. *Miscellaneous:* Tetanus, tetany, laryngismus stridulus.

(f) *Trachea and bronchi:*

1. *Congenital:* Atresia, stenosis, tracheomalacia.
2. *Inflammatory:* Tracheobronchitis.
3. *Neoplastic:* Tumours of trachea.
4. *Traumatic:* Foreign body, stenosis trachea (e.g. following prolonged intubation or tracheostomy).

(g) *Lesions outside respiratory tract:*

1. *Congenital:* Vascular rings (cause stridor and dysphagia), oesophageal atresia, tracheooesophageal fistula, congenital goitre, cystic hygroma.
2. *Inflammatory:* Retropharyngeal and oesophageal abscess.
3. *Traumatic:* FB oesophagus (secondary tracheal compression).
4. *Tumors:* Masses in neck.

CHAPTER 10 OPHTHALMOLOGY

1. Which of the following treatment is given in a child 2 years age with keratomalacia?

A. Vitamin A 2 lac IU orally at the day 0 and 14

B. Vitamin A 2 lac IU orally at the day 1, 14 and 30

C. Vitamin A 2 lac IU orally at the day 0, 1, 14

D. Vitamin A 2 lac IU orally at the day 1, 14

Answer: Option C. Vitamin A 2 lac IU orally at the day 0, 1, 14

Explanation:

Vitamin A therapy: Treatment schedules apply to all stages of active xerophthalmia viz. XN, X1A, X1B, X2, X3A and X3B. Oral administration is the recommended method of treatment. However, in the presence of repeated vomiting and severe diarrhea, intramuscular injections of water-miscible preparation should be preferred. The WHO recommended schedule is as given below:

i. ***All patients above the age of 1 year*** **(except women of reproductive age): 200,000 IU of vitamin A orally or 100,000 IU by intramuscular injection should be given immediately on diagnosis and repeated the following day and 2 weeks later.**

ii. *Children under the age of 1 year and children of any age who weigh less than 8 kg* should be treated with half the doses for patients of more than 1 year of age.

iii. **Women of reproductive age, pregnant or not:** (a) *Those having night blindness* (XN), conjunctival xerosis (X1A) and Bitot's spots (X1B) should be treated with a daily dose of 10,000 IU of vitamin A orally (1 sugar coated tablet) for 2 weeks. (b) *For corneal xerophthalmia,* administration of full dosage schedule (described for patients above 1 year of age) is recommended.

Age	Immediately on diagnosis	Next day	2 weeks later
<6 months	50,000 IU	50,000 IU	50,000 IU
6-12 months	100,000 IU	100,000 IU	100,000 IU
> 12 months	200,000 IU	200,000 IU	200,000 IU
Women of reproductive age	200,000 IU	200,000 IU	200,000 IU

2. Following chemotherapy regimen is used in treatment of retinoblastoma:

A. Cyclophosphamide, vincristin, chlorambucil

B. Carmustine, vincristine, etoposide

C. Etoposide, carboplatin, vincristine

D. Chlorambucil, etoposide, carboplatin

Answer: Option C. Etoposide, carboplatin, vincristine

Explanation:

Chemotherapy is a mainstay of treatment in most cases, and may be used in conjunction with local treatments. Intravenous **carboplatin, etoposide and vincristine (CEV)** are given in three to six cycles according to the grade of retinoblastoma. Single-(carboplatin alone) or dual-agent therapy has also given favourable results in some circumstances, such as bridging therapy to allow deferral of more aggressive measures. Selective ophthalmic artery infusion has shown promising outcomes and study is ongoing. Intravitreal melphalan seems to be effective for vitreous seeding, though carries a very small risk of extraocular dissemination. Sub-tenon carboplatin injection is now less commonly used given the availability of effective alternatives. Chemoreduction may be followed by focal treatment with cryotherapy or TTT to consolidate tumour control.

3. Which of the following operation uses a valve implant used in a patient of glaucoma?

A. Zedon

B. Decon

C. Reton

D. Seton

Answer: Option D. Seton

Explanation:

The operation using glaucoma valve implant is also known as **Seton operation.**

Glaucoma valve implants commonly used include Molteno Krupin-Denver and AGV.

Shunts Using Episcleral Explants

Introduction

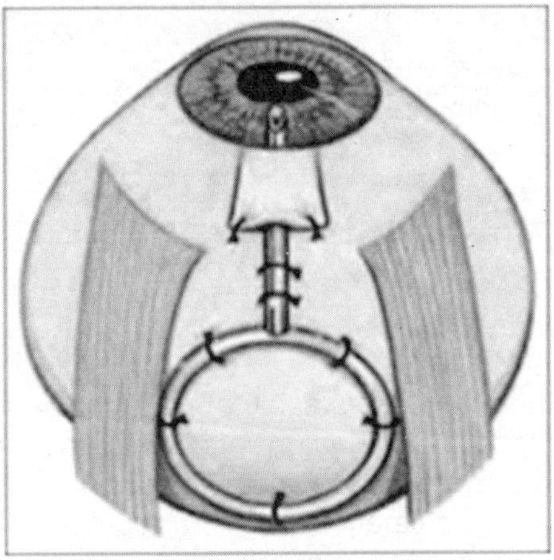

Single-plate Molteno drainage device

Glaucoma drainage devices (GDD) create a communication between the anterior chamber and the sub-Tenon space via a tube attached to a posteriorly explanted episcleral reservoir. Some contain pressure-sensitive valves for the regulation of aqueous flow. Reduction of IOP is due to passive, pressure-dependent flow of aqueous, limited by the wall of a tissue capsule that forms around the explant over the course of several weeks postoperatively. Over recent years the use of GDD has increased, with a large trial, the Tube Versus Trabeculectomy Study, providing good-quality evidence of their safety and comparability to mitomycin C-enhanced trabeculectomy. In practice the threshold for GDD implantation has been lowered, though the number of trabeculectomies being performed remains significantly higher than the rate of GDD implantation.

Examples of GDD implants include:

- **Molteno:** This consists of a silicone tube connected to one or two polypropylene plates 13 mm in diameter.
- **Baerveldt:** This implant consists of a silicone tube connected to a silicone plate of large area; silicone may elicit little tissue reaction in comparison with polypropylene.
- **Ahmed:** This is a valved implant consisting of a silicone tube connected to a silicone sheet valve held in a polypropylene body. The valve mechanism consists of two thin silicone elastomer membranes, with the aim of reducing early postoperative hypotony and its complications.

  Indications: The circumstances under which GDD may be superior to trabeculectomy are incompletely defined, and many factors must be taken into account, including an individual surgeon's experience and expertise. The introduction of the Ex-PressTM mini-shunt implant modification may have extended the repertoire of trabeculectomy to include some of the previously clearly defined indications for GDD implantation such as ICE syndrome.

GDD may be considered in the following cases, though the list is not exhaustive:

- Eyes with severe conjunctival scarring precluding accurate dissection of the conjunctiva.
- Uncontrolled glaucoma despite previous trabeculectomy with adjunctive antimetabolite therapy.
- Secondary glaucoma where routine trabeculectomy, with or without adjunctive antimetabolites, is less likely to be successful. Examples include neovascular glaucoma and glaucoma following traumatic anterior segment disruption.
- Certain congenital glaucomas where conventional procedures have failed.

Complications

- The rate of serious complications is similar to that of mitomycin trabeculectomy.
- **Excessive drainage**, resulting in hypotony and a shallow anterior chamber.
- **Malposition** may result in endothelial or lenticular touch with corneal decompensation and cataract respectively.

Ciliary sulcus or pars plana tube placement can be used in some eyes to negate the possibility of corneal touch.

- **Tube erosion** through the sclera and conjunctiva.
- **Corneal decompensation** due to endothelial cell loss.
- **Double vision** due to extraocular muscle interference; this may be a higher risk with some implants than others.
- **Early drainage failure** may occur as a result of blockage of the end of the tube by vitreous, blood or iris.
- **Late drainage failure** occurs in about 10% of cases per year and is comparable to, or perhaps slightly better than, that following trabeculectomy.

Results

The results depend on the type of glaucoma. In general, an IOP in the mid-teens is achieved, though as with trabeculectomy topical medication is frequently required in the medium and longer term. The success rate in some conditions such as neovascular glaucoma is often disappointing. Adjunctive mitomycin C may enhance the success rate of drainage shunt surgery but is associated with a higher complication rate.

5. Which of the following surgery is used in a patient having ptosis with poor levator function?

A. Fasanela–Servat operation

B. Frontalis sling operation

C. Levator resection

D. Levator advancement

Answer: Option B. Frontalis sling operation

Explanation:

Frontalis sling operation (Brow suspension) is performed in patients having severe ptosis with no or poor levator function.

Treatment

Congenital ptosis: It almost always needs surgical correction. In severe ptosis, surgery should be performed at the earliest to prevent stimulus deprivation amblyopia. However, in mild and moderate ptosis, surgery should be delayed until the age of 3-4 years, when accurate measurements are possible. Congenital ptosis can be treated by any of the following operations:

1. **Fasanella-Servat operation:** It is performed in cases having mild ptosis (1.5-2 mm) and good levator function. In it, upper lid is everted and the upper tarsal border along with its attached Muller's muscle and conjunctiva are resected.
2. **Levator resection:** It is a very commonly performed operation for moderate and severe grades of ptosis. It is contraindicated in patients having severe ptosis with poor levator function.

   Amount of levator resection required: Most of the surgeons find it out by adjusting the lid margin in relation to cornea during operation on the table in individual case. However, a rough estimate in different grades of ptosis is as follows:

   - *Moderate ptosis:* Level of LPS Amount of LPS to be Function resected Good 16-17 mm (minimal) Fair 18-22 mm (moderate) Poor 23-24 mm (maximum).
   - *Severe ptosis:* Fair levator 23-24 mm (maximum function LPS resected).

   Techniques: Levator muscle may be resected by either conjunctival or skin approach.

   i. *Conjunctival approach* (Blaskowics' operation): This technique is comparatively easy but not suitable for large amount of resection. In it LPS muscle is exposed by an incision made through the conjunctiva near the tarsal border, after the upper lid is doubly everted over a Desmarre's lid retractor.
   ii. *Skin approach (Everbusch's operation)*: It is a more frequently employed technique. It allows comparatively better exposure of the LPS muscle through a skin incision along the line of future lid fold.
3. **Frontalis sling operation (Brow suspension):** This is performed in patients having severe ptosis with no levator function. In this operation, lid is anchored to the frontalis muscle via a sling. Fascia lata or some non-absorbable material (e.g., supramide suture) may be used as sling (See Figure).

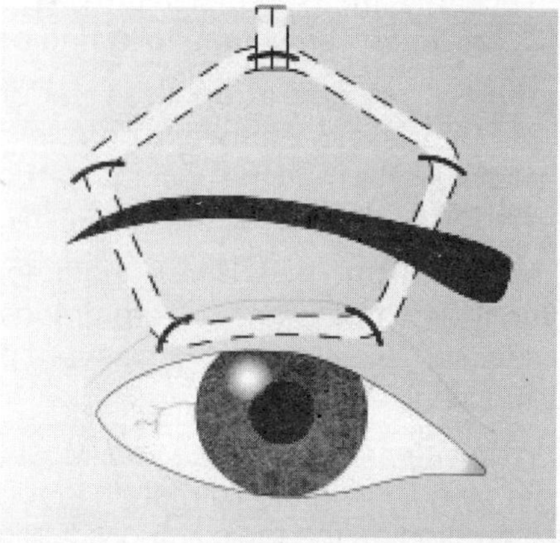

6. Which of the following is the cause from below given image of a patient having reduced visual axis?

A. Astigmatism
B. Keratomalacia
C. Foreign body
D. Leukocoria

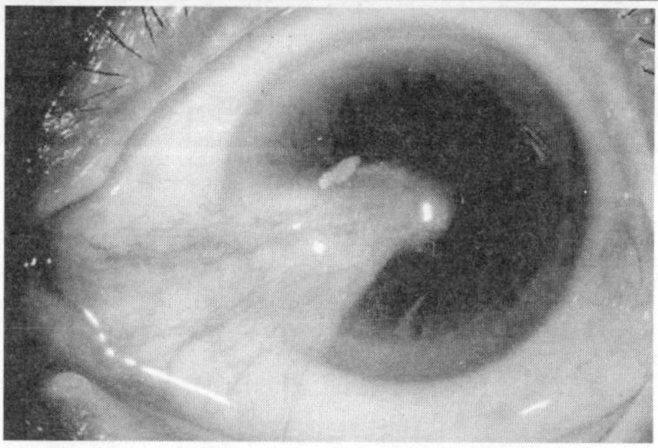

Answer: Option A. Astigmatism

Explanation:

Above given image showing wing-shaped fold of conjunctiva encroaching upon the cornea from either side–pterygium which causes **corneal astigmatism** resulting in reduced visual axis.

PTERYGIUM

Pterygium (L. Pterygion = a wing) is a wing-shaped fold of conjunctiva encroaching upon the cornea from either side within the interpalpebral fissure.

Etiology: Etiology of pterygium is not definitely known. But the disease is more common in people living in hot climates. Therefore, the most accepted view is that it is a response to prolonged effect of environmental factors such as exposure to sun (ultraviolet rays), dry heat, high wind and abundance of dust.

Pathology: Pathologically pterygium is a degenerative and hyperplastic condition of conjunctiva. The subconjunctival tissue undergoes elastotic degeneration and proliferates as vascularised granulation tissue under the epithelium, which ultimately encroaches the cornea. The corneal epithelium, Bowman's layer and superficial stroma are destroyed.

Clinical features: Pterygium is more common in elderly males doing outdoor work. It may be unilateral or bilateral. It presents as a triangular fold of conjunctiva encroaching the cornea in the area of palpebral aperture, usually on the nasal side, but may also occur on the temporal side. Deposition of iron seen sometimes in corneal epithelium anterior to advancing head of pterygium is called *stocker's line.*

Parts: A fully developed pterygium consists of three parts:

i. *Head* (apical part present on the cornea), ii. *Neck* (limbal part) and iii. *Body* (scleral part) extending between limbus and the canthus.

Types: Depending upon the progression it may be progressive or regressive pterygium.

Progressive pterygium is thick, fleshy and vascular with a few infiltrates in the cornea, in front of the head of the pterygium (called cap of pterygium).

Regressive pterygium is thin, atrophic, attenuated with very little vascularity. There is no cap. Ultimately it becomes membranous but never disappears.

Symptoms: Pterygium is an asymptomatic condition in the early stages, except for *cosmetic intolerance.* **Visual disturbances occur when it encroaches the pupillary area or due to corneal astigmatism induced due to fibrosis in the regressive stage.** Occasionally *diplopia* may occur due to limitation of ocular movements.

Complications like cystic degeneration and infection are infrequent. Rarely, neoplastic change to epithelioma, fibrosarcoma or malignant melanoma, may occur.

Differential diagnosis: Pterygium must be differentiated from pseudopterygium. *Pseudopterygium* is a fold of bulbar conjunctiva attached to the cornea. It is formed due to adhesions of chemosed bulbar conjunctiva to the marginal corneal ulcer. It usually occurs following chemical burns of the eye.

Treatment: Surgical excision is the only satisfactory treatment, which may be indicated for: (1) cosmetic reasons, (2) continued progression threatening to encroach onto the pupillary area (once the pterygium has encroached pupillary area, wait till it crosses on the other side), (3) diplopia due to interference in ocular movements.

Recurrence of the pterygium after surgical excision is the main problem (30-50%). However, it can be reduced by any of the following measures:

1. Transplantation of pterygium in the lower fornix (McReynold's operation) is not performed now.
2. Postoperative beta irradiations (not used now).
3. Postoperative use of antimitotic drugs such as mitomycin-C or thiotepa.
4. Surgical excision with bare sclera.
5. Surgical excision with free conjunctival graft taken from the same eye or other eye is presently the preferred technique.
6. In recurrent recalcitrant pterygium, surgical excision should be coupled with lamellar keratectomy and lamellar keratoplasty.

7. Esotropia is seen in which of the following condition?

A. Presbyopia
B. Hypermetropia
C. Myopia
D. Glaucoma

Answer: Option B. Hypermetropia

Explanation:

Refractive accommodative **esotropia is seen hypermetropia.**

Esotropia is a form of strabismus in which one or both eyes turns inward. The condition can be constantly present, or occur intermittently, and can give the affected individual a "cross-eyed" appearance.

TYPES

1. **Accommodative esotropia:** It occurs due to over action of convergence associated with accommodation reflex. It is of three types: refractive, non-refractive and mixed.
   i. ***Refractive accommodative esotropia:*** It usually develops at the age of 2 to 3 years and is associated with high hypermetropia (+4 to +7 D). Mostly it is for near and distance (marginally more for near) and fully correctable by use of spectacles.
   ii. ***Non-refractive accommodative esotropia:*** It is caused by abnormally AC/A (accommodative convergence/accommodation) ratio. This may occur even in patients with no refractive error. Esotropia is greater for near than that for distance (minimal or no deviation for distance). It is fully corrected by adding +3 DS for near vision.
   iii. ***Mixed accommodative esotropia***: It is caused by combination of hypermetropia and high AC/A ratio. Esotropia for distance is corrected by correction of hypermetropia; and the residual esotropia for near is corrected by an addition of +3 DS lens.
2. **Non-accommodative esotropias:** This group includes all those primary esodeviations in which amount of deviation is not affected by the state of accommodation. It includes:
   i. ***Essential infantile esotropia:*** It usually presents at 1-2 months of age. However, it may be detected shortly after birth or any time within the first 6 months of life. Previously, it was known as *congenital esotropia.* It is characterised by fairly large angle of squint (> 30°), alternate fixation in primary gaze and crossed fixation in lateral gaze.
   ii. ***Essential acquired or late onset esotropia:*** It is a common variety of concomitant convergent squint. It typically occurs during first few years of life. It is of three types:
      - *Basic type:* In it the deviation is usually equal at distance and near.

- *Convergence excess type*: In it the deviation is large for near and small or no deviation for distance.
- *Divergence insufficiency type:* It is characterized by a greater deviation for distance than near.

3. **Secondary Esotropia:**

It includes:

- *Sensory deprivation esotropia:* It results from monocular lesions (in childhood) which either prevent the development of normal binocular vision or interfere with its maintenance. Examples of such lesions are: cataract, severe congenital ptosis, aphakia, anisometropia, optic atrophy, retinoblastoma, central chorioretinitis and so on.
- *Consecutive esotropia:* It results from surgical overcorrection of exotropia.

8. Which of the following test is shown in below given image?

A. Maddox wing test B. Prism cover test

C. Cover test D. Maddox rod test

Answer: Option C. Cover test

Explanation:

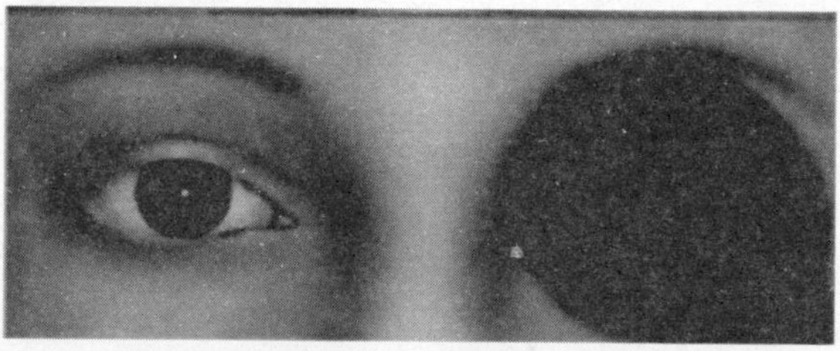

Here above given image is showing completely covered one eye with black disc, which is done in Cover test to diagnose concomitant strabismus.

EVALUATION OF A CASE OF CONCOMITANT STRABISMUS

Cover Tests

i. ***Direct cover test:*** It confirms the presence of manifest squint. To perform it, the patient is asked to fixate on a point light. Then, the normal looking eye is covered while observing the movement of the uncovered eye. In the presence of squint the uncovered eye will move in opposite direction to take fixation, while in apparent squint there will be no movement. This test should be performed for near taxation (i.e., at 33 cm) distance taxation (i.e., at 6 meters).

ii. ***Alternate cover test:*** It reveals whether the squint is unilateral or alternate and also differentiates concomitant squint from paralytic squint (where secondary deviation is greater than primary).

Cover-Uncover Test

The cover-uncover test consists of two parts:

Cover test to detect a heterotropia. It is helpful to begin the near test using a light to observe the corneal reflections and to assess fixation in the deviating eye. It should then be repeated for near using an accommodative target and for distance as follows:

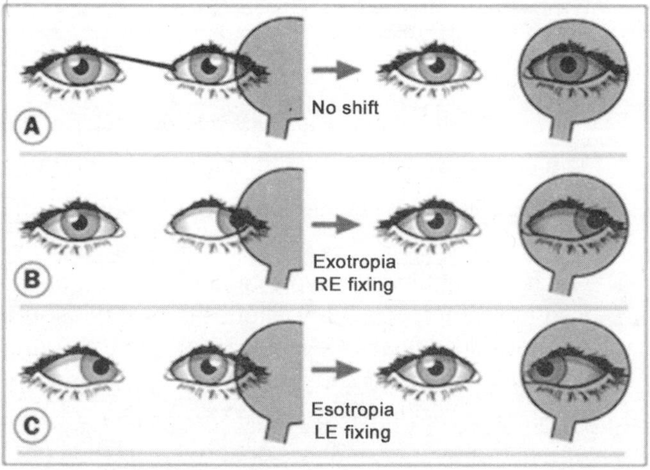

Possible result of cover test

- The patient fixates on a straight ahead target.
- If a right deviation is suspected, the examiner covers the fixing left eye and notes any movement of the right eye to take up fixation.
- No movement indicates orthotropia or left heterotropia.

- Adduction of the right eye to take up fixation indicates right exotropia and abduction, right esotropia.
- Downward movement indicates right hypertropia and upward movement right hypotropia.
- The test is repeated on the opposite eye.

The uncover test detects heterophoria. It should be performed both for near (using an accommodative target) and for distance as follows:

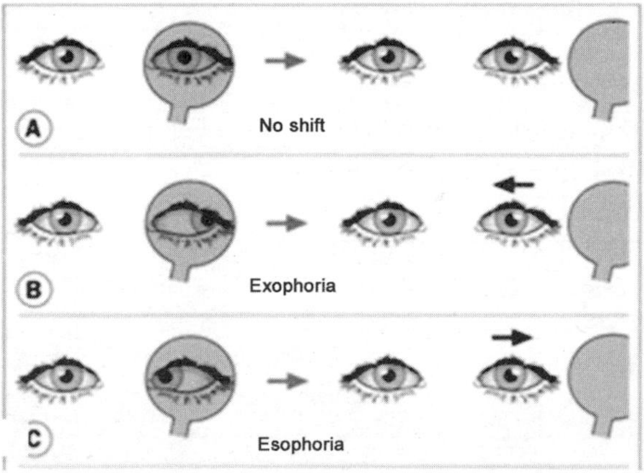

Possible results of the uncover test

- The patient fixates a straight ahead distant target.
- The examiner covers the right eye and, after 2–3 seconds, removes the cover.
- No movement indicates orthophoria; a keen observer will frequently detect a very slight latent deviation in most normal individuals, as few individuals are truly orthophoric, particularly on near fixation.

If the right eye had deviated while under cover, a re-fixation movement (recovery to BSV) is observed on being uncovered.

- Adduction (nasal recovery) of the right eye indicates exophoria and abduction esophoria.
- Upward or downward movement indicates a vertical phoria.
- After the cover is removed, the examiner notes the speed and smoothness of recovery as evidence of the strength of motor fusion.
- The test is repeated for the opposite eye.

- Most examiners perform the cover test and the uncover test sequentially, hence the term cover-uncover test.

Alternate Cover Test

The alternate cover test induces dissociation to reveal the total deviation when fusion is disrupted. It should be performed only after the cover-uncover test.

- The right eye is covered for several seconds.
- The occluder is quickly shifted to the opposite eye for 2 seconds, then back and forth several times. After the cover is removed, the examiner notes the speed and smoothness of recovery as the eyes return to their pre-dissociated state.
- A patient with a well-compensated heterophoria will have straight eyes before and after the test has been performed whereas a patient with poor control may decompensate to a manifest deviation.

Prism Cover Test

- The prism cover test measures the angle of deviation on near or distance fixation and in any gaze position. It combines the alternate cover test with prisms and is performed as follows:
- The alternate cover test is first performed to establish the direction and approximate extent of deviation.
- Prisms of increasing strength are placed in front of one eye with the base opposite the direction of the deviation (i.e. the apex of the prism is pointed in the direction of the deviation). For example, in a convergent strabismus the prism is held base out, and in a right hypertropia, base down before the right eye.
- The alternate cover test is performed continuously as stronger prisms are introduced, typically using a prism bar consisting of a column of prisms of progressive strength. The amplitude of the refixation movement should gradually decrease as the strength of prism approaches the extent of deviation.
- The end-point is approached when no movement is seen. To ensure the maximum angle is found, the prism strength can be increased further until a movement is observed

in the opposite direction (the point of reversal) and then reduced again to find the neutral value; the angle of deviation is then taken from the strength of the prism.

9. Which of the following test is shown in below given image?

A. Cover-uncover test
B. Prism cover test
C. Maddox rod test
D. Maddox wing test

Answer: Option C. Maddox rod test

Explanation:

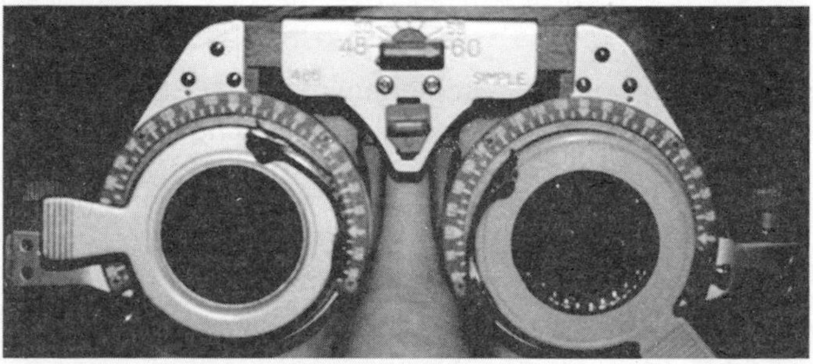

Here above image is showing red color glass rods set together in a metallic disc in front of one eye, this is a Maddox road test.

Patient is asked to fix on a point light in the center of Maddox tangent scale at a distance of 6 meters. A Maddox rod is placed in front of one eye with axis of the rod parallel to the axis of deviation.

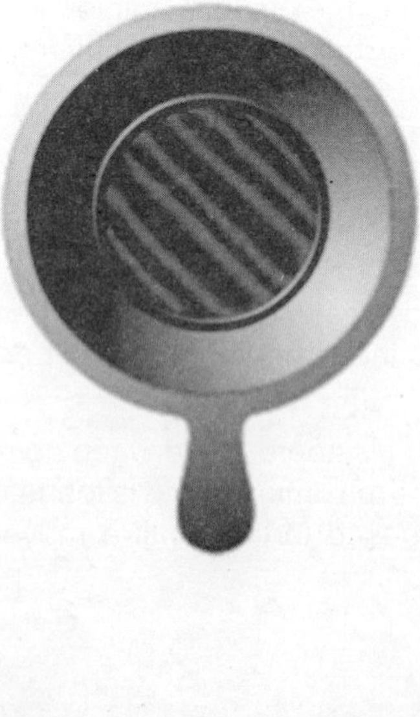

Maddox Rod

The Maddox rod converts the point light image into a line. Thus, the patient will see a point light with one eye and a red line with the other. Due to dissimilar images of the two eyes, fusion is broken and heterophoria becomes manifest. The number on Maddox tangent scale where the red line falls will be the amount of heterophoria in degrees. In the absence of Maddox tangent scale, the dissociation between the point light and red line is measured by the superimposition of the two images by means of prisms placed in front of one eye with apex towards the phoria.

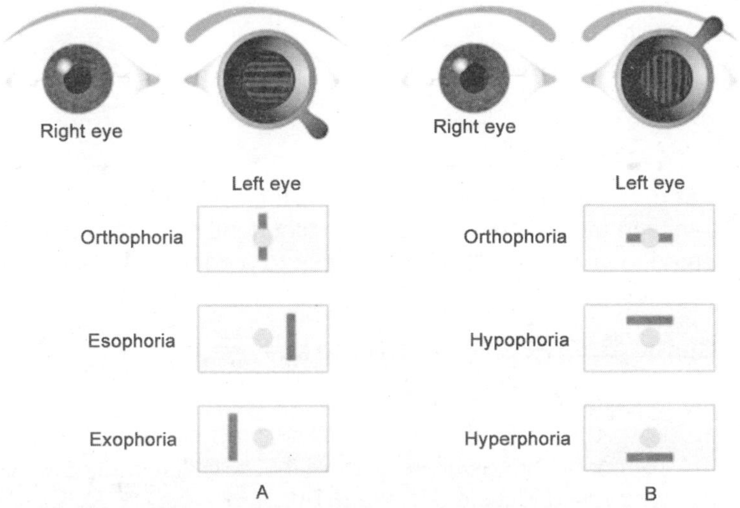

Maddox rod test for horizontal (A) and vertical (B) heterophorias

10. Write down the prescription for against the rule astigmatism.

A. – 1.0 D cyl. in 180-degree axis

B. – 4.0 D cyl. and + 2.5 D spherical in 180-degree axis

C. – 1.5 D cyl. in 90-degree axis

D. + 1 D cyl. in 90-degree axis

Answer: Option C. –1.5 D cyl. in 90-degree axis

Explanation:

Against the rule astigmatism is corrected by minus cylindrical lenses in 90-degree axis, so from above given options our answer is – 1.5 D cyl. in 90-degree axis.

Corneal astigmatism

- Against the rule
  - Vertical meridian flatter than horizontal
  - Corrected with (-) cyl. × 90°

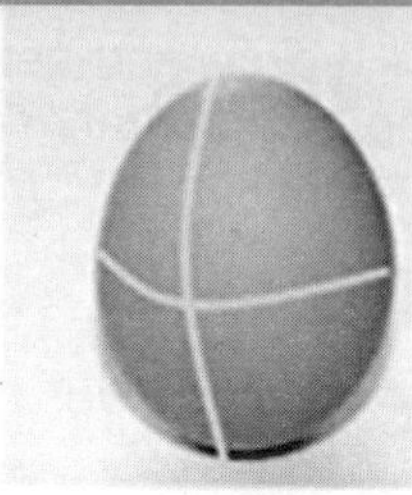

- With the rule
  - Vertical meridian steeper than horizontal
  - Corrected with (-) cyl. × 180°

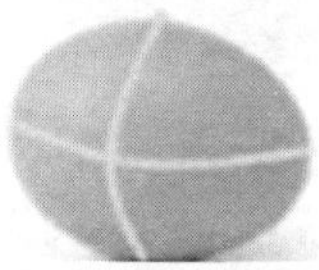

Astigmatism is a type of refractive error, wherein the refraction varies in the different meridia. Consequently, the rays of light entering in the eye cannot converge to a point focus but form focal lines.

CLINICAL TYPES OF ASTIGMATISM

Types of Regular Astigmatism

1. **With-the-rule astigmatism:** This type of astigmatism is common among children where the vertical meridian is the steepest and it stays close to 90˚.
2. **Against-the-rule astigmatism:** In this type of astigmatism, the horizontal meridian stays close to 180˚. It is steeper than the vertical meridian. Against-the-rule astigmatism is common in the elderly.
3. **Oblique astigmatism:** If the principal meridians are not at 90˚ and 180˚, it is categorized as oblique astigmatism. Here, the shape of the eyeball resembles a tilted American football with its prime meridians lying between 30˚–60˚ and 120°–150°.
4. **Bioblique astigmatism**, wherein the two principal meridia are not at right angle to each other, e.g., one may be at 30° and the other at 100°.

Irregular Astigmatism: In it refraction varies in multiple meridia which admits no geometrical analysis. It commonly follows corneal scarring.

When eyewear prescriptions are written, they can be classified into different areas depending on the power or refractive error.

There are **seven categories** to which prescriptions can fall:

1. **Simple Hyperopia, requires minus or concave glasses.**
2. **Simple Myopia, requires plus or convex glasses.**
3. **Simple Myopic Astigmatism, requires cylindrical glass and it has minus power (of glass) in only one meridian.**
4. **Simple Hyperopic Astigmatism, requires cylindrical glass and it has plus power (of glass) in only one meridian.**
5. **Compound Hyperopic Astigmatism:** It has **+ in one and – in another meridian but major meridian power will be (+) (+) on both 90 and 180 degree axis.**
6. **Compound Myopic Astigmatism:** It has **+ in one and – in another meridian but major meridian power will be (–) (–) on both 90 and 180 degree axis.**
7. **Mixed Astigmatism, major meridian powers will be opposites (–)(+) (+)(–) on both 90 and 180 degree axis.**

CHAPTER 11

MEDICINE

1. Polyuria is defined as urine output more than:

A. 20 ml/kg/day
B. 30 ml/kg/day
C. 50 ml/kg/day
D. 70 ml/kg/day

Answer: Option C. 50 ml/kg/day

Explanation:

Polyuria: Urine volume above 3 L/day or 50 ml/kg/day, with the recognition that normal individuals who drink a large amount of fluid intake, form large volumes of urine.

Causes: Diabetes insipidus, diabetes mellitus, salt losing nephritis, diuretic phase of ATN, diuretic therapy, hypercalcaemia, hypokalaemia, psychogenic polydipsia (thirst), chlorpromazine and anticholinergic agents (↑thirst).

Oliguria: This refers to a urine output insufficient to sustain life, usually < 400 ml/day in an adult of average size.

Anuria: This refers to absence of urine flow (< 50 ml/day) and is caused usually by urinary obstruction, total renal arterial or venous occlusion or renal cortical necrosis or RPGN.

Nocturia: Nocturnal urine volume equals or exceeds diurnal urine volume. It is a common symptom of diabetes mellitus, diabetes insipidus, early stages of chronic renal failure, cardiac failure (with treatment), insomnia, prostatic obstruction and other causes of polyuria.

2. Which is the cause of tender hepatomegaly with jaundice in a patient of hematopoeitc stem cell transplantation?

A. Cirrhosis
B. Hepatitis
C. Veno-occlusive disease
D. Cholecystitis

Answer: Option C. Veno-occlusive disease

Explanation:

Veno-occlusive diseases, occurs most commonly as a complication of myeloablative regimens that are used to prepare patients for haematopoietic stem cell transplantation and present with tender hepatomegaly with jaundice.

Veno-Occlusive Disease

Veno-occlusive diseases, also known as sinusoidal obstruction syndrome, occurs most commonly as a complication of myeloablative regimens that are used to prepare patients for haematopoietic stem cell transplantation. Other causes include chemotherapeutic agents in conventional doses, chronic immunosuppression with azathioprine or 6-thioguanine, and ingestion of herbal teas made with pyrrolizidine alkaloids.

Occurs due to circulatory obstruction at the level of central hepatic veins.

Presents with weight gain with or without ascites, right upper quadrant pain of liver origin, hepatomegaly and jaundice.

May develop multiorgan failure, particularly pulmonary and renal failure.

Management includes control of fluid overload, ascites and supportive treatment. TIPSS is contraindicated.

3. Osborn wave is seen in case of:

A. Hyperthermia
B. Hypothermia
C. Metabolic acidosis
D. Metabolic alkalosis

Answer: Option B. Hypothermia

Explanation:

ECG Features of Hypothermia

It is characterised by ***J-wave or junctional wave or 'Osborne' wave***, a hump like deflection which occurs at the junction of the distal limb of QRS complex with the S-T segment. There is a delay in the inscription of the intrinsicoid deflection (> 0.06 sec), that might be an early sign of impending VF.

Sinus bradycardia and prolonged QT interval may also occur.

HYPOTHERMIA

J Wave or Osborne wave

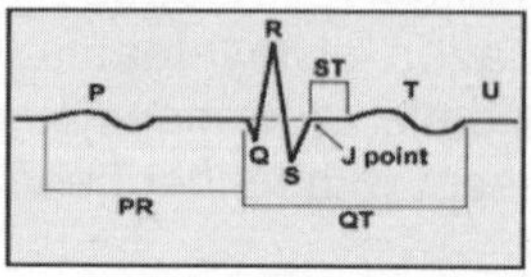

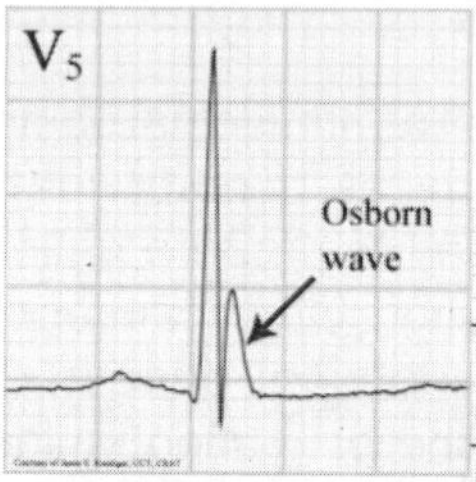

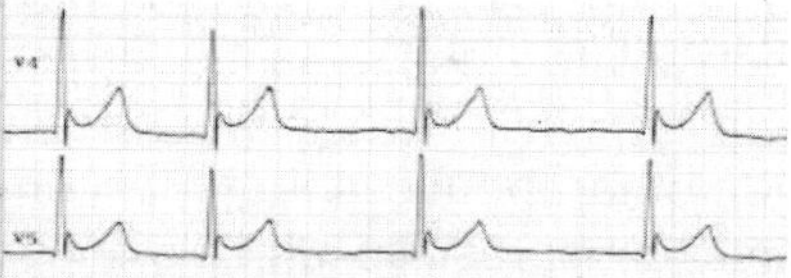

4. Which of the following is not an AIDS defining illness?

A. Pneumocystis jiroveci pneumonia

B. Extrapulmonary tuberculosis

C. Tertiary syphilis

D. Oesophageal candidiasis

Answer: Option C. Tertiary syphilis

Explanation:

Tertiary syphilis is not an AIDS defining illness.

Following are AIDS defining conditions and include:

Recurrent, severe infections (meningitis, pneumonia, septicaemia, etc.)
Oesophageal/pulmonary candidiasis
Cryptosporidiosis
CMV/toxoplasmosis disease of more than 1 month of age
Recurrent non-typhoidal salmonella septicaemia
Disseminated/extrapulmonary mycobacterial tuberculosis
Atypical mycobacterial infections
Wasting syndrome
Pneumocystis jiroveci pneumonia
HIV encephalopathy

5. Which of the following syndrome occurs due to blockage of PICA ?

A. Weber's syndrome

B. Parinaud syndrome

C. Medial medullary syndrome

D. Wallenberg syndrome

Answer: Option D. Wallenberg syndrome

Explanation:

Occlusion of the posterior inferior cerebellar artery or one of its branches, or of the vertebral artery leads to lateral medullary syndrome also called Wallenberg syndrome.

Lateral Medullary Syndrome

This syndrome is characterised by:

Vestibulocerebellar symptoms: Vertigo, falling towards the side of lesion, diplopia, and multidirectional nystagmus (inferior cerebellar peduncle and vestibular nucleus).

Autonomic dysfunction: Ipsilateral Horner's syndrome, hiccups.

Sensory symptoms: Initially abnormal stabbing pain over the ipsilateral face then loss of pain and temperature sensation over the contralateral side of body (spinal trigeminal nucleus involvement).

Ipsilateral bulbar muscle weakness: Hoarseness, dysphonia, dysphagia, and dysarthria, decreased gag reflex (nucleus ambiguus).

Weber's syndrome (superior alternating hemiplegia) is a form of stroke characterized by the presence of an ipsilateral oculomotor nerve palsy and contralateral hemiparesis or hemiplegia. It is caused by midbrain infarction as a result of occlusion of the paramedian branches of the **posterior cerebral artery.**

Medial medullary syndrome, also known as inferior alternating syndrome, hypoglossal alternating hemiplegia, lower alternating hemiplegia, or Dejerine syndrome, is a type of alternating hemiplegia resulting from occlusion of **the anterior spinal artery** which results in the infarction of medial part of the medulla oblongata.

Parinaud syndrome, also known as the dorsal midbrain syndrome, is a supranuclear vertical gaze disturbance caused by compression of the tectal plate, most frequently due to a posterior commissure.

It is characterised by a classic triad of findings:

- Upward gaze palsy, often manifesting as diplopia.
- Pupillary light-near dissociation (pupils respond to near stimuli, but not light).
- Convergence-retraction nystagmus.

6. In which of the following condition cardiac mumur is increased on standing position?

A. Hypertrophic obstructive cardiomyopathy

B. Mitral regurgitation

C. Aortic regurgitation

D. Mitral stenosis

Answer: Option A. Hypertrophic obstructive cardiomyopathy

Explanation:

In Hypertrophic obstructive cardiomyopathy (HOCM), Harsh ejection systolic murmur best heard at the lower-left sternal border as well as at the apex due to left ventricular outflow tract obstruction. This murmur increases during standing and Valsalva maneuver (which reduce ventricular preload) but decreases during squatting and sustained hand grip (which increase afterload), and also by leg raising (which increases preload). This situation is in contrast to a murmur of aortic stenosis, in which these manoeuvres decrease the intensity of the murmur.

HYPERTROPHIC OBSTRUCTIVE CARDIOMYOPATHY

Features

- There is left ventricular hypertrophy that may be generalised, but usually involving the interventricular septum predominantly. The upper portion of the interventricular septum is more hypertrophied (asymmetrical septa hypertrophy–ASH) and may result in left ventricular outflow tract obstruction (in 25%).

- Cases with outflow tract obstruction are referred to as hypertrophic obstructive cardiomyopathy (HOCM) and those without obstruction as HCM. However, since obstruction is dynamic, the term HOCM is not used now-a-days.
- The overall annual death rate in patients with HCM is estimated at–1%/year, whereas that in patients with obstruction is–2%/year.
- The disease is familial and transmitted as an autosomal dominant trait.

Clinical Features

- Many patients are asymptomatic.
- Family history of sudden death may be positive.
- Dyspnoea, fatigue, angina (due to ventricular hypertrophy which increases myocardial oxygen demand, particularly during exertion), syncope or near syncope. Sudden death during or after physical exertion. Arrhythmias are common.

Auscultation

Rapidly rising carotid pulse ("jerky"). Bisferiens pulse (two systolic peaks). Double apical impulse. Loud fourth heart sound.

Harsh ejection systolic murmur best heard at the lower-left sternal border as well as at the apex due to left ventricular out-flow tract obstruction. This murmur increases during standing and Valsalva manoeuvre (which reduce ventricular preload) but decreases during squatting and sustained hand grip (which increase afterload), and also by leg raising (which increases preload). This situation is in contrast to a murmur of aortic stenosis, in which these maneuvers decrease the intensity of the murmur.

Pansystolic murmur at mitral area due to mitral regurgitation.

Investigations

- Electrocardiogram shows left ventricular hypertrophy, and widespread deep and broad Q waves.
- Chest radiograph is normal or shows mild-to-moderate cardiac enlargement.

- Echocardiography is diagnostic. It may also show systolic anterior motion of anterior leaflet of mitral valve, which is a major contributor to left ventricular outflow tract obstruction and the accompanying mitral regurgitation.

Treatment

- β-blockers in angina and syncope. Treatment with β-blockers improves ventricular relaxation, increases diastolic filling time, and reduces susceptibility to ventricular and supraventricular arrhythmias.
- Amiodarone for controlling arrhythmias.
- Calcium channel blockers that do not have significant vasodilatory action are also beneficial because of their negative inotropic and chronotropic effects. They should not be used in presence of left ventricular outflow tract obstruction.
- If β-blockers alone are not sufficient, disopyramide (which also has a negative inotropic effect) along with β-blockers are helpful to reduce outflow tract obstruction.
- Surgical myotomy or myectomy of the hypertrophied septum.
- Digoxin, diuretics, nifedipine, nitrates and β-agonists should be avoided since they increase outflow tract obstruction.
- Implantable cardioverter-defibrillator in high-risk patients (cardiac arrest survivors, spontaneous sustained or non-sustained ventricular tachycardia, family history of premature sudden death, unexplained syncope, left ventricular thickness; $\geq$ 30 mm and abnormal blood pressure during exercise).
- Septal alcohol ablation is being increasingly used.
- Evaluation of family members.

7. Alzheimer's disease is associated with which of the following Apo Enzyme?

A. Apo E 2 B. Apo E 4

C. Apo E 3 D. Apo E 1

Answer: Option B. Apo E 4

Explanation:

Apo E4 gene is associated with the risk of development of Alzheimer's disease.

Alzheimer's disease is a progressive neurodegenerative disease resulting in decline in cognitive functions together with declining activities of daily living (ADL) and behavioural disturbances.

It is the most common cause of cognitive impairment in elderly persons. From the age of 60 onwards up to 80 years, incidence and prevalence of AD increases exponentially with age, doubling every 5 years.

Pathology

- The pathological process consists principally of neuronal loss, principally in the temporoparietal cortex but also in the frontal cortex, together with an inflammatory response to the deposition of senile plaques and neurofibrillary tangles.
- Senile plaques and neurofibrillary tangles are regarded as hallmark of Alzheimer's disease, though they may also be present with normal aging.
- Senile plaques consist of extracellular deposition of congophilic, insoluble material that is amyloid-β (Aβ). It is derived from the enzymatic cleavage of a larger membrane protein, the amyloid precursor protein (APP).
- Neurofibrillary tangles represent intracellular paired helical filaments of hyperphosphorylated protein known as tau protein. Tau protein is expressed in neurons and normally acts to stabilise microtubules in the cells.
- Other pathologic features include synaptic degeneration, accumulation of abnormal lysosomes and mitochondria, neuronal loss and glia-mediated inflammation.

Aetiology

- The exact aetiopathogenesis is not known.
- Three hypotheses include cholinergic hypothesis (reduced acetylcholine), amyloid hypothesis and tau hypothesis.
- Genes that increase the probability of sporadic Alzheimer's disease include the allele E4 of apolipoprotein E (APOE) and the sortilin-related receptor I (SORLI) gene (which is involved in cholesterol transport, β-amyloid formation

and APP processing). Early onset of Alzheimer's disease (onset < 60 years) is uncommon and is usually autosomal dominant. Three gene mutations have been identified: APP gene located on the chromosome 21; the presenilin-1 (PSI) and presenilin-2 (PS2) genes located on chromosomes 14 and 1 respectively.

- Moderate consumption of red wine, increased dietary intake of fruits and vegetables, and the use of nonsteroidal anti-inflammatory drugs are associated with a lower risk.

Potential acquired risk factors for Alzheimer's disease are shown below:

- Ageing
- Family history of Alzheimer's disease
- Reduced reserve capacity of brain
- Low educational and occupational attainment
- Low mental ability in early life
- Reduced mental and physical activity during late life.
- Diet
- Reduced consumption of fish
- Increased consumption of dietary fat.
- Head injury
- Risk factors associated with vascular disease
- Hypercholesterolaemia
- Hypertension
- Smoking
- Obesity
- Diabetes

Clinical Features

- It is an insidious onset disease with symptoms in 3 domains: cognitive, behavioural and functional. Mild cognitive impairment is characterized as a transitional stage between normal ageing and Alzheimer's disease.
- The patient has disturbances of memory, language and visual skills.
- There is an impaired ability to learn new things and recall previously learnt information. An inability to retain recently acquired information is typically the initial symptom, whereas memory for remote events is relatively spared until late. Episodic memory impairment (memory for personally

experienced events in a particular temporal and spatial context) is an important cognitive deficit. This can be tested by the three words recall item and the orientation items of the mini-mental state examination (MMSE).

- Impairment of semantic memory (knowledge of public events, words and of the associations between concepts), working memory (ability to manipulate short-term memory representations) and executive functions (coordination of multiple cognitive processes) are often present.
- A decline in language function and increased difficulty with names and understanding what is being said (nominal and comprehensive dysphasia). The first manifestations of language dysfunction usually include word finding difficulties, circumlocution, and reduced vocabulary in spontaneous speech and anomia.
- An impaired ability to carry out motor activities despite intact motor function (dyspraxia).
- Failure to recognize or identify objects despite intact sensory function (agnosia).
- There is a gradual decline in ADL that ultimately leads to profound disability and dependence on others.
- Other features include behavioral problems, psychotic symptoms and depression. Psychotic symptoms are not the presenting features but develop later during the course of disease. Occurrence of psychosis during the initial stages of dementia suggests other diagnoses such as dementia with Lewy bodies. Persecutory delusions occur in nearly 50% of the patients.
- It is important to differentiate between Alzheimer's disease and other treatable causes of dementia.
- Pneumonia is a common cause of death because aspiration is common due to impaired swallowing mechanisms in the later stages. Other common causes of death include complications from urinary tract infections and falls.

Laboratory Investigations

- These are carried out to exclude a treatable cause of dementia.
- Common investigations are blood chemistry, a complete blood count, tests for syphilis, serum levels of vitamin B_{12} and thyroid functions.

- A CT head is usually done to exclude an intracranial pathology. An MRI may show atrophy in the hippocampus, mesial and lateral temporal, isthmus cingulate and orbitofrontal areas. It can help exclude normal pressure hydrocephalus. Focal frontal or anterior temporal atrophy suggests a diagnosis of frontotemporal dementia. Large white matter abnormalities indicate a vascular dementia, particularly if the history is one of a stepwise decline in cognitive function.
- High resolution functional MRI may distinguish AD from normal aging.
- Cerebrospinal fluid is normal but may show slight elevation in protein content. There is an increase in total tau and phosphorylated tau but a decrease in amyloid-beta (Aβ).
- Functional neuroimaging studies such as PET and SPECT scans can provide a supporting role in diagnosis. PET shows decreased FDG uptake in hippocampus, parietotemporal cortex and posterior cingulate cortex.

Diagnosis

- Criteria for a diagnosis of clinically probable Alzheimer's disease are the presence of an episodic memory deficit in combination with impairment of at least one other cognitive domain. Frequently affected domains at an early stage are executive functions and word finding. There must be a significant impact on ADL and no alternative explanations (delirium, medication, comorbidity and depression).
- MMSE is useful in the initial evaluation of patients with suspected dementia.
- Cognitive aging (age-related cognitive decline) refers to age-related decline that selectively affects specific cognitive processes, including delayed recall, processing speed and executive functions. Familiarity of past objects and persons is usually not affected in age-related cognition decline.

MANAGEMENT

Cognitive Deficits

- Cholinesterase inhibitors provide modest improvement in symptoms and reduction in the rate of cognitive decline. They inhibit acetylcholinesterase, the enzyme that degrades acetylcholine in the synaptic cleft, thereby increasing the availability of acetylcholine. These drugs include donepezil, rivastigmine and galantamine. Common side effects include nausea, vomiting, diarrhoea and weight loss. Donepezil is started at a dosage of 5 mg daily at bedtime and increased to 10 mg daily after 1-4 weeks. Galantamine is started at a dosage of 4 mg twice daily and gradually titrated to 12 mg twice daily with step-ups at 1-4 week intervals. Rivastigmine is started at a dosage of 1.5 mg twice daily and titrated over 1-3 months to 6 mg twice daily.

- In moderate to severe cases, memantine, an N-methyl-D-aspartate (NMDA) antagonist maybe added to cholinesterase inhibitors. It is believed to protect neurons from glutamate-mediated excitotoxicity.
- Other agents include vitamin E, statins and NSAIDs, though their exact role is not clear.

8. Bundle of KENT is involved in which of the following disease?

A. WPW syndrome

B. Takotsubo cardiomyopathy

C. Arrythmogenic right ventricular dysplasia

D. HOCM

Answer: Option A. WPW syndrome

Explanation:

Wolff-Parkinson-White syndrome (WPW) is the most common type of ventricular pre-excitation syndrome. It occurs due to an abnormal fast accessory pathway from the atria to the ventricles, the bundle of Kent, which bypasses the atrioventricular node. This causes the ventricles to partially depolarize earlier, leading to a widened QRS complex on ECG with a slurred upstroke, the delta wave. The PR interval is shortened as well. Supraventricular tachycardia may occur if a reentry circuit develops, and may necessitate hospitalization. Catheter ablation of the bundle of Kent is the definitive treatment for the condition.

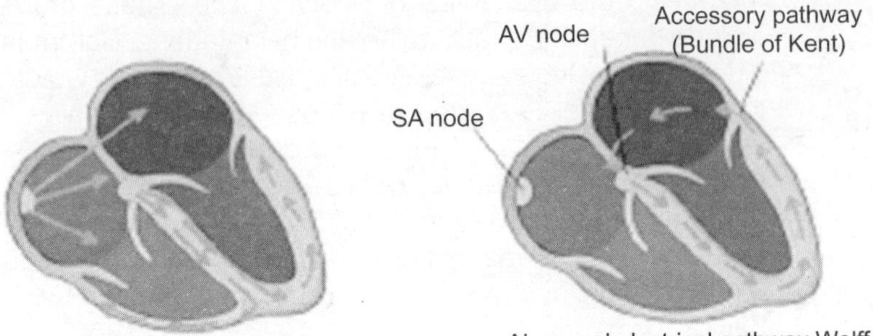

Normal electrical pathways

Abnormal electrical pathway Wolff-Parkinson-White syndrome

Cause: Presence of an abnormal band of atrial tissue connecting the atria and ventricles and bypassing the AV node.

During sinus rhythm conduction takes place partly through the AV node and partly through the bypass tract. This results in a short PR interval (<0.12 seconds), a delta wave in the beginning of QRS complex due to activation of ventricles via the accessory pathway, and prolonged QRS complex (>0.12 seconds) due to fusion of excitation via two pathways.

This tract can act as a re-entry pathway and the patient may develop supraventricular tachycardia.

Complications

Supraventricular tachycardia, atrial fibrillation, ventricular tachycardia, ventricular fibrillation (VF) and death.

Treatment

Narrow complex tachycardia is treated in the same way as PSVT.

For broad-complex tachycardia, isopyramide, quinidine, flecainide, propafenone and amiodarone are useful as these drugs increase the refractory period and reduce the conduction rate through the bypass tract. In selected cases radiofrequency ablation of the bypass tract can be done. In patients with WPW syndrome and atrial fibrillation, cardioversion is the treatment of choice. Caution should be employed when using digitalis, adenosine or verapamil in patients of WPW syndrome and atrial fibrillation because increase in AV nodal refractory period produces increased conduction through the accessory pathway which may precipitate ventricular fibrillation.

9. All of the following are true regarding GBS:

A. It is a predominant sensory neuropathy

B. It causes ascending paralysis

C. It is a chronic demyelinating polyneuropathy

D. It is an inflammatory disorder of peripheral nerves

Answer: Option B. It causes ascending paralysis

Explanation:

In Guillain-Barré syndrome (GBS), Motor paralysis is more striking and is symmetrical, involving proximal muscles more than distal. It begins in the legs, progressing over several days to involve arms, face and eyes (ascending paralysis).

GB syndrome (GBS) is the most common **acute demyelinating polyneuropathy** that is presumed to be autoimmune in nature. It affects people at any age. It usually follows viral infection, rarely after surgery or immunisation.

Pathogenesis

GB syndrome is a **monophasic immunologically mediated inflammatory disorder of peripheral nerves**. Multifocal demyelination with inflammation results in conduction block. Severe forms show secondary axonal degeneration. GB syndrome commonly follows an infection. Antiganglioside antibodies are seen in at least one-third of GBS patients. These antibodies appear to cross-react with antigens in the lipopolysaccharides of some antecedent infective agents. These antibodies act against gangliosides, such as GM1, distributed throughout the myelin in the peripheral nervous system. Both cellular and humoral immune mechanisms probably play a role in its development. Since inflammation is important in its pathogenesis, GB syndrome is also known as acute inflammatory demyelinating polyneuropathy (AIDP).

Clinical Features

It is an acute disorder. It usually progresses for a few days and rarely up to 1 month. **It is a predominant motor neuropathy. Sensory findings are minimum and consist of distal paranesthesias with mildly disturbed joint position sense.**

- Motor paralysis is more striking and is symmetrical, involving proximal muscles more than distal. It begins in the legs, progressing over several days to involve arms, face and eyes (ascending paralysis).
- Reflexes are absent.
- 50% show bifacial weakness.
- Some show bulbar muscular weakness.
- Respiratory paralysis occurs in a few.
- Autonomic disturbances occur in a few, resulting in sudden fluctuations in BP and heart rate.
- Bladder involvement is rare, and even when seen is mild and hardly lasts longer than 1 week.
- Clear sensory level and marked bladder involvement are against the diagnosis of GB syndrome.
- Similarly, extensor plantar response is extremely rare.

Miller Fisher Syndrome

It is a variant of GB syndrome and is characterized by a reflexia, ataxia and ophthalmoplegia without significant limb weakness. Often preceded by Campylobacter jejuni infection (usually producing diarrhoea).

Other Variants

- Acute motor axonal neuropathy.
- Progresses more rapidly and has an earlier peak than demyelinating GBS.
- Tendon reflexes are relatively preserved or even exaggerated.
- Autonomic dysfunction is rare.
- Acute motor and sensory axonal neuropathy.

Course

Muscle weakness gradually progresses over 1-3 weeks and then plateaus over next several days to weeks before gradual recovery. On recovery, nearly 15% patients do not have any deficit while minor deficit and major deficits occur in nearly 70% and 5-10% cases, respectively.

Investigations

- CSF becomes abnormal after I week of illness and shows raised proteins (> 45 mg/dL), normal sugar and cell count (generally < 10/mm^3 ; rarely cell count may go up to 50 cells/ mm^3, but never above that). This is known as albuminocytological dissociation.
- Nerve conduction velocity studies show slowing of velocities (demyelination pattern).
- Acute intermittent porphyria, post-diphtheritic neuritis and drug-induced acute polyneuropathies will need to be ruled out.

Treatment

- Immediate management of a patient with GB syndrome consists of maintenance of airway, breathing and circulation. Ventilate if patient develops respiratory failure.
- Monitor pulse, BP and cardiac activity using a cardiac monitor as these patients have autonomic instability.
- Steroids are of little value in these patients.
- Plasmapheresis and intravenous immunoglobulin (0.4 g/kg/day for 5 days or 2 g/day for 2 days) have been shown to accelerate recovery.

10. A 23 years old patient presented with headache, fever, convulsion and altered sensorium. CSF histological shows Cowdry A body. What will be the diagnosis?

A. HSV

B. CMV

C. Japanese encephalitis

D. Pneumococcal meningitis

Answer: Option A. HSV

Here, 23 years old patient presented with headache, fever, convulsion and altered sensorium. These are feature of meningitis. Now, CSF histological shows Cowdry A body which is seen in herpes virus infection. So here diagnosis is HSV infection.

INCLUSION BODIES

It is the most characteristic histological feature in virus infected cells. It is of following types:

A. Intracytoplasmic eosinophilic inclusions:

Negri bodies–rabies

Guarnieri bodies – variola (smallpox), vaccinia

Bollinger bodies – fowlpox

Henderson - Peterson bodies – molluscum contagiosum

B. Intranuclear acidophilic inclusion bodies:

Cowdry type A – Herpes, chickenpox, CMV, yellow fever

Torres bodies – yellow fever

Cowdry type B – polio virus

C. Both nuclear and cytoplasmic:

Warthin Finkeldey – measles

D. Intranuclear basophilic inclusion bodies:

Cowdry type B – adenovirus.

Herpes Simplex Viral Encephalitis

Herpes simplex (HSV) encephalitis is the most common cause of fatal sporadic fulminant necrotizing viral encephalitis. It is important to suspect this condition as it is potentially treatable. Although there are no clinical features that are pathognomonic for HSVE, predilection of the virus for temporal and orbitofrontal lobes results in characteristic clinical picture that should alert the clinician to the condition. A 1 to 4-day history of gradually increasing headache and fever is followed by alteration of consciousness, memory loss, personality changes, confusion, disorientation and olfactory hallucinations. Focal neurologic signs such as hemiparesis, aphasia, focal or generalised seizures and signs of meningeal irritation may also be present.

Epidemiology

Childhood and adult herpes encephalitis are usually due to HSV-1 (90%) with the rest due to HSV-2 .

Clinical Presentation

The presentation is unfortunately relatively non-specific consisting of fever, headaches, focal neurological deficits, seizures, and altered or decreased level of consciousness.

Diagnosis is established with PCR of CSF, although the combination of the clinical scenario, CSF demonstrating pleocytosis and elevated protein, and appropriate imaging is usually highly suggestive and permits commencement of treatment.

Pathology

HSV is an obligatory intracellular virus that enters via infecting nasopharyngeal cells into the sensory branch of lingual nerve then ascends to trigeminal ganglion and remains latent for a lifetime. Reactivation in the case of immunosuppression, trauma, or other stresses can result in fulminant hemorrhagic necrotizing encephalitis. HSV has a high affinity for limbic systems with bilateral but asymmetric involvement.

Microscopic Appearance

Perivascular cuffs of lymphocytes, large inclusions in neurones and glial cells called "owl's eye", neuronophagia, necrosis and hemorrhage are characteristics of herpes simplex encephalitis.

Cerebrospinal Fluid:

- Clear.
- Increased pressure.
- Protein levels are mildly elevated (70-700 mg/dL; values >800 mg/dL rarely seen).
- Sugar is normal or mildly reduced.
- Cell count is increased (usually 5-500/mm^3) and is lymphocytic. RBSs are common in herpes simplex encephalitis.
- Antibodies to specific virus in increasing titres are seen if serial examinations are done. It is useless for immediate diagnosis. IgM antibodies are important for early diagnosis.
- PCR of CSF is the diagnostic method of choice for viral encephalitis including HSE and therapy should be instituted pending the results of PCR.

Radiographic Features

In the immunocompetent adult patient, the pattern is quite typical and manifests as a bilateral asymmetrical involvement of the limbic system, medial temporal lobes, insular cortices and inferolateral frontal lobes. The basal ganglia are typically spared, helping to distinguish it from a middle cerebral artery infarct.

Extralimbic involvement is more prevalent in children than in adults, seen most commonly in the parietal lobe, with sparing of basal ganglia. Eventually, it results in marked cystic encephalomalacia and volume loss in affected areas.

In immunocompromised patients, involvement can be more diffuse, and more likely to involve the brainstem.

11. A 52 years old female patient presented with headache while eating. What will be the most probable diagnosis from below given options?

A. Subarachnoid hemorrhage

B. Takayasu disease

C. Migrane

D. Giant cell arteritis

Answer: Option D. Giant cell arteritis

Explanation:

Here, a 52 years old female patient presented with headache while eating – jaw claudication which is a common feature of Giant cell arteritis.

Jaw claudication in the muscles of the tongue and jaw, e.g., while chewing, occurs in approximately one-quarter of people with giant cell arteritis. In severe cases, this may lead to numbness or infarction of the scalp or the tongue. It is important to specifically ask patients about jaw claudication, as patients may not connect this with their headache or other symptoms. Pain while chewing and the presence of jaw claudication strongly indicates giant cell arteritis. Distinguishing between jaw pain from other causes (such as temporomandibular joint dysfunction) and true jaw claudication is important – the pain in jaw claudication is a cramping pain occurring after prolonged chewing or talking.

Giant Cell Arteritis

Giant cell arteritis is an immune-mediated, ischaemic condition caused by inflammation in the wall of medium to large arteries. While it can affect all medium to large arteries in the head, neck and upper torso, the involvement of the temporal artery is usually the only artery in which physical changes are clinically apparent (giving rise to the alternative name of temporal arteritis). It is the most common form of vasculitis in adults.

Most significant risk factors for giant cell arteritis are:

- Age > 50 years.
- A previous or current diagnosis of polymyalgia rheumatica.
- Female gender.
- This is a disease of the elderly, occurring almost exclusively in people over the age of 55 years. It is closely associated with polymyalgia rheumatica.
- Arteritis can occur in any large and medium artery although it has a predilection for the extracranial carotid artery and its branches such as the superficial temporal, occipital, ophthalmic, posterior ciliary arteries and vertebral arteries.
- The disease is characterised by the classic complex of fever, anaemia, high ESR and headache (usually temporal) in an elderly patient.
- The temporal artery may become tender, thickened and cordlike or nodular.
- Scalp pain, claudication of tongue and jaw are frequent.
- Visual symptoms including diplopia and even sudden blindness may result from ischaemic optic neuritis. The contralateral eye is often affected within one to two weeks making prompt recognition and treatment critical.
- Involvement can extend to the aorta, its primary and secondary branches including subclavian and axillary arteries, which leads to upper extremity ischaemia, absent or asymmetrical pulses and blood pressure readings.
- Neurological manifestations occur in about 30% of patients and include mononeuropathies, peripheral polyneuropathies of upper or lower extremities, and occasionally, transient ischaemic attacks and strokes.
- Thoracic aortic aneurysm or dissection is typically a late complication.
- The diagnosis is confirmed by biopsy of the temporal artery.
- Duplex ultrasonography can detect the characteristic appearance of a hypoechoic "halo", occlusions and stenosis of temporal artery.
- This condition is exquisitely sensitive to corticosteroid

therapy. Prednisolone is given at a dose of 40-60 mg/day. Dramatic response to a trial of prednisolone can confirm the diagnosis other than a temporal artery biopsy.

12. Which of the following is the most common presentation in a patient with myasthenia gravis?

A. Upper limb paralysis B. Ptosis

C. Lower limb paralysis D. Dysarthria

Answer: Option B. Ptosis

Explanation:

In about two-thirds of individuals, the initial symptom of MG is related to the muscles around the eye. There may be **eyelid drooping (ptosis due to weakness of levator palpebrae superioris)** and double vision (diplopia, due to weakness of the extraocular muscles).

- Myasthenia gravis (MG) is an autoimmune disorder where antibodies are produced against acetylcholine receptors located at motor end plates in myoneural junctions.
- Antibodies are produced by B lymphocytes that are defectively regulated by T lymphocytes. T lymphocyte tolerance to self-antigens is established in the thymus, but in MG this tolerance is lost those results in production of autoantibodies against acetylcholine receptors.
- Thymic hyperplasia is observed in about 65% of MG patients, and thymomas are present in about 10% of MG patients.

Signs and Symptoms

The initial, main symptom in MG is painless weakness of specific muscles, not fatigue. The muscle weakness becomes progressively worse during periods of physical activity and improves after periods of rest. Typically, the weakness and fatigue are worse toward the end of the day. MG generally starts with ocular (eye) weakness; it might then progress to a more severe generalized form, characterized by weakness in the extremities or in muscles that govern basic life functions.

Eyes

In about two-thirds of individuals, the initial symptom of MG is related to the muscles around the eye. There may be eyelid drooping (ptosis due to weakness of levator palpebrae superioris) and double vision (diplopia, due to weakness of the extraocular muscles). Eye symptoms tend to get worse when watching television, reading, or driving, particularly in bright conditions. Consequently, some affected individuals choose to wear sunglasses. The term "ocular myasthenia gravis" describes a subtype of MG where muscle weakness is confined to the eyes, i.e., extraocular muscles, levator palpebrae superioris, and orbicularis oculi. Typically, this subtype evolves into generalized MG, usually after a few years.

Eating

The weakness of the muscles involved in swallowing may lead to swallowing difficulty (dysphagia). Typically, this means that some food may be left in the mouth after an attempt to swallow, or food and liquids may regurgitate into the nose rather than go down the throat (velopharyngeal insufficiency). Weakness of the muscles that move the jaw (muscles of mastication) may cause difficulty chewing. In individuals with MG, chewing tends to become more tiring when chewing tough, fibrous foods. Difficulty in swallowing, chewing, and speaking is the first symptom in about one-sixth of individuals.

Speaking

Weakness of the muscles involved in speaking may lead to dysarthria and hypophonia. Speech may be slow and slurred, or have a nasal quality. In some cases, a singing hobby or profession must be abandoned.

Head and Neck

Due to weakness of the muscles of facial expression and muscles of mastication, facial weakness may manifest as the inability to hold the mouth closed (the "hanging jaw sign") and as a snarling expression when attempting to smile. With drooping eyelids, facial weakness may make the individual appear sleepy or sad. Difficulty in holding the head upright may occur.

Other

The muscles that control breathing (dyspnea) and limb movements can also be affected; rarely do these present as the first symptoms of MG, but develop over months to years. In a myasthenic crisis, a paralysis of the respiratory muscles occurs, necessitating assisted ventilation to sustain life. Crises may be triggered by various biological stressors such as infection, fever, an adverse reaction to medication, or emotional stress.

INVESTIGATIONS

Tensilon Test (Edrophonium Test)

- Edrophonium is a rapidly acting acetylcholinesterase inhibitor. It has a short duration of action and reverses the muscular weakness dramatically in myasthenia. In adults, a 2 mg injection is given as a test dose (to check for tolerance) followed by another 8 mg that results in dramatic improvement in ptosis, diplopia, nasal voice, etc. within 30 seconds and persists up to 1-2 minutes. Positive test is highly suggestive of MG. Borderline or mild improvement may occur in other neuromuscular disorders. Side effects like abdominal cramps can be relieved by atropine.

Others

- Chest radiography and CT scan for thymic enlargement.
- Thyroid function tests (10% may have associated hyperthyroidism).
- Acetylcholine receptor antibody levels (present in >90% patients with generalised myasthenia).
- Anti-muscle-specific protein (tyrosine) kinase (anti-MuSK) antibodies in many patients who are negative for ACh receptor antibodies.
- Patients with MuSK-antibody associated MG are usually younger women who present with predominant facial, bulbar and respiratory weakness, lingual atrophy and relatively mild limb weakness.
- Electrodiagnostic studies (nerve conduction testing, repetitive nerve stimulation, exercise testing and in certain instances single-fibre EMG).
- **Ice test:** In a patient with ptosis a small cube of ice is placed over the eyelid for about 2 minutes. Improvement of the ptosis after this procedure suggests a disorder of neuromuscular transmission.

Management

- Anticholinesterases are effective in providing symptomatic relief. Neostigmine (15 mg) 1-2 tablets, three to six times a day or pyridostigmine 60-120 mg three to six times a day may be used. Dosage is titrated to the need of the patient. Cholinergic systemic side effects like abdominal cramps and increased salivation are managed with propantheline 15 mg 2-3 times a day. Pyridostigmine is generally better tolerated than neostigmine due to fewer gastrointestinal side effects. Excessive dosage of anticholinesterase can result in cholinergic muscular weakness associated with excessive sweating, salivation, lacrimation, diarrhoea and small pupils. It can be differentiated from myasthenic weakness by edrophonium test. Treatment response with anticholinesterases is much less favourable in anti-MuSK MG, with a significantly increased risk of myasthenic crisis.
- Corticosteroids are useful in induction and maintenance of remission. However, in about 15% patients corticosteroids may worsen symptoms transiently during initial periods of treatment and may precipitate myasthenic crisis.
- Thymectomy can induce remission when the disease is generalised and has not been chronic. It is also recommended in patients with thymoma. Thymectomy may or may not reduce requirement of steroids.
- Immunosuppression with azathioprine, cyclophosphamide, cyclosporine, tacrolimus or mycophenolate mofetil is recommended when the dosage of steroid requirement is too high to maintain remission. Rituximab has also been used in refractory cases.
- Plasma exchange and intravenous irnmunoglobulin are useful for inducing a short-term remission like prior to surgery or during myasthenic crisis.

13. A 67 years old patient is presented with dyspnea. His PFT reveals elevated FEV_1/FVC. What is the diagnostic pattern he had?

A. Asthma
B Restrictive disease
C. Obstructive pattern
D. Mixed pattern

Answer: Option B. Restrictive disease

Explanation:

Restrictive lung disease (reduced FVC, reduced FEV_1, normal or elevated FEV_1: FVC ratio, reduced total lung capacity and reduced diffusion capacity).

Restrictive lung diseases can be due to poor breathing mechanics, as a result of conditions like myasthenia gravis, obesity, and scoliosis. They may also be caused by interstitial lung disease. In restrictive lung disease, the lung volume decreases and the FEV_1/FVC ratio is normal to increased (greater than 80%).

Categories of Disease			
	Obstructive	**Mixed**	**Restrictive**
FEV_1/FVC	↓ 70%	↓ 70-79%	Normal or ↑
FEV_1	↓ (marked)	↓	Normal or ↓ (slight)
FVC	Normal or ↓	↓	↓
PEFR	↓	↓	N or ↑ with linear decrease in flow versus lung volume
MVV	↓	↓	Normal or ↓
TLC	Normal or ↑	↓	↓

Restrictive Diseases (PAINT)

- Pleural disease
- Alveolar
- Interstitial lung diseases
- Neuromuscular diseases, Diaphragmatic paralysis, Myasthenia gravis, Guillain-Barré syndrome, Muscular dystrophies, Cervical spine injury.
- Thoracic cage abnormalities, Kyphoscoliosis, Obesity, Ankylosing spondylitis.

Obstructive Diseases

- Bronchial asthma
- Chronic obstructive lung disease
- Bronchiectasis
- Cystic fibrosis
- Bronchiolitis.

14. Which of the following is a drug of choice in a patient with ventricular tachycardia with myocardial infarction?

A. Dopamine

B. Lignocaine

C. Digoxin

D. Dobutamine

Answer: Option B. Lignocaine

Explanation:

Drug of choice for sustained ventricular tachycardia after myocardial infarction is lignocaine.

Cardiac arrhythmias and conduction disturbances are commonly observed in patients with myocardial infarction. The available data suggest the administration of lidocaine, either through a large intramuscular dose (300 mg), which is particularly suited for outpatient situations, or through intravenous loading doses followed by a constant lidocaine infusion. **Routine prophylaxis is not recommended.**

- Patients with ventricular arrhythmia should be treated with direct-current countershock if hemodynamic deterioration is present. Drug therapy for patients with ventricular arrhythmias who are resistant to lidocaine include procainamide, bretylium, or intravenous amiodarone (experimental drug).
- Ventricular arrhythmias who are resistant to shock should be treated with amiodarone followed by repeat cardioversion.

15. Which of the following is treatment of choice in a patient with given ECG image with hypotension?

A. Bupivacaine

B. DC cardioversion

C. Amiodarone

D. Lignocaine

Answer: Option B. DC cardioversion

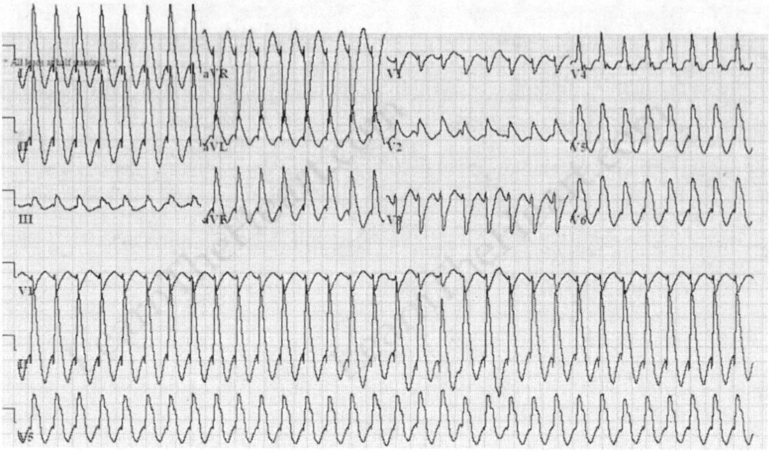

Explanation:

Above ECG image is showing ventricular tachycardia and patient is present with hypotension with these ECG changes that suggest patient is hemodynamically unstable.

If the patient is haemodynamically unstable in the form of hypotension, angina, heart failure or altered sensorium, immediate cardioversion in synchronised mode is required as a treatment.

Ventricular Tachycardia

It is a wide complex tachycardia (rate >100/minute) with regular rate and single QRS morphology. Non-sustained ventricular tachycardia (VT) is a series of repetitive ventricular beats that have a duration of less than 30 seconds; sustained VT lasts for more than 30 seconds.

Causes

- It usually occurs in the presence of some underlying heart disease and is rarely seen in normal hearts.

Clinical Features

- The patient may be asymptomatic or may present with palpitations or haemodynamic collapse.
- The assumption that a haemodynamically stable patient cannot have VT is erroneous.

Electrocardiogram

- The width of the QRS complex is generally >0.16 second.
- Positive or negative concordance of the QRS complex across the pre-cordial leads (e.g. R waves or S waves only).
- A monophasic "Rr" pattern in lead V_1 (termed rabbit ears) with a taller left ear.
- An indeterminate axis (between -90° and -180°).
- In severe underlying heart disease the QRS morphology may be variable (polymorphic VT). The basal QT interval before onset of polymorphic VT is normal as compared to torsade de pointes.

Treatment

- If the patient is haemodynamically unstable in the form of hypotension, angina, heart failure or altered sensorium, immediate cardioversion in synchronised mode is required. If the patient is stable, amiodarone and lidocaine are the drugs of choice.
- Amiodarone 150 mg intravenously over 10 minutes, then 1 mg/minute for 6 hours and then 0.5 mg/minute for next 18 hours. Lidocaine 1-1.5 mg/kg IV over 1 minute followed by infusion at 10-40 μg/kg/minute. A repeat bolus of 50 mg may be required during the first 30 minutes to avoid sub-therapeutic blood levels.
- Lidocaine is safe if given by slow I.V. injection; is used to suppress VT and prevent VF. It is ineffective in atrial arrhythmias. Because of rapidly developing and titratable action it is a good drug in the emergency setting, e.g., arrhythmias following acute MI or during cardiac surgery. In acute MI, I.V. infusion of lidocaine can prevent VF, but a metaanalysis has shown that it fails to improve survival; may even increase short term mortality. Therefore, lidocaine is no longer administered prophylactically to all MI patients, but may be used in selected cases, and to treat ventricular arrhythmias when they occur.
- Efficacy of lidocaine in chronic ventricular arrhythmia is poor, but it suppresses VT due to digitalis toxicity, for which it is used because it does not worsen A-V block.

16. Which of the following is treatment of choice in a patient with given ECG image ?

A. DC cardioversion B. Lignocaine

C. Digoxin D. Adenosine

Answer: Option D. Adenosine

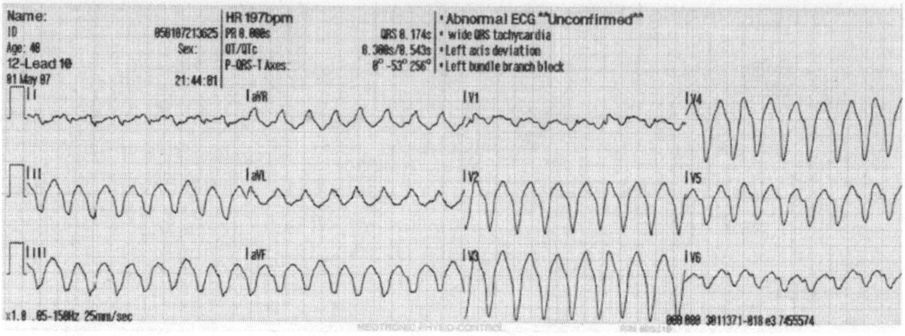

Explanation:

Treatment of PSVT (*Harrison, page 4336, 20th edition*)

Carotid sinus massage is reasonable provided the risk of carotid vascular disease is low, as indicated by absence of carotid bruits and no prior history of stroke. A Valsalva maneuver should be attempted in cooperative individuals, and if effective, the patient can be taught to perform this maneuver as needed. If vagal maneuvers fail or cannot be performed, **intravenous adenosine will terminate the vast majority of PSVT episodes by transiently blocking conduction in the AV node**. Adenosine may produce transient chest pain, dyspnea and anxiety. It is contraindicated in patients with prior cardiac transplantation due to potential hypersensitivity. It can theoretically aggravate bronchospasm. Adenosine precipitates AF, which is usually brief, in up to 15% of patients, so it should be used cautiously in patients with WPW syndrome in whom AF may produce hemodynamic instability. Intravenous beta blockers and calcium channel blockers (verapamil or diltiazem) are also effective but may cause hypotension before and after arrhythmia termination and have a longer duration of action.

PSVT

It is usually paroxysmal and recurrent, and has a rate of 140-220 beats/minute with 1 : 1 conduction.

It usually results from re-entry of an atrial ectopic in the AV node (AV nodal re-entry tachycardia–AVNRT). PSVT can also result from re-entry in the accessory pathways [AV re-entry tachycardia (AVRT)]. Occasionally, it results from increased atrial automaticity.

Usually, AVRT is orthodromic with activation transmitted from atria to ventricles via the AV node and back via the accessory pathway ("orthodromic" because the AV node is conducting in the "correct direction"). Less commonly, the direction of activation is antidromic that leads to aberrant ventricular activation and broad QRS complexes.

It is often difficult to differentiate AVNRT and AVRT on the basis of ECG.

Causes

- Idiopathic in healthy individuals
- Excessive coffee, tea, alcohol or tobacco
- Anxiety
- Hyperthyroidism
- Organic heart disease (ischaemic, valvular or congenital).

Clinical Features

- The onset and termination of the arrhythmia are sudden.
- Patients most commonly complain of palpitations, an odd feeling in the chest and on occasion, light headedness or syncope.
- Those with significant heart disease may have additional symptoms during the arrhythmia such as dyspnoea and chest pain.
- Some patients have polyuria and experience diuresis during or after PSVT.

Electrocardiogram

- The P wave is usually buried in the QRS complex or occurs slightly before or after the QRS complex.
- The QRS complexes occur at regular intervals (there is constant RR cycle length) and are similar to those seen during sinus rhythm since activation of the ventricular myocardium is unaltered and is via the His-Purkinje system.
- Significant ST segment depression during tachycardia has been observed in 25-50% of patients. Majority of these patients do not have underlying coronary artery disease.

Treatment

Vagal manoeuvres like carotid sinus massage, Valsalva manoeuvre and gag reflex are useful. These manoeuvres delay conduction in AV node in a patient with circuit tachycardia. If vagal manoeuvres are unsuccessful, drug therapy is warranted.

Adenosine is administered as an initial bolus of 6 mg rapidly over 1-3 seconds followed immediately by 20 mL of saline. If required, a second and third dose of 12 mg is repeated in 1-2 minutes. Synchronised cardioversion is performed if patient is haemodynamically compromised. Long-term control can be achieved by radiofrequency ablation of the re-entrant pathway.

Other drugs include propranolol, esmolol, verapamil, diltiazem and adenosine. They prolong the AV refractory period.

17. Which of the following is an endogenous pyrogen?

A. IL-1 B. IL-2

C. IL-4 D. Bacterial toxin

Answer: Option A. IL-1

Explanation:

Pyrogene

Pyrogene are substances that cause fever.

Pyrogens may be exogenous or endogenous

Exogenous → **Bacterial toxins**

Endogenous → **IL-1β, TNF-α, IL-6, Interferons, Ciliary neurotrophic factor.**

These pyrogene affects the thermoreceptor in the hypothalamus that elevates the thermoregulatory set point and causes fever.

18. Which of the following is true about Brown Sequard syndrome?

A. C/L loss of joint sense and position

B. I/L loss of complete sensory functions

C. There is loss of kinesthesia on same side

D. C/L motor functions

Answer: Option C. There is loss of kinesthesia on same side

Explanation:

In Brown Sequard syndrome, there is loss of kinesthesia (awareness of the position and movement of the parts of the body by means of sensory organs–proprioceptors in the muscles and joints) on ipsilateral side.

Brown Sequard Syndrome

- **If the spinal cord is completely transected** – All the sensations and motor functions distal to segment of transection are blocked.
- **Transection of spinal cord on single side results in "Brown Sequard Syndrome".**
- **Functions affected:**

Ipsilateral side	Contralateral side
• **Loss of dorsal column sensations** • *Complete loss of motor functions below the level of transection*	**Loss of anterior and lateral spinothalamic pathway**
Vibration, fine touch, proprioception and joint position	*Loss observed 2 to 6 segments below the level of transection* **Pain, Pressure Crude touch, Temperature**

19. Which of the following heart chamber enlargement causes oesophageal displacement?

A. Right ventricle
B. Left ventricle
C. Right atrium
D. Left atrium

Answer: Option D. Left atrium

Explanation:

Left atrial enlargement causes posterior displacement of a barium-filled esophagus on chest X-ray.

Left atrial enlargement may result from many conditions, either congenital or acquired. It has some characteristic findings on a frontal chest radiograph. CT or MRI may also be used for diagnosis.

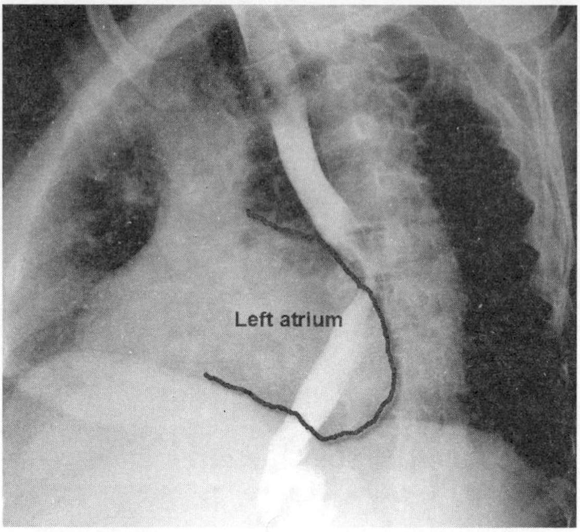

Clinical Presentation

An enlarged left atrium can have many clinical implications, such as:

- **Ortner syndrome:** Left recurrent laryngeal nerve palsy secondary to compression from enlarged left atrium.
- **Dysphagia megalatriensis:** Compression of esophagus between the enlarged left atrium and vertebral bodies.
- **Atrial fibrillation:** Via a multiple wavelet mechanism.
- **Thromboembolic events (e.g., ischemic stroke):** Due to stasis of blood in the enlarged left atrium (especially the left atrial appendage) and/or atrial fibrillation.

Pathology

Broadly speaking, the causes of left atrial enlargement can be divided into congenital and acquired causes:

- Acquired
  - Mitral stenosis
  - Mitral regurgitation
  - Left ventricular failure
  - Left atrial myxoma
  - Atrial fibrillation
    - ◊ It is uncertain if this is a cause or only a consequence

- Congenital
  - Ventricular septal defect (VSD)
  - Patent ductus arteriosus (PDA)

The common mechanism is increased atrial wall tension due to increased filling pressures, which eventually leads to atrial enlargement.

There are associations between left atrial enlargement and atrial fibrillation, stroke, and mortality after myocardial infarction. With a reduced incidence of mitral valve disease from rheumatic fever, the incidence of left atrial enlargement has also decreased.

Radiographic Features

Cardiac chamber enlargement is best assessed volumetrically with echocardiography and more recently (but less widespread) with CT and MRI. Chest X-rays, however, are so frequently obtained, and formed the mainstay of chest imaging for decades, that a great deal has been written about the various appearances of chamber enlargement. It is, therefore, essential to be familiar with normal cardiomediastinal outlines.

Plain Radiograph

As the left atrium enlarges, it may become directly visible, or displace adjacent structures.

Direct visualization of the enlarged atrium includes:

- Double density sign
  - When the right side of the left atrium pushes into the adjacent lung, and becomes visible superimposed or even beyond the normal right heart border (known as atrial escape).
  - A similar appearance can be caused by the right superior pulmonary vein in patients without atrial enlargement.
- Oblique measurement of greater than 7 cm
  - Measured from midpoint of left main bronchus to the right border of the left atrium (this requires a double density sign of course).

- Thought to be the most reliable sign on chest radiography.

- Convex left atrial appendage (third mogul sign): Normally the left heart border just below the pulmonary outflow track should be flat or slightly concave.

Indirect signs include:

- Splaying of the carina, with the increase of the tracheal bifurcation angle to over 90 degrees
  - This refers to both the interbronchial angle (i.e., angle formed by the central axis of the left and right main bronchi) and the subcarinal angle.
  - Both are inaccurate and dependent on radiographer technique, inspiration and body habitus.
  - The mean and range of both measurements vary widely in normal individuals
    - ◊ Interbronchial angle: Normal mean 67-77° (range 34-109°).
    - ◊ Subcarinal angle: Normal mean 62-73° (range 34-90°).
- Posterior displacement of the left mainstem bronchus on the lateral radiograph
  - Right and left bronchi, therefore, do not overlap, but rather form an upside down “V”, sometimes referred to as the walking man sign.
- Superior displacement of the left mainstem bronchus on frontal view.
- Posterior displacement of a barium-filled esophagus or nasogastric tube.

20. What is the most effective mode of prevention in case of nosocomial infection with MRSA?

A. Prophylactic antibiotic

B. Prophylactic immunoglobulin

C. Hand washing

D. Rom and clothes disinfection

Answer: Option C. Hand washing

Explanation:

- Most common mode of spread of S. aureus infection is via hands of health care workers.
- S. aureus is most common cause of surgical wound infection and can cross infect wound of other patient.
- **Most effective mode of prevention of nosocomial S. aureus infection is hand washing.**

21. Which of the following is not correct about Duke's major criteria?

A. Two positive culture for HACEK

B. One positive culture for streptococcus viridans

C. Two positive culture for staphylococcus

D. One positive culture for Coxiella burnetii

Answer: Option B. One positive culture for streptococcus viridans.

Explanation:

Duke's major criteria include **two positive** cultures for **streptococcus viridans.**

Modified Duke Criteria for Infective Endocarditis

Has a mean sensitivity of 80% for diagnosing infective endocarditis.

MAJOR CRITERIA

1. **Blood Cultures Positive**

   Typical microorganisms consistent with infective endocarditis from **two blood cultures**:

   Viridans streptococci, Streptococcus bovis, **HACEK group** (Haemophilus, Actinobacillus, Cardiobacterium, Eikenella, Kingella), or Community-acquired **Staphylococcus aureus** or enterococci in the absence of a primary focus.

   OR

   Other microorganisms consistent with IE from persistently positive blood cultures defined as: Two positive cultures of blood samples drawn >12 hours apart, or All of three or a majority of four separate cultures of blood (with first and last sample drawn 1 hour apart).

OR

Single positive blood culture for Coxiella burnetii or positive serology for Q fever, Bartonella species and Chlamydia psittaci or phase I IgG antibody titer of >1:800.

2. **Evidence of endocardial involvement**

   Echocardiogram positive for IE:

   Oscillating intracardiac mass without alternative explanation, or Abscess, or New partial dehiscence of prosthetic valve, or New valvular regurgitation (worsening or changing of preexisting murmur not sufficient).

Minor Criteria

- Predisposition to infective endocarditis: Predisposing heart condition, injection drug use, previous infective endocarditis, or prosthetic valve or material.
- Fever, temperature >38°C.
- Vascular phenomena: Major arterial emboli, septic pulmonary infarcts, mycotic aneurysm, intracranial haemorrhages, subconjunctival petechiae, Janeway lesions.
- Immunologic phenomena: Glomerulonephritis, Osler's nodes, Roth's spots, positive rheumatoid factor.
- Microbiological evidence: Positive blood culture but does not meet a major criterion or serological evidence of active infection with organisms consistent with infective endocarditis.
- Pathological criteria.
- Positive microbiology or histology of pathologic tissue material attained at surgery or autopsy (vegetations, valve tissue, embolic fragments or tissue/pus from intracardiac abscesses).

Diagnosis of IE is definite in the presence of:

- Pathological criteria, or
- Two major criteria, or
- One major and two minor criteria, or
- Five minor criteria.

Diagnosis of IE is possible in the presence of one major and one minor criteria, or three minor criteria.

22. A 56 years old female presented with signs of meningitis. Her smear shows presence of gram positive diplococci. Which of the following is the diagnosis?

A. Staphylococcus

B. H. Influenza

C. Pneumococcus

D. Neisseria meningitis

Answer: Option C. Pneumococcus

Explanation:

Here, 56 years old female presented with signs of meningitis. Her smear shows presence of gram positive diplococcic–pneumococcus are gram positive diplococcic which is the most common cause of meningitis in adult.

PNEUMOCOCCUS

- Gram positive Lanceolate diplococci.
- It is most common cause of Lobar pneumonia, sinusitis, otitis media.
- It is most common cause of bacterial meningitis in adults.
- **Capsulated, lanceolate, diplococcic, bile soluble, optochin sensitive, possess specific polysaccharide capsule and shows quelling reaction.**
- Type 3 pneumococci has abundant capsular material, so more virulent.
- Austrain syndrome: Concurrence of pneumococcal pneumonia, endocarditis and meningitis. Diagnosis.

MENINGITIS

Introduction

Acute bacterial meningitis is an inflammation of the leptomeninges (arachnoid and pia), and fluid residing in the space that it encloses and also that in the ventricles of the brain. As the subarachnoid space is continuous around the brain, the spinal cord and the optic nerves, an infective agent gaining entry to any part of it may extend immediately to all of it, even its most remote recesses. Therefore, meningitis is always cerebrospinal. It also reaches the ventricles, either directly or by reflux through the basal foramens of Magendie and Luschka.

Meningitis may be acute meningitis (with onset over hours to days) or chronic meningitis (syndrome persisting more than 4 weeks). Partially treated pyogenic meningitis may present with chronic meningitis.

Inflammation of the meninges sometimes extends into the parenchyma with resultant symptoms and signs of cerebral or spinal cord involvement, often termed meningoencephalitis or meningoencephalomyelitis.

PREDISPOSING FACTORS

Pneumococcal Meningitis

Acute otitis media

Mastoiditis

Pneumonia

Diabetes mellitus

Recent head injury

Sickle-cell disease

Hodgkin's lymphoma

Multiple myeloma

Immunoglobulin deficiency

Splenectomy

Renal transplantation

Bone marrow transplantation

Pathogenesis

All three important organisms are normal inhabitants of nasopharynx. Antecedent viral infections of the upper respiratory tract or lungs predispose the colonised patient to bloodstream invasion, which is the usual route by which bacteria reach the meninges. Once blood-borne, pneumococcus, meningococcus and H. influenzae have a predilection for meninges. Transnasal spread through cribriform plate to subarachnoid space may be important.

Disruption of blood-CSF barrier by trauma, circulating endotoxin or an initial viral infection of the meninges also facilitates the entry of bacteria into subarachnoid space.

Clinical Features

Fever, headache and vomiting are the cardinal features. Seizures, impairment of consciousness, photophobia, stiff neck and stiff back.

Three patterns of onset are documented:

- Fulminant onset-patient becomes seriously ill within 24 hours, without antecedent respiratory tract infections (25%).
- Meningitis developing over 1-7 days and associated with respiratory symptoms (50%).
- Meningeal symptoms after 1-3 weeks of respiratory symptoms (20%).

In elderly, immunocompromised and debilitated patients, the classic signs of meningitis may be minimal, where low-grade fever and changes in mental status may occur without headache or neck rigidity.

Meningococcal meningitis usually occurs as outbreaks. The evolution is extremely rapid and the onset is attended by petechial or purpuric skin eruptions, large ecchymoses and lividity of the skin of the lower parts of the body. Circulatory collapse may occur.

Pneumococcal meningitis is usually preceded by an infection in the lung, ear or sinuses. Heart valves may be affected.

H. influenzae meningitis follows upper respiratory tract infections and ear infections in young.

Signs of Meningeal Irritation

Neck stiffness (neck rigidity).

Kernig's sign.

Brudzinski's neck sign.

Brudzinski's leg sign.

Investigations

- Increased total leucocytes, polymorphonuclear leucocytosis and raised ESR.
- Cerebrospinal fluid studies shown in the box.
- Appearance is turbid.

- Pressure is elevated above 180 mm H20.
- Cell count is raised, ranging from 5000 to 20,000/ml, neutrophil leucocytes predominate. Protein level is elevated (more than 45 mg/dl).
- Sugar level is decreased (less than 40 mg/dl or less than 40% of blood sugar).
- Gram's stain of the sediment of CSF may show meningococci as Gram-negative, kidney-shaped, intracellular diplococci (inside neutrophils), and pneumococci as Gram-positive diplococci.
- Culture of CSF grows the pathogen in 70-80% of cases.
- Measurement of bacterial antigen in the CSF (Latex agglutination test).
- Limulus amoebocyte lysate assay detects Gram-negative endotoxin in CSF and is highly sensitive.

23. Which of the following best test, used for diagnosis of neurosyphilis?

A. TPHA
B. RPR
C. VDRL test
D. EIA

Answer: Option C. VDRL test

Explanation:

The gold standard for diagnosis of neurosyphilis is **VDRL from CSF**, which is highly specific but only 30-70% sensitive for neurosyphilis. CSF FIA-ABS is more sensitive but not specific because false positives are common.

The organism (Treponema pallidum) invades nervous system within 3-18 months after primary infection. Initial event is asymptomatic meningitis. This may remain so and cause more damage later on. All forms of neurosyphilis have meningitis as a component, in variable severity. Vascular changes occur secondary to meningitis as endarteritis obliterans.

Asymptomatic Neurosyphilis

- Asymptomatic invasion of CNS by Treponema is common within a few months of primary infection.
- Diagnosis is made by demonstrating CSF lymphocytosis with elevated protein and positive VDRL test.

- This is found in nearly 25% of cases with late latent form of syphilis. Many of these patients may go onto develop **symptomatic neurosyphilis**.
- These patients should be treated with penicillin.

Symptomatic Neurosyphilis

Although mixed features are common, the major categories are:

- Meningeal syphilis.
- Meningovascular syphilis.
- Parenchymatous syphilis that includes general paralysis of insane and tabes dorsalis.

Meningeal Syphilis

- Symptoms of meningitis may occur at any time after infection, but appears usually within 2 years.
- Symptoms consist of headache, stiff neck, cranial nerve palsies, convulsions and mental confusion.
- Papilloedema with symptoms of increased ICP may occur.
- Patient is afebrile. CSF is abnormal.
- May have skin rash on palms and soles.

Meningovascular Syphilis

- Presents usually 6-7 years after initial infection, but can be as early as 6 months to as late as 10-12 years.
- Should be suspected whenever a young patient presents with stroke resulting in hemiparesis, aphasia, visual loss, etc.

  Features of stroke are generally subacute in nature. Other features are headache, vertigo, insomnia and psychological abnormalities.

CSF Findings

- Pressure may be normal or raised.
- Fluid is clear.
- Protein is elevated (100-200 mg%).
- Sugar is normal.
- Cell count is mildly elevated and is lymphocytic.

- Gamma globulin levels are elevated.
- VDRL and FTA-ABS (fluorescent treponemal antibody absorption) are positive.

Investigation of Choice

- For primary syphilis–DGM (Dark Ground Microscopy).
- For secondary syphilis–all are equal.
- For Latent syphilis–EIA >TPPA.
- For tertiary–TPPA.
- For neurosyphilis–VDRL.

24. Which of the following is a true mechanism of action of tetanus toxin?

A. Presynaptically blocks release of glycine and GABA in cerebral cortex

B. Postsynaptically blocks release of glycine and GABA in cerebral cortex

C. Presynaptically blocks release of glycine and GABA in brainstem and spinal cord

D. Postsynaptically blocks release of glycine and GABA in brainstem and spinal cord

Answer: Option C. Presynaptically blocks release of glycine and GABA in brainstem and spinal cord

Explanation:

Tetanus toxin presynaptically blocks release of glycine and GABA in brainstem and spinal cord.

TETANUS TOXIN

Tetanolysin

- O_2 labile hemolysin
- No role in tetanus

Tetanospasmin

- O_2 stable, plasma coded, single chain zinc-metalloprotease
- Release in wound with low redox potential, devitalised tissue.

Heavy chain

Mediates binding and entry of light chain into nerve cells

↓ Cleavage Light chain

(Active moiety)

↓

Binds to motor neuron

↓

Enters axon

↓

Transported to nerve cell body in the **brainstem and spinal cord** by retrograde intraneural transport (do not cross BBB)

↓

Blocks cleavage of synaptobrevin (a protein essential for function of synaptic apparatus)

↓

Presynaptically blocks release of glycine and GABA (strychinine acts post synaptically)

Tetanus toxin is intraaxonally transported to motor nuclei of the cranial nerves or ventral horns of the spinal cord. This toxin is produced as a single 150-kDa protein that is cleaved to produce heavy (100-kDa) and light (50-kDa) chains linked by a disulfide bond and noncovalent forces. The carboxy terminal of the heavy chain binds to specific membrane components in presynaptic α-motor nerve terminals; evidence suggests binding to both polysialogangliosides and membrane proteins. This binding results in toxin internalization and uptake into the nerves. Once inside the neuron, the toxin enters a retrograde transport pathway, whereby it is carried proximally to the motor neuron body in what appears to be a highly specific process. Unlike other components of the endosomal contents, which undergo acidification following internalization, tetanus toxin is transported in a carefully regulated pH-neutral environment that prevents an acid-induced conformational change that would result in light-chain expulsion into the surrounding cytosol.

The next stage in toxin traicking is less clearly understood but involves tetanus toxin's escaping normal lysosomal degradation processes and undergoing translocation across the synapse to the GABA-ergic presynaptic inhibitory interneuron terminals. Here the light chain, which is a zinc-dependent endopeptidase, cleaves vesicle-associated membrane protein 2 (VAMP2, also known as synaptobrevin). This molecule is necessary for presynaptic binding and release of neurotransmitter; thus tetanus toxin prevents transmitter release and effectively blocks inhibitory interneuron discharge. The result is unregulated activity in the motor nervous system. Similar activity in the autonomic system accounts for the characteristic features of skeletal muscle spasm and autonomic system disturbance. The increased circulating catecholamine levels in severe tetanus are associated with cardiovascular complications.

Clinical Manifestations

- Contraindicated tetani has little invasive property.
- Most common from of tetanus is generalized tetanus in which toxins enters the lymphatics and blood stream.
- Median time of onset after injury is 7 days.
- First symptom – increase tone in masseter muscles called as trismus or lock jaw, followed by sequential involvement of nerves of head, trunk and extremities (Descending tetanus) since short nerves are affected earlier. Hands and feet are relatively spared. Sustained contraction of facial muscles results in sinus sardonius.
- Mentation is unimpaired.
- Deep tendon reflex increase.
- Autonomic dysfunction (sympathetic increase), sudden cardiac death may occur.
- Short incubation period = Grave prognosis.
- Neonatal tetanus usually occurs as generalized form.
- In local tetanus, only the nerves supplying the affected muscles are involved. Remember: Tetanus patients are not infectious and there is no person to person transmission.

25. Which of the following is a most common mechanism of ventricular aneurysm following Myocardial infarction?

A. Anterior wall transmural

B. Inferior wall transmural

C. Posterior wall transmural

D. Subendocardial

Answer: Option A. Anterior wall transmural

Explanation:

A Left Ventricular Aneurysm (LVA) is most commonly the result of MI, usually involving the anterior wall. Other causes of LVA include hypertrophic cardiomyopathy and Chagas disease, both of which can lead to the formation of an apical aneurysm.

True LVA is defined as a well delineated, thin, scarred, or fibrotic wall, devoid of muscle or containing necrotic muscle, that is a result of **a healed transmural myocardial infarction (MI).** The involved wall segment is either akinetic (without movement) or dyskinetic (with paradoxical ballooning) during systole, and collapses inward when the ventricle is fully vented during surgery. Aneurysms of the apex and anterior wall are more than four times as common as those of the inferior or inferoposterior walls.

Massive anterior infarction complicated by a dyskinetic left ventricular LV aneurysm.

Left Ventricular Aneurysm

The term *ventricular aneurysm* is usually used to describe *dyskinesis* or local expansile paradoxical wall motion. Normally functioning myocardial fibers must shorten more if stroke volume and cardiac output are to be maintained in patients with ventricular aneurysm; if they cannot, overall ventricular function is impaired. True aneurysms are composed of scar tissue and neither predispose to nor are associated with cardiac rupture.

The complications of LV aneurysm do not usually occur for weeks to months after STEMI; they include CHF, arterial embolism, and ventricular arrhythmias. Apical aneurysms are the most common and the most easily detected by clinical examination. The physical finding of greatest value is a double, diffuse, or displaced apical impulse. Ventricular aneurysms are readily detected by two-dimensional echocardiography, which may also reveal a mural thrombus in an aneurysm.

Rarely, myocardial rupture may be contained by a local area of pericardium, along with organizing thrombus and hematoma. Over time, this *pseudoaneurysm* enlarges, maintaining communication with the LV cavity through a narrow neck. Because a pseudoaneurysm often ruptures spontaneously, it should be surgically repaired if recognized.

The term ventricular aneurysm applies to a circumscribed, thin-walled, noncontractile outpouching of the ventricle. The vast majority develop in the setting of atherosclerotic occlusive coronary artery disease following a transmural myocardial infarction. Other causes such as Chagas disease, sarcoid, blunt chest trauma, and congenital malformations are distinctly uncommon! These aneurysms may be true aneurysms when a well-delineated fibrous scar develops, which is almost devoid of myocardial tissue and in which the characteristic fine trabecular pattern of the inner surface has been replaced by smooth fibrous tissue. Less commonly, a narrow necked false/ pseudoaneurysm develops following a ruptured heart, in which the resultant hemorrhage is contained circumferentially by fibrous pericardial adhesions and laterally by the pericardium itself. In this circumstance the wall is avascular and is composed of fibrous tissue and pericardium without myocardial elements.

Although inferior and anterior myocardial infarctions occur with almost equal frequency, 85% of true LV aneurysms are located apically and anteroseptally. Only 5-10% are inferoposterior, near the base of the heart, or involve the lateral wall. This predilection for the apical site may be explained by the fact that there are only three layers of muscle at the apex compared with four layers at the base. When extensive inferior infarction large enough to cause an aneurysm does occur, the additional complications of mitral regurgitation, right ventricular infarction, and heart block may limit survival and, therefore, subsequent aneurysm formation. In addition, the inferior wall tends to have a dual blood supply from the right and left circumflex coronary arteries and, as such, is better collateralized. Pseudoaneurysms tend to involve the posterior or diaphragmatic surface more commonly than the apical or lateral wall. Most LV aneurysms result from an occluded or markedly stenosed left anterior descending coronary (LAD) artery without an adequate collateral blood supply. It is speculated that these collaterals tend to increase the number and size of viable myocardial cell islands within the area of infarction, reducing the probability of infarct expansion and subsequent thin walled scar formation.

26. Which of the following infection is strict requirement for Isolation?

A. Rubella

B. Pneumococcal meningitis

C. Influenza

D. Leprosy

Answer: Option C. Influenza

Explanation:

Droplet precautions/isolation should be implemented for patients with suspected or confirmed influenza for 7 days after illness onset or until 24 hours after the resolution of fever and respiratory symptoms, whichever is longer, while a patient is in a healthcare facility.

Isolation period of various other diseases

Disease	Isolation period
Chickenpox	6 days after onset of rash
Measles	Onset of catarrhal to 3rd day of rash
German Measles	NONE (except Ist trimester of pregnancy)
Cholera, Diphtheria	3 days after tetracyclines started till 48 hours of antibiotics
Shigellosis, Salmonellosis	Until 3 consecutive negative stool cultures
Hepatitis A	3 weeks
Polio	2 weeks adult, 6 weeks paediatric
Tuberculosis	Until 3 weeks of effective chemotherapy
Herpes Zoster	6 days after onset of rash
Mumps	Until swelling subsides
Pertussis	4 weeks or until paroxysms cease
Meningococcal meningitis	Until first 6 hours antibiotics completed
Streptococcal pharyngitis	Until first 6 hours antibiotics completed

Isolation is the separation for the period of communicability, of infected persons from others in such places/conditions as to prevent/limit transmission to those susceptible–It applies to persons who are known to be ill with a contagious disease.

Solation: Separation for the period of communicability of persons/animals from others to prevent disease transmission.

INFLUENZA

- **Incubation period:** 2–3 days.
- **Clinical Features:**
  - *Uncomplicated influenza:* Influenza like illness (Fever, cough, sore throat, rhinorrhoea, headache, muscle pain), GIT illness (diarrhoea WITHOUT dehydration).
  - *Complicated/severe influenza:* Pneumonia, CNS involvement, Severe diarrhoea, Secondary complications.
  - Exacerbation of chronic diseases.
  - *Progressive disease:* Oxygen impairment/cardiopulmonary insufficiency, CNS complications, Invasive secondary bacterial infection, Severe dehydration.
- **Risk factors of severe disease:**
  - Infants and children < 2 years.
  - Pregnant females.
  - COPD.
  - Chronic cardiac disease.
  - Metabolic disorders.
  - Chronic renal/hepatic/neurological/hemoglobinopathies/immunosuppression (including HIV) disorders.
  - Children on aspirin therapy.
  - Persons aged > 65 years.
  - Morbid obesity.
- **Laboratory diagnosis:**
  - *Most timely and sensitive detection:* RT-PCR test.
  - *Samples:* Nasopharyngeal + throat swabs [Tracheal/bronchial aspirates in lower respiratory tract infection cases].
  - *Point-of-care/Rapid diagnostic tests:* Not recommended.
- **Duration of isolation:** For 7 days after onset of illness OR 24 hours after resolution of fever/respiratory symptoms whichever is longer.

- **Antiviral therapy:**
  - *Severe/progressive clinical illness:* Oseltamivir (if not available or resistance, use Zanamivir).
  - *High risk of severe/complicated illness:* Oseltamivir OR Zanamivir.
  - *Not high risk OR Uncomplicated confirmed/suspected illness:* No need of treatment.
  - *Dosage:*
    - Oseltamivir 75 mg BD × 5 days.
    - Zanamivir 2 inhalations (2 × 5 mg) BD × 5 days.

27. Which of the following is a most common type of alcohol induced cardiomyopathy?

A. Hypertrophic cardiomyopathy

B. Dilated cardiomyopathy

C. HOCM

D. Restrictive cardiomyopathy

Answer: Option B. Dilated cardiomyopathy

Explanation:

Alcohol is one of the most common causes of dilated cardiomyopathy.

Causes of dilated cardiomyopathy

Major Causes of Dilated Cardiomyopathy (with Common Examples)
Inflammatory myocarditis
Noninfective
Granulomatous inflammatory disease
Sarcoidosis
Giant cell myocarditis
Eosinophilic myocarditis
Polymyositis, dermatomyositis
Collagen vascular disease
Checkpoint inhibitor chemotherapy
Transplant rejection
Toxic
Alcohol
Catecholamines: amphetamines, cocaine
Chemotherapeutic agents (anthracyclines, trastuzumab)

Contd.

Contd.

Interferon
Other therapeutic agents (hydroxychloroquine, chloroquine)
Drugs of misuse (emetine, anabolic steroids)
Heavy metals: lead, mercury
Occupational exposure: hydrocarbons, arsenicals
Metabolic
Nutritional deficiencies: thiamine, selenium, carnitine)

Features of various cardiomyopathy			
	Dilated	**Restrictive**	**Hypertrophic**
Ejection fraction (normal >55%)	Usually <30% when symptoms severe	25–50%	>60%
Left ventricular diastolic dimension (normal <55 mm)	≥60 mm	<60 mm (may be decreased)	Decreased
Left ventricular wall thickness	Normal or decreased	Normal or increased	Markedly increased
Atrial size	Increased, may also be primarily affected	Increased; may be massive	Increased; related to elevated filling pressures
Valvular regurgitation	Related to annular dilation; mitral appears earlier during decompensation; tricuspid regurgitation with right ventricular dysfunction	Related to endocardial involvement; frequent mitral and tricuspid regurgitation, rarely severe	Related to valve-septum interaction; mitral regurgitation
Common first symptoms	Exertional intolerance	Exertional intolerance, fluid retention early, may have dominant right-sided symptoms	Exertional intolerance; may have chest pain
Congestive symptoms	Left before right, except right prominent in young adults	Right dominates	Left-sided congestion at rest may develop late

Contd.

Contd.

Arrhythmias	Ventricular tachyarrhythmia; conduction block in Chagas' disease, and some families. Atrial fibrillation.	Ventricular uncommon except in sarcoidosis, conduction block in sarcoidosis and amyloidosis. Atrial fibrillation.	Ventricular tachyarrhythmias; atrial fibrillation.

28. A 40 years female presented with hepatosplenomegaly, arthritis and elevated ferritin level, what is the diagnosis?

A. Gout

B. Adult onset Still's disease

C. Reiter's disease

D. Rheumatoid arthritis

Answer: Option B. Adult onset Still's disease

Explanation:

Here, 40 years female presented with hepatosplenomegaly, arthritis and elevated ferritin level–all these features are seen in adult onset Still's disease.

Adult Onset Still's Disease

- It is a form of Still's disease that occurs in adults and is characterised by a triad of high spiking fever, a characteristic evanescent skin rash and **arthritis/arthralgias**.
- Fever is transient, lasting typically under 4 hours and is most commonly quotidian or double quotidian in pattern.
- Rash is maculopapular, predominantly found on the proximal limbs and trunk.
- Joints affected most frequently are the knees, wrists and ankles. Other manifestations include lymphadenopathy, **hepatomegaly, splenomegaly,** pleuritis and pericarditis.
- Macrophage activation syndrome can occur in some patients.

Investigations show anaemia, neutrophilic leucocytosis, thrombocytosis, raised ESR and CRP elevated liver enzymes.

Ferritin levels usually higher than those found in patients with other autoimmune or inflammatory diseases. A more useful marker is reduced level (<20%) of glycosylated fraction of ferritin.

Course

- Self-limited or monocyclic pattern characterised by remission within 1 year from the onset.
- Intermittent or polycyclic systemic pattern recurrent flares, with or without articular symptomatology.
- Chronic articular pattern dominant articular manifestations that can lead to joint destruction.

Treatment is with NSAIDs and steroids. Role of DMARDs (biological and non-biological) is not clear but may be used in refractory cases.

Still's disease is systemic-onset, seronegative RA [juvenile idiopathic arthritis (ITA)] occurring in children.

- Characteristically, the disease presents with high fever, arthralgia and arthritis, myalgia and also hepato-splenomegaly, lymphadenopathy, evanescent skin rashes, anaemia and leucocytosis. Pleurisy and pericarditis may occur.
- Approximately, 10% of children develop overt clinical features of macrophage activation syndrome, a life-threatening condition characterised by fever, organomegaly, cytopenia, hyperferritinemia, hypertriglyceridemia, hypofibrinogenemia and coagulopathy, The diagnostic hallmark is the presence on bone marrow examination of numerous, well-differentiated macrophages that are engaged actively in the phagocytosis of haematopoietic elements.
- Tests for rheumatoid factor are negative, but there is neutrophilia, thrombocytosis and elevated ESR.

- The disease has a good prognosis and most of the patients respond to NSAIDs or steroids.

29. A 52 years old male patient presented with multiple short lasting episodes of unilateral headache accompanying conjunctival congestion and lacrimation. Which of the following is the diagnosis of this patient?

A. SUNCT

B. Primary stabbing headache

C. Cluster headache

D. Trigeminal neuralgia

Answer: Option A. SUNCT

Explanation:

Here, 52 years old male patient presented with multiple short lasting episodes of unilateral headache accompanying conjunctival congestion and lacrimation. So presence of short episode of headache rule out option C–cluster headache and presence of autonomic symptoms such as conjunctival congestion and lacrimation rule out primary stabbing headache and trigeminal neuralgia. So answer by exclusion is SUNCT.

	Typical length of attack	**Associated ipsilateral autonomic activation**	**Typical effective treatment**
SUNCT/SUNA	1–600s	Yes	Lidocaine infusion
Trigeminal neuralgia	Fraction of a second to 2 min	No	Anticonvulsants
Paroxysmal hemicrania	2–30 min	Yes	Indomethacin
Primary stabbing headache	A few seconds	No	Indomethacin, gabapentin
Cluster headache	15–180 min	Yes	Oxygen

Prominent autonomic features	Sparse or no autonomic features
Cluster headache	Trigeminal neuralgia
Chronic paroxysmal hemicrania	Idiopathic stabbing headache
Episodic paroxysmal hemicrania	Cough headache
SUNCT syndrome	Benign exertional headache
Clustertic syndrome	Headache associated with sexual activity Hypnic headache

TRIGEMINAL AUTONOMIC CEPHALALGIAS, INCLUDING CLUSTER HEADACHE

The TACs describe a grouping of primary headaches including cluster headache, paroxysmal hemicrania (PH), SUNCT (short-lasting unilateral neuralgiform headache attacks with conjunctival injection and tearing)/SUNA (short-lasting unilateral neuralgiform headache attacks with cranial autonomic symptoms), and hemicrania continua. TACs are characterized by relatively short-lasting attacks of head pain associated with cranial autonomic symptoms, such as lacrimation, conjunctival injection, aural fullness, or nasal congestion. Pain is usually severe and may occur more than once a day. Because of the associated nasal congestion or rhinorrhea, patients are often misdiagnosed with "sinus headache" and treated with decongestants, which are ineffective.

SUNCT (Short-lasting Unilateral Neuralgiform headache attacks with Conjunctival injection and Tearing)

Short-lasting Unilateral Neuralgiform headache attacks with Conjunctival injection and Tearing (SUNCT) is a syndrome predominant in males, with a mean age of onset around 50 years. The attacks are strictly unilateral, generally with the pain persistently confined to the ocular/periocular area. Most attacks are moderate to severe in intensity and burning, stabbing or electrical in character. The mean duration of paroxysms is 1 minute, with a usual range of 10 to 120 seconds (total range 5 to 250 seconds). Prominent, ipsilateral conjunctival injection and lacrimation regularly accompany the attacks.

Nasal stuffiness/rhinorrhoea are frequently noted. In addition, there is subclinical forehead sweating. During attacks, there is increased intraocular pressure on the symptomatic side and swelling of the eyelids. No changes in pupil diameter have been observed. Attacks can be triggered mostly from trigeminally innervated areas, but also from the extratrigeminal territory. There are also spontaneous attacks. An irregular temporal pattern is the rule, with symptomatic periods alternating with remissions in an unpredictable fashion. During active periods, the frequency of attacks may vary from <1 attack/day to >30 attacks/hour. The attacks predominate during the daytime, nocturnal attacks being seldom reported.

The International Headache Classification established by the **International Headache Society** criteria for diagnosing SUNCT for therapeutic purposes is:

(i) Type of attack – Attacks of unilateral orbital, supraorbital, or temporal areas from stabbing or pulsating pain accompanied by ipsilateral conjunctival injection and lacrimation.

(ii) Number of attacks per day – 3 to 200 attacks per day.

(iii) Attack load in minutes per day – 5–240 seconds.

DIAGNOSIS

SUNCT is a rare primary headache syndrome characterized by severe, unilateral orbital or temporal pain that is stabbing or throbbing in quality. Diagnosis requires at least 20 attacks, lasting for 5–240s; ipsilateral conjunctival injection and lacrimation should be present. In some patients, conjunctival injection or lacrimation is missing, and the diagnosis of SUNA can be made.

The pain of SUNCT/SUNA is unilateral and may be located anywhere in the head. Three basic patterns can be seen: single stabs, which are usually short-lived; groups of stabs; or a longer attack comprising many stabs between which the pain does not completely resolve, thus giving a "saw-tooth" phenomenon with attacks lasting many minutes. Each pattern may be seen in the context of an underlying continuous head pain. Characteristics that lead to a suspected diagnosis of SUNCT are the cutaneous (or other) triggers of attacks, a lack of refractory period to triggering between attacks, and the lack of a response to indomethacin. Apart from trigeminal sensory disturbance, the neurologic examination is normal in primary SUNCT/SUNA.

The diagnosis of SUNCT/SUNA is often confused with TN particularly in first-division TN. Minimal or no cranial autonomic symptoms and a clear refractory period to triggering indicate a diagnosis of TN.

Secondary (Symptomatic) SUNCT

SUNCT can be seen with posterior fossa or pituitary lesions. All patients with SUNCT/SUNA should be evaluated with pituitary function tests and a brain MRI with pituitary views.

TREATMENT

Treatment SUNCT/SUNA Abortive Therapy

Therapy of acute attacks is not a useful concept in SUNCT/SUNA because the attacks are of such short duration. However, IV lidocaine, which arrests the symptoms, can be used in hospitalized patients.

Preventive Therapy

Long-term prevention to minimize disability and hospitalization is the goal of treatment. The most effective treatment for prevention is lamotrigine, 200–400 mg/d. Topiramate and gabapentin may also be effective. Carbamazepine, 400–500 mg/d, has been reported by patients to offer modest benefit.

Surgical approaches such as microvascular decompression or destructive trigeminal procedures are seldom useful and often produce long-term complications. Greater occipital nerve injection has produced limited benefit in some patients. Occipital nerve stimulation is probably helpful in a subgroup of these patients. For intractable cases, short-term prevention with IV lidocaine can be effective.

	Cluster Headache	**Paroxysmal Hemicrania**	**SUNCT/SUNA**
Gender	M>F	F=M	F~M
Pain			
Type	Stabbing, boring	Throbbing, boring, stabbing	Burning, stabbing, sharp
Severity	Excruciating	Excruciating	Severe to excruciating
Site	Orbit, temple	Orbit, temple	Periorbital

Contd.

Contd.

Attack frequency	1/alternate day–8/d	1–20/d (>5/d for more than half the time)	3–200/d
Duration of attack	15–180 min	2–30 min	5–240s
Autonomic features	Yes	Yes	Yes (prominent conjunctival injection and lacrimation)
Migrainous features	Yes	Yes	Yes
Alcohol trigger	Yes	No	No
Cutaneous triggers	No	No	Yes
Indomethacin	—	Yes	—
Abortive treatment	Sumatriptan injection or nasal spray Oxygen	No effective treatment	Lidocaine (IV)
Prophylactic treatment	Verapamil Topiramate Melatoinin	Indomethacin	Lamotrigine Topiramate
	Lithium		Gabapentin

30. In a patient of lipoprotein deficiency, which of the following substance will increase after fatty meal?

A. VLDL B. HDL

C. Chylomicron D. LDL

Answer: Option C. Chylomicron

Explanation:

Lipoprotein lipase deficiency causes increase chylomicrons in plasma after fatty meal, often leading to acute pancreatitis therefore the mainstay of treatment is a specialized very-low-fat diet.

Other name of lipoprotein lipase deficiency:

- Apolipoprotein C II Deficiency
- Burger Grutz Syndrome
- Chylomicronemia Syndrome

Familial Lipoprotein Lipase deficiency is an inherited condition that is usually present during infancy or early childhood.

- Familial Lipoprotein Lipase Deficiency is an inherited disorder caused by a defective gene responsible for an enzyme called lipoprotein lipase. As a result, the affected individuals lack the ability to produce lipoprotein lipase enzyme that is needed to breakdown the fat molecules.
- The disorder is characterized by a massive accumulation of fatty particles (chylomicrons) in blood and a corresponding increase of fatty substances called triglycerides.
- The signs and symptoms associated with Familial Lipoprotein Lipase Deficiency include recurrent attacks of pancreatitis resulting in abdominal pain, nausea, vomiting, and loss of appetite. Also, there may be a formation of yellow skin deposits, called xanthomas, on the eyelid, hands, elbows and knees.
- Complications of Familial Lipoprotein Lipase Deficiency are recurrent episodes of abdominal pain due to inflammation of the pancreas, xanthomas causing cosmetic concerns, enlargement of the organs (liver and spleen), and occlusion of blood vessels in the retina.
- The deficiency disorder is treated by controlling blood triglyceride levels and through symptomatic treatment. Restriction to a very low-fat diet can dramatically improve the symptoms of Familial Lipoprotein Lipase Deficiency.
- Since it is an inherited disorder, there are no preventive measures available. Awareness of the risk factors, such as a positive family history, can allow early detection.
- When the individuals adhere to a fat-free diet, the symptoms are considerably improved and this can bring about a favorable outcome.

The signs and symptoms of include:

- Failure to thrive in infancy
- Episodes of abdominal pain due to inflammation of the pancreas. Abdominal pain is usually the first sign of the condition.
- Loss of appetite.
- Nausea, vomiting.

- Pain in the muscles and bones.
- Xanthomas: Yellow fatty skin deposits appearing on the eyelids, hands, or on the knees and elbows.
- Pale retina (in the back of the eye), white-colored blood vessels in the retina.
- Recurrent pancreatitis (inflammation of the pancreas).
- Yellowing of the eyes and skin (jaundice).

CHAPTER 12

SURGERY

1. In a case of retrosternal goiter, which of the following approach is used?

A. Trans sternal through via anterior mediastinum

B. Transcervical approach

C. Transthoracic approach via fourth intercostal space

D. Transthoracic approach via second intercostal space

Answer: Option B. Transcervical approach

Explanation:

Virtually all retrosternal goiter with intrathoracic extension can be removed via a cervical incision.

Retrosternal Goiter

A goiter is said to be retrosternal, substernal or mediastinal if **more than half** of **thyroid tissue** is **below** the **opening** of **thoracic cage.**

Usually arises from **lower pole** of a **nodular goiter**.

Often symptomless, **discovered** on a routine **chest X-ray**.

Tracheal deviation and **scabard trachea** (flattening of trachea caused by compression).

Surgical removal of intrathoracic goiter.

A goiter is considered **mediastinal** if **at least 50%** of the **thyroid tissue** is **located intrathoracically**.

Primary Mediastinal Goiters	Secondary Mediastinal Goiters
• Constitute approximately **1%** of all mediastinal goiters • **Arise from accessory (ectopic) thyroid tissue located in the chest** • **Supplied by intrathoracic blood vessels** • **Do not have any connection to thyroid tissue in the neck.**	• Constitute **majority** of mediastinal goiters • Arise from **downward extension** of **cervical thyroid tissue** along the fascial planes of the neck and • Derive their **blood supply from** the **superior** and **inferior thyroid arteries**.

Removal

Virtually **all intrathoracic goiters** can be **removed via a cervical incision**.

Indications of Median Sternotomy
Patients who have: **1. Invasive thyroid cancers** 2. Had **previous thyroid operations** and may have developed **parasitic mediastinal vessels** **3. Primary mediastinal goiters** with **no thyroid tissue in the neck**

The **chest** should be **prepared in most cases** in the event it is necessary to perform a median sternotomy to control mediastinal bleeding or completely remove an unsuspected invasive cancer.

The goiter is **approached via a neck incision**.

When sternotomy is indicated, **the sternum usually should be divided** to the level of **the third intercostal space** and then laterally on one side at the **space between** the **third** and **fourth ribs.**

2. Parathyroid gland is found after surgery which is accidentally removed during surgery. At which of the following site, it will be implanted?

A. Tensor fascia lata
B. Biceps
C. Quadriceps femoris
D. Brachioradialis

Answer: Option D. Brachioradialis

Explanation:

PARATHYROID AUTOTRANSPLANTATION

Whenever **multiple parathyroids** are **resected**, it is preferable to **cryopreserve tissue**, so that it may be autotransplanted should the patient become hypoparathyroid.

Approx. 12-14 pieces of 1 mm are transplanted into the nondominant forearm in belly of brachioradialis muscle.

Total parathyroidectomy with autotransplantation removes all identified glands and uses an easily accessible area, most commonly the forearm or the sternocleidomastoid muscle, as the site for implantation. The gland to be transplanted is minced into 1 mm pieces and 12 to 18 pieces are embedded in well-vascularized muscle and marked with a stitch or clip. Some groups use a technique of injection into subcutaneous tissue. Neovascularization occurs over a period of several weeks. The principal advantage of this technique is that residual parathyroid function is easily monitored and recurrences can be treated by partial resection under local anesthesia without the need for cervical reexploration. There are several disadvantages. More aggressive medical treatment is necessary postoperatively to maintain adequate serum calcium levels and avoid serious hypocalcemic complications. Autograft failure can lead to hypoparathyroidism, which can be profound. Retrieval of all small grafts may be difficult at reoperation. Implantation into muscle may interfere with hemodialysis access in the future; invasive growth of autografts into muscle and adjacent tissue requiring radical resection has been described. Finally, supernumerary glands may still be present in the neck, thereby resulting in two potential sites of recurrence.

3. In a case of 'Omphalocele', which of the following pathological abnormality is noted?

A. It is a physiological hernia

B. Herniation of liver

C. Failure of intestine to return into abdomen

D. Covering sac is absent

Answer: Option C. Failure of intestine to return into abdomen

Explanation:

Abdominal Wall Defects

Omphalocele
• **Intestine fails to return, abdominal contents protruding directly through the umbilical ring with a sac covering the bowel.**
• **Abdominal contents are covered with peritoneum on the inside and amnion on the outside.**
• Size of the defect is variable, ranging from a small opening through which a small portion of the intestine is herniated to a large one in which the entire bowel and liver are included.

Contd.

Contd.

• Chromosomal abnormalities are present in roughly 30% of infants, including trisomies 13, 18 and 21. • More than half of infants have other major or minor malformations, with cardiac being the most common, followed by musculoskeletal, gastrointestinal and genitourinary. • Close association with Beckwith-Wiedemann syndrome (omphalocele, hyperinsulinemia and macroglossia). • Poor prognosis due to associated abnormalities.

Gastroschisis
• Fetal gut is extruded through a defect in the abdominal wall. • Defect is always on the right side of the umbilical ring with an intact umbilical cord. • Covering sac is absent. • Risk for associated anomalies is low. • Association with intestinal atresia in up to 15%. • Atresias may involve the small and large intestine. • Babies are more often small for gestational age and born to mothers with a history of cigarette, alcohol, and recreational drug use and intake of aspirin, ibuprofen, and pseudoephedrine during the first trimester. • Increased risk in mothers younger than 20 years. • In patients with gastroschisis, the intestine is often thickened, edematous, matted together and foreshortened. • Good prognosis.

Exomphalos (Omphalocele)

Incidence: 1 in 5000 live births.

- Due to failure of all or part of the midgut to return to the coelom during early fetal life.
- Sac is very thin, consists an outer layer of amniotic membrane and inner layer of peritoneum.
- Intestine lies freely mobile within the intact sac without evidence of adhesions or inflammation.
- In contrast, the liver has dense adhesions to the sac.

Omphalocele/exomphalos: Congenital herniation of abdominal contents at the umbilicus (i.e. into the umbilical cord). Occasionally divided into:

< 4 cm—Umbilical cord hernia.

> 4 cm—Omphalocele.

- In smaller defects a single loop of intestine may not be obvious.

- In large defects, the liver, spleen, stomach, pancreas, colon or bladder may be seen through the membrane.

Moore's classification of omphalocele	
Type	**Diameter of Defect**
Type 1	<2.5 cm
Type 2	2.5 to 5 cm
Type 3	>5 cm

Treatment

Small defects may be **closed primarily soon after birth.**

Indications of Surgery in Umbilical Hernia	
• Persisting **beyond 5 years** • **Symptomatic** • **Strangulated**	• Defect **size >2 cm** • **Progressive enlarging hernia after the age 1-2 years**

Small defects: Closed primarily.

Defects >3 cm: Closed using prosthetic mesh.

Mayo's repair
Vest-over-pants repair proposed by Mayo employs **imbrication of superior** and **inferior fascial edges**.
Because of **increased tension** on the **repair** and **recurrence rates** of 30%, it is **rarely performed today**.

4. Gall stones are made of which of the following biochemical structure?

A. Crystalline cholesterol dihydrate
B. Crystalline cholesterol monohydrate
C. Amorphous cholesterol monohydrate
D. Amorphous cholesterol monohydrate

Answer: Option B. Crystalline cholesterol monohydrate

Explanation:

Cholesterol monohydrate crystal agglomerate to become macroscopic crystal by nucleation ultimately forms gallstone.

PATHOGENESIS OF CHOLESTEROL GALLSTONES

- **Cholesterol** is **insoluble** in **water** (**water** is major constituent of bile, **85-95%**).
- **Bile acid** and **phospholipids** in bile keep cholesterol in solution by the formation of **micelles**.

- An **excess of cholesterol** relative to bile acids and phospholipids allows cholesterol to form crystals and such bile is called **Lithogenic** or **supersaturated bile.**

Factors Responsible for Formation of Gallstones		
Lithogenic bile	**Nucleation**	**Stasis or GB hypomotility**
• **Increased Biliary Cholesterol:** – **Obesity** Cholesterol rich diet **Clofibrate** therapy • **Decreased Bile Acids:** – Primary biliary cirrhosis – **OCPs** Mutation of **CYP7A1** gene **Impaired entero-hepatic circulation** of bile acids: **Ileal disease** or **resection, cholestyramine** or **colestipol** (bile acid sequestrants) • **Decreased Biliary Lecithin**: – **MDR-3** gene **mutation** leads to defective	Cholesterol monohydrate crystal agglomerate to become macroscopic crystal by nucleation • **Pro-nucleating** Factors: – **Mucin** – Non-mucin glycoprotein – Infection • **Anti-nucleating Factors:** • Apolipoprotein **A-I** and **A-II** **Excess of pro-nucleating factors or deficiency of anti-nucleating factors results in formation of gallstones**	• Prolonged **TPN** • Prolonged **fasting** • **Pregnancy** • **Octreotide** • **OCPs** • Massive **burns**

Black stones are composed of **insoluble bilirubin pigment polymer** mixed with **calcium phosphate** and calcium **bicarbonate.**

Brown pigment stones contain calcium bilirubinate, calcium palmitate and calcium stearate as well as cholesterol.

5. Degloving injury involves which part of skin to be avulsed?

A. Skin only

B. Skin and subcutaneous fat region

C. Skin and subcutaneous fat region with underlying fascia

D. Skin and subcutaneous fat region with underlying fascia and tendon

Answer: Option B. Skin and subcutaneous fat region

Explanation:

Degloving occurs when the skin and subcutaneous fat are stripped by avulsion from its underlying fascia, leaving neurovascular structures, tendon or bone exposed.

Degloving Injuries

It occurs due to shearing force between tissue planes as traction—avulsion injury. It usually occurs between subcutaneous tissue and deep fascia or between muscle and bone. It can be localised or circumferential.

Avulsion injury strips off the superficial tissues exposing the neurovascular bundle, muscles, tendons and bone. Degloving injury can be open or closed. It can be in one plane or multiple planes. It is commonly observed in machinery injuries or major road traffic accidents. It is much more extensive than of on initial presentation. Under anaesthesia fluoroscein is injected intravenously and viable skin is visible as fluorescent yellowish—green colour under ultraviolet light. As injection of fluoroscein is not fully safer, serial excision is better to look for dermal punctate bleeding. It needs examination under general anaesthesia, wound excision/radical excision, flap coverage, micro flap surgeries, skin grafting, with proper asepsis, and blood transfusion as there is significant blood loss in these injuries.

6. Which of the false regarding deep venous thrombosis?

A. Clinical evaluation is most reliable

B. Some people may present first time with pulmonary embolism

C. It is common on both sides

D. Leg pain and edema are most common presenting feature

Answer: Option A. Clinical evaluation is most reliable

Explanation:

The clinical signs of DVT are unreliable in the most of the ICU patients and most patients with ultrasound-proven DVT will have no subjective complaints or physical findings.

Most common presentation of DVT: Pain and swelling, especially in the calf of one lower limb.

Bilateral DVT is common, occurring in up to 30%.

Many patients have no symptoms of thrombosis and may first present with signs of a pulmonary embolism, e.g., pleuritic chest pain, hemoptysis and shortness of breath.

Deep Venous Thrombosis in ICU

ICU patients typically manifest all three components of Virchow's triad that contribute to risk for venous thrombosis—stasis, endothelial injury and hypercoagulability. Surveillance ultrasonography and venography studies in trauma and medical ICUs have determined the incidence of deep venous thrombosis (DVT) in 30% to 40% of patients; in these patients, DVTs that extend to the thigh in approximately 40% to 50% will result in a PE. The mortality rate of an untreated PE is 25%; thus, it is prudent for every institution to have a formal prevention strategy for venous thromboembolism (VTE) and PE. High-risk factors that justify prophylaxis include the following: major general surgery (thoracic or abdominal operations under general anesthesia, lasting ≥30 minutes), neurosurgical procedures, coronary artery bypass surgery, surgery for gynecologic malignancies, major urologic surgery, multiple trauma, hip fracture, spinal cord injury, surgery or chemotherapy for malignancy, congestive heart failure and respiratory failure.

The clinical signs and symptoms of DVT (e.g., leg pain, swelling, rubor, fever) are unreliable in the ICU and most patients with ultrasound-proven DVT will have no subjective complaints or physical findings. On the other hand, duplex ultrasonography is noninvasive, portable, and has sensitivity and specificity of more than 95%, making it an excellent screening tool; however, its usefulness for detecting proximal clot is limited. Literature has supported use of the D-dimer assay, noting its high negative predictive value, but D-dimer is insufficient to exclude DVT in patients who have a moderate to high clinical probability based on pretest assessment. However, the combination of a normal D-dimer concentration and low pretest probability is likely adequate to rule out VTE.

Treatment of DVT has typically been with IV unfractionated heparin (UFH) but because of its more consistent and predictable response, favorable dosing, and equivalent efficacy, with fewer bleeding complications, LMWH is now preferred.

Deep Venous Thrombosis

DVT of the leg is complicated by the immediate risk of pulmonary embolus and sudden death.

Patients are at risk of developing a post-thrombotic limb and venous ulceration.

Calf veins are the most common site of DVT in post-operative period, but risk of embolism from calf venous thrombosis is extremely low.

Most common site of DVT: Calf veins (soleal veins).

DVT of femoropopliteal veins are the most common site of pulmonary thromboembolism.

Most important predisposing factor: Hospital admission for the treatment of a medical or surgical condition.

Clinical Features

Physical signs: Mild pitting edema of the ankle, dilated surface veins, a stiff calf and tenderness over the course of the deep veins.

Earliest sign of DVT: Calf tenderness, Low-grade fever may be present, especially in a patient who is having repeated pulmonary emboli.

Homan's sign: Resistance (not pain) of the calf muscles to forcible dorsiflexion is not discriminatory and should be abandoned.

Homan's sign	Resistance (not pain) of the calf muscles to forcible dorsiflexion
Phlegmasia alba dolens	Painful white leg Obstruction of major deep venous channel
Phlegmasia cerulea dolens	Painful blue leg Obstruction of both collaterals and deep venous channel
Moses sign	Calf tenderness on direct pressure on the calf
Pratt's sign	Calf tenderness on squeezing the calf from the sides

Diagnosis

D-dimer measurement: If normal, no indication for further investigation but, if raised, a duplex ultrasound examination of the deep veins should be performed.

Duplex ultrasound: Investigation of choice for diagnosis of DVT (Filling defects in flow and lack of compressibility indicate the presence of a thrombosis).

Ascending venography: Shows thrombus as a filling defect, is now rarely required.

Treatment

Confirmed DVT on duplex imaging: Start subcutaneous LMWH and rapid anticoagulation with warfarin unless there is a specific contraindication.

Thrombolysis: In iliac vein thrombosis, especially if seen early and limb is extremely swollen.

A minimum treatment time of anticoagulation advocated in DVT is 3 months.

Duration of heparin should be at least 5 days.

Warfarin is usually started at a dose of 10 mg on day one, 10 mg on day two and 5 mg on day three.

PT on day 3 guides the maintenance dose of warfarin.

Risk of DVT in Relation to Age and Duration of Surgery

High Risk
• General **urological surgery** in patient **>40 years** • **Extensive pelvic** or **abdominal surgery** • **Major orthopaedic surgery** of lower limbs
Moderate Risk
• **General surgery** in patients **≥40 years** • **Surgery** lasting for **≥30 minutes** • **General surgery** in patients **<40 years** on **OCPs**
Low Risk
• **Uncomplicated surgery** in patients **<40** years **without additional risk** • **Minor surgery** (**<30 minutes**) in patients **<40 years** without additional risk

Mechanical Prophylaxis
Early ambulation: Simplest method of prophylaxis–Acts by activating calf-pump mechanism **Pneumatic compression devices:**Most common method of prophylaxis– Pneumatic compression prevents stasis
Pharmacological Prophylaxis
Unfractionated heparin: Replaced by LMWH **Fractionated low molecular weight heparin (LMWH):** Better efficacy than unfractionated heparin. No laboratory monitoring is necessary

7. Which of the following triangle is shown in below given image?

A. Doom's triangle

B. Gastrinoma triangle

C. Calot's triangle

D. Cholecystohepatic triangle

Answer: Option B. Gastrinoma triangle

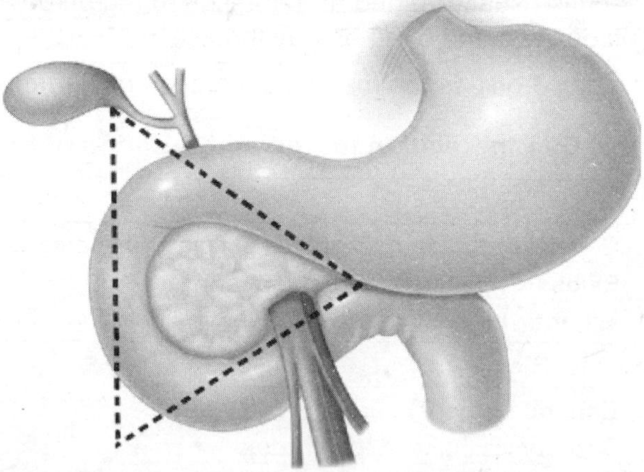

Explanation:

Ninety percent of gastrinomas are located within the gastrinoma triangle, bounded by the lines connecting the cystic duct, the junction between the second and third portions of the duodenum, and the junction between the neck and body of the pancreas.

Boundaries of Gastrinoma/Passaro's Triangle
• **Junction** of the **cystic** and **CBD**
• **Junction** of **2nd** and **3rd part** of **duodenum**
• **Junction** of **neck** and **body** of **pancreas**

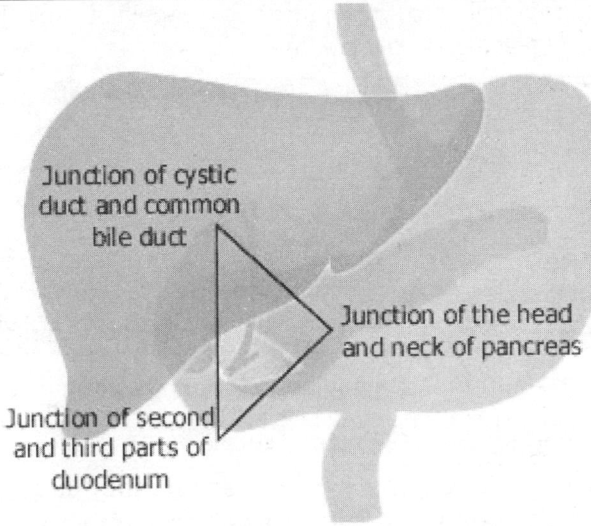

The **hepatobiliary triangle** (or **cystohepatic triangle**)/ **Calot's triangle** is an anatomic space bordered by the cystic duct inferiorly, common hepatic duct medially and the inferior (visceral) surface of the liver superiorly. The cystic artery lies within the cystohepatic triangle, which is used to locate it during a laparoscopic cholecystectomy.

Calot's Triangle

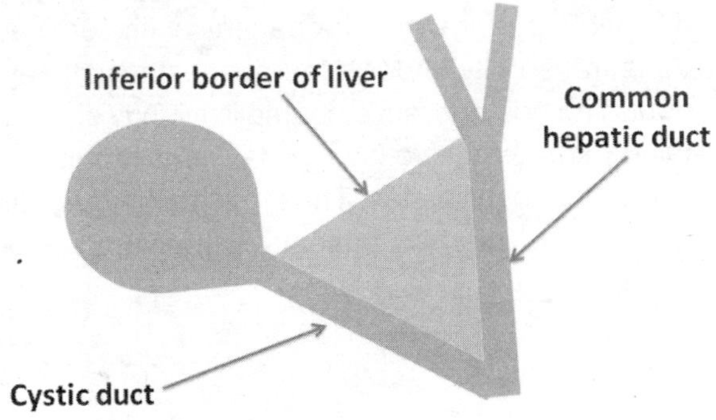

The **Triangle of Doom** is an anatomical triangle defined by the vas deferens medially, spermatic vessels laterally and peritoneal fold inferiorly. This triangle contains external iliac artery and vein, the deep circumflex iliac vein, the genital branch of genitofemoral nerve and hidden by fascia, the femoral nerve. It bears significance in laparoscopic repair of groin hernia. Surgical staples are avoided here.

8. Which of the following is true regarding Dohlman surgery used in Zenker's diverticulum?

A. It is laser excision of diverticula

B. Open surgical resection of pouch

C. It is endoscopic excision of poch

D. It uses endoscopic stapling of septum

Answer: Option D. It uses endoscopic stapling of septum

Explanation:

An alternative to open surgical repair is **the endoscopic Dohlman procedure**, which has become more popular. **Endoscopic division of the common wall/septum between the esophagus and diverticulum using a laser or stapler has also been successful**. Because of the configuration of the inline stapling device, this approach has been advocated for larger diverticula. The risk for an incomplete myotomy increases with smaller diverticula, smaller than 3 cm. This method divides the distal cricopharyngeus muscle while obliterating the sac. The esophagus and diverticulum form a common channel. The technique requires maximal extension of the neck and can be difficult to perform in older patients with cervical stenosis. It is done transorally under general anesthesia in approximately 1 hour. The postoperative course is slightly shorter, with patients taking liquids the following day and requiring only a single overnight hospital stay. Thus, this technique has gained favor and is advocated for patients with diverticula between 2 and 5 cm.

Treatment options for Zenker's diverticula
Surgical therapy **(Cricopharyngeal myotomy + Diverticulopexy)** is **treatment of choice** • **Cricopharyngeal myotomy**–a myotomy alone is sufficient for small diverticula • **Myotomy with excision of sac**–done for large (>4 cm) diverticula • **Diverticulopexy** • **Diverticulo-esophagostomy** using a linear cutting staple gun – The septum between the esophagus and the diverticula is divided–Also known as **Dohlman procedure**

9. Which of the following surgical knot is shown in below given image?

A. Reef knot
B. Surgeon knot
C. Alberdeen knot
D. Granny knot

Answer: Option D. Granny knot

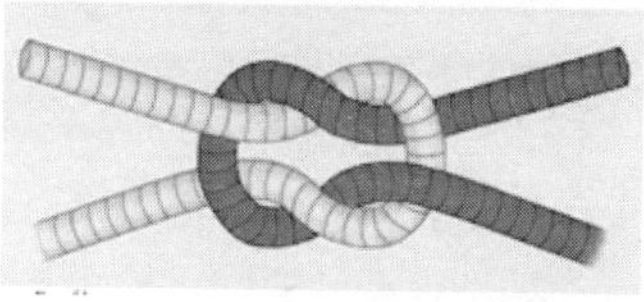

Explanation:

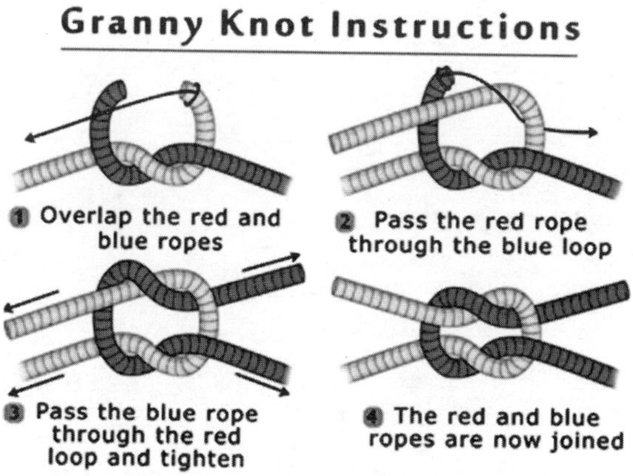

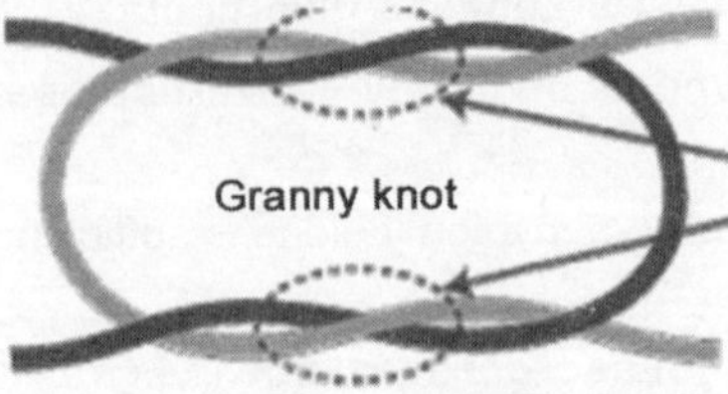

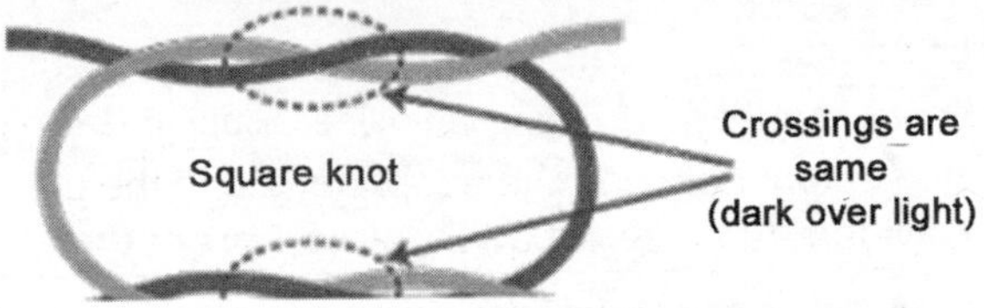

Surgeon's knot

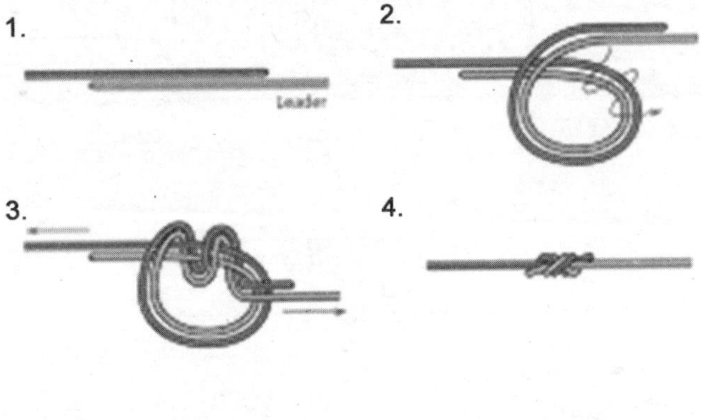

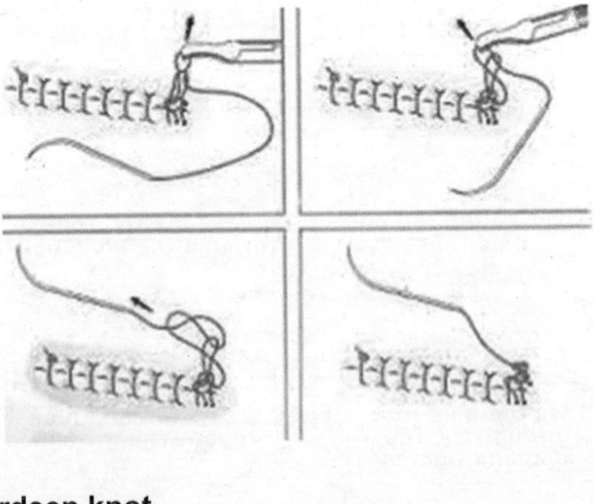

Alberdeen knot

10. Which of the following size of scalpel blade is given in below image, that is used for incision and drainage?

A. 21
B. 15
C. 13
D. 11

Answer: Option D. 11

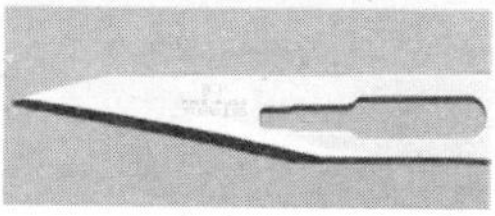

Explanation:

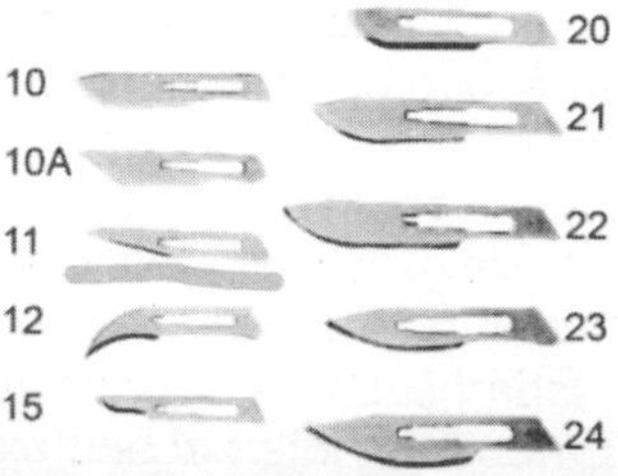

11. A 52 years old patient presented with hard, painless, non-fluctuant and non-progressive swelling in the neck as shown in below image. There is no evidence of lymphadenopathy. Which of the following is diagnosis of the patient?

A. Sternomastoid tumor
B. Branchial cyst
C. TB lymphadenitis
D. Dermoid cyst

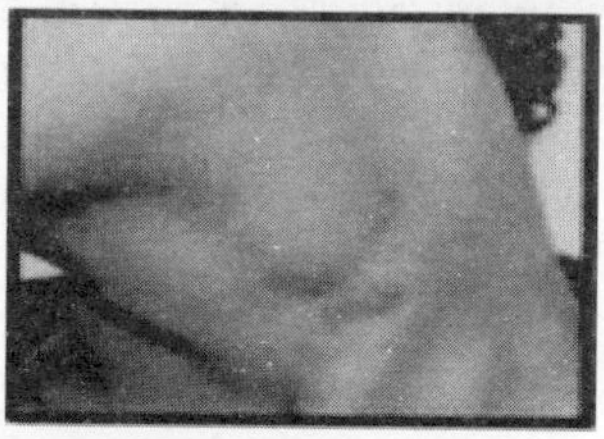

Answer: Option B. Branchial cyst

Explanation:

Here, answer is given by exclusion. 52 years old patient presented with hard, painless, non-fluctuant and non-progressive swelling in the neck as shown in above image. There is no evidence of lymphadenopathy. So one option TB lymphadenitis can be ruled out. Now swelling is not in midline, so dermoid cyst also can be ruled out. Here, lesion appears separated and anterior to sternocleidomastoid muscle so Sternomastoid tumor is also ruled out. Now remaining option Branchial cyst generally presents as a swelling in the upper part of the neck anterior to sternocleidomastoid muscle. Therefore our answer in this case is branchial cyst.

Branchial Cyst

It is common in the second decade of life but can occur at any age with equal frequency in both sexes. Cyst presents as a swelling in the upper part of the neck anterior to sternocleidomastoid muscle. Mass is smooth, round, fluctuant, nontender and nontransilluminant. A painful increase in size at the time of upper respiratory infection can occur. Anomalies of the second branchial arch are the most common. A branchial cyst may be associated with a sinus or a fistula. A second arch branchial sinus has an external opening at the junction of lower and middle of the anterior border of sternomastoid and may exude mucoid discharge. It may have an internal opening in the tonsillar fossa. When both internal and external openings are present, it is called a branchial fistula. Treatment of branchial cyst is surgical excision along with its tract, if present.

Sternomastoid Tumor

Mostly seen in the newborns due to birth trauma. Fibrosis and later shortening of the sternocleidomastoid muscle causes torticollis. Face is turned to opposite side but the head is tilted on the ipsilateral shoulder. A mass can be palpated in the sternocleidomastoid muscle on physical examination. In long-standing cases, asymmetry of face and head can develop as a sequel.

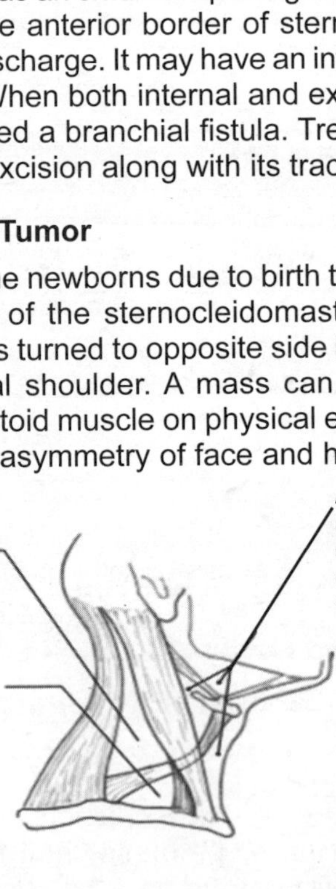

Lateral swellings of neck as seen in different triangles of neck

12. According to CEAP classification, 46 years female presenting with visible 0.5 mm dilated superficial tortuous varicose veins without significant edema is classified under which group?

A. C1 B. C2

C. C3 D. C4

Answer: Option C. C2

Explanation:

Here, patient presented with visible 0.5 mm dilated superficial tortuous varicose veins without edema which included in C2 group which include **development of varicose veins** (visible and palpable varicose veins).

CEAP classification is used to evaluate severity of the disease and the progression of the disease on the basis of the clinical signs present.

C for clinical signs (grade 0-6) Supplemented by (A) for asymptomatic and (S) for symptomatic. 0 No visible or palpable signs of venous disease 1 Presence of telangiectasia or reticular veins 2 **Varicose veins** 3 Oedema 4 Skin changes (trophic changes): pigmentation,eczema, lipodermatosclerosis 5 Trophic changes indicated in 4 with healed ulcer 6 Trophic changes indicated in 4 with active ulcer
E for the etiological classification, the following categories are used: C for congenital P for primary S for secondary (post-thrombotic, post-traumatic, other) N for No venous cause identified
A for the anatomical distribution, depending on the sector involved: S for superficial D for deep P for perforating N for No venous location identified
P for the pathophysiological dysfunction responsible: R for reflux O for obstruction R,O for reflux and obstruction N for No venous pathophysiology identified

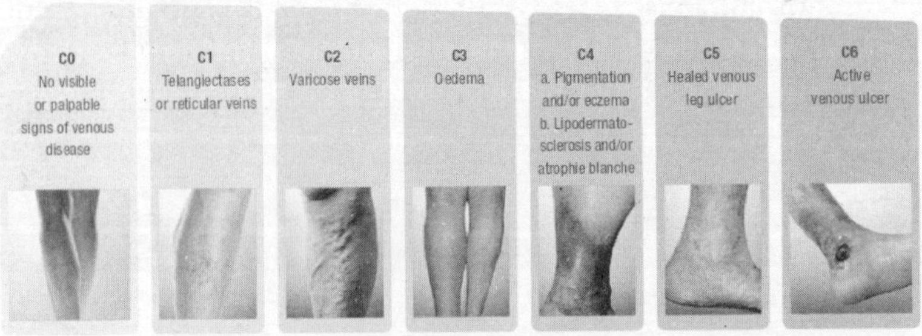

13. A 32 years old female presented with cystic neck swelling in midline neck region as shown in below image. Which of the following is diagnosis of the patient?

A. Thyroglossal cyst

B. Branchial cyst

C. Secondaries in neck

D. Dermoid cyst

Answer: Option D. Dermoid cyst

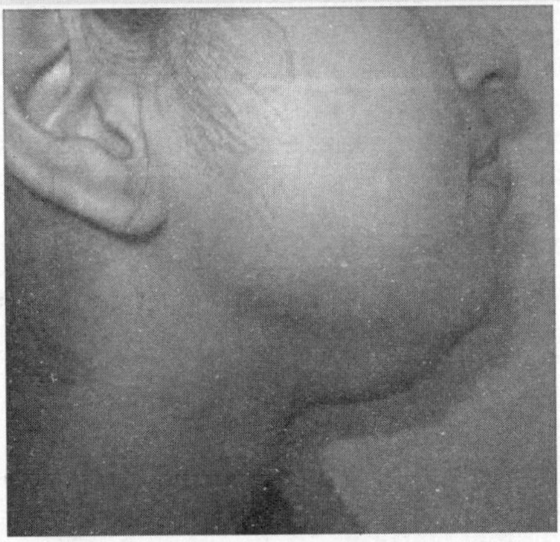

Explanation:

Here, 32 years old female presented with cystic neck swelling in midline neck region as shown in above image. Two of the most common types of cyst that occur under the skin surface in the region of submental triangle are sebaceous cyst and dermoid cyst. These are true cyst, line by epithelium. So, here answer is dermoid cyst.

It presents as a midline submental swelling but does not move on protrusion of the tongue as it is not attached to foramen caecum. Sometimes it arises from the floor of mouth and needs differentiation from ranula. Treatment is surgical excision. A midline dermoid is also seen just above the suprasternal notch.

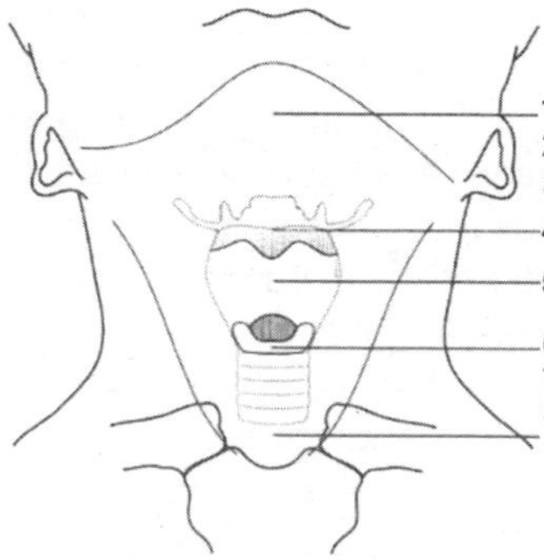

They are composed of multiple tissue elements derived from the three primitive embryonic layers foreign to the area in which they occur. The peak incidence is in the second and third decades of life. There is no gender predisposition. Radiographic evidence of normal tissue (e.g., well-formed teeth or globular calcifications, a fatty mass) in an abnormal location can be considered specific. The teratodermoid (dermoid) cyst is the simplest form of a teratoma and composed of derivatives of the epidermal layer, including dermal and epidermal glands, hair, and sebaceous material. Teratomas are histologically more complex. The solid component of the tumor often contains well-differentiated elements of bone, cartilage, teeth, muscle, connective tissue, fibrous and lymphoid tissue, nerve, thymus, mucous and salivary glands, lung, liver, or pancreas. Malignant tumors are differentiated from benign tumors by the presence of primitive (embryonic) tissue or of malignant components. Immature teratomas/dermoid contain combinations of mature epithelial and connective tissues, with immature areas of mesenchymal and neuroectodermal tissues. Teratomas / dermoid with malignant components are divided into categories based on the elements present.

Diagnosis and therapy rely on surgical excision. For benign tumors that are so large or with involvement of adjacent structures so that complete resection is impossible, partial resection can lead to the resolution of symptoms, frequently without relapse. For malignant dermoid, chemotherapy and radiation therapy, combined with surgical excision, are individualized for the type of malignant components contained in the tumors. The overall prognosis is poor for malignant dermoid.

THYROGLOSSAL DUCT CYST

It presents as a cystic midline swelling, usually affecting young children but can occur at any age. It is usually rounded with a diameter of 2–4 cm. It increases in size with upper respiratory tract infection. Sometimes it presents as a draining sinus if it has burst due to infection or has been surgically drained. Because of the attachment of thyroglossal duct to foramen caecum at the base of tongue, it moves with tongue protrusion.

Structures Moving with Deglutition	
Thyroid gland	Pre and paratracheal nodes
Thyroglossal cyst	Sub-hyoid bursa

14. A 40 years old female presented with painless, gradually progressive swelling for 10 years. It appears firm to nodular and shows variable consistency. Which of the following diagnosis of the patient, based on below given image?

A. Branchial cyst
B. Sebaceous cyst
C. Pleomorphic adenoma
D. Dermoid cyst

Answer: Option C. Pleomorphic adenoma

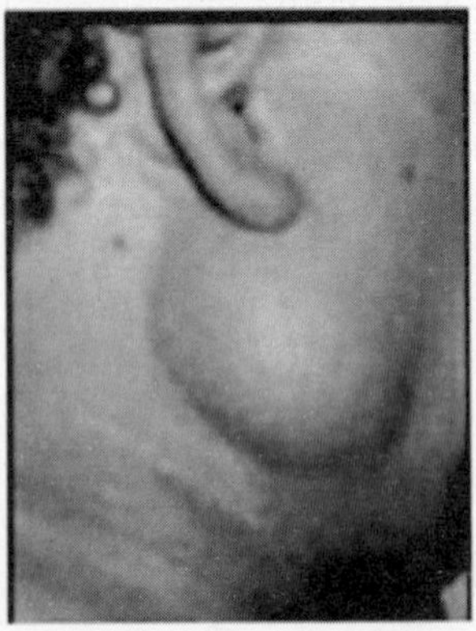

Explanation:

Here a 40 years old female presented with painless, gradually progressive swelling for 10 years. It appears firm to nodular and shows variable consistency. Based on above given image swelling is located at parotid region and so most probable site of origin of this tumor is parotid gland and **pleomorphic adenoma is the most common (≈50%) tumor of the parotid.**

TUMORS OF PAROTID GLAND

Benign

- *Epithelial*
  - Pleomorphic adenoma: This is the most common (≈50%) tumor of the parotid.
  - Warthin tumor: Essentially only found in the parotid, in older, usually male, patients; it is bilateral in 10-15%.
  - Intraductal papilloma of salivary glands.
  - Oncocytoma of salivary glands.
  - Myoepithelioma: Until recently considered a subtype of pleomorphic adenoma; they can also originate in breast and bronchus.
- *Non-epithelial*
  - Hemangioma
  - Lymphangioma
  - Lipoma.

Malignant

- Mucoepidermoid carcinoma: Most of the malignant lesions
- Adenoid cystic carcinoma
- Myoepithelioma
- Adenocarcinoma (not otherwise specified)
- Acinic cell carcinoma of salivary glands
- Squamous cell carcinoma of salivary glands
- Malignant mixed tumors of the salivary glands
  - Carcinoma ex pleomorphic adenoma
  - Carcinosarcoma (true mixed tumor of the salivary glands)
  - Metastasizing pleomorphic adenoma

- Salivary duct carcinoma
- Metastases (mostly to intraparotid lymph nodes)
  - Cutaneous squamous cell carcinoma
  - Malignant melanoma
- Lymphoma (rare)
  - Primary: Arising from the parotid gland as a MALToma.
  - Secondary: Involving the intraparotid lymph nodes.

PLEOMORPHIC ADENOMA OF THE SALIVARY GLANDS

Pleomorphic adenomas, also known as **benign mixed tumors (BMTs)**, are the most common salivary gland tumors.

Epidemiology

Pleomorphic adenomas account for 70-80% of benign salivary gland tumors and are especially common in the parotid gland. Patients are typically middle aged and prior head and neck irradiation is a risk factor for the development of these tumors.

Clinical Presentation

Patients typically present with a smooth, painless, enlarging mass.

Distribution

- Parotid gland: 84%
  - Commoner in the superficial lobe
- Submandibular gland: 8%
- Minor salivary glands: 6.5%
  - Widely distributed including the nasal cavity, pharynx, larynx, trachea
- Sublingual glands: 0.5%

They are less common in salivary glands other than the parotid but remain the most common benign tumor of each gland.

Pleomorphic adenomas are also commonly found in the lacrimal glands where they account for approximately 50% of lacrimal gland tumors.

Pathology

As the name suggests, pleomorphic adenomas are composed of a mixture of variable histology. They contain both epithelial and myoepithelial (mesenchymal) tissues, with mixed histology. They appear encapsulated and well circumscribed however the pseudocapsule is delicate and incomplete with microscopic extensions reaching beyond it, accounting for the high risk of recurrence when these tumors are enucleated.

The gross appearance depends upon the relative proportion of epithelial elements and a stromal component which may range from myxoid to cartilage. Tumors with a prominent cartilaginous matrix have a bluish-grey opalescent appearance.

Three histological types have been described:

1. Myxoid (hypocellular): Most common, highest rate of recurrence
2. Cellular
3. Classic

Radiographic Features

On all modalities, these tumors typically appear as rounded masses with well-defined, "bosselated" or "polylobulated" borders (many small undulations, not truly lobulated). They are most commonly located within the parotid gland, particularly the superficial lobe.

When they arise from the deep lobe of the parotid they can appear entirely extraparotid, seen in the prestyloid parapharyngeal space, without a fat plane between it and the parotid, and widen the stylomandibular tunnel. Pleomorphic adenomas can also arise from salivary rest cells in the parapharyngeal space itself without connection to the parotid gland.

On imaging, they commonly present as well circumscribed rounded masses, most commonly located within the parotid gland, hypoechogenic on ultrasound and bright on T2WI with homogeneous enhancement on MRI.

15. Which of the following condition shows increased serum calcitonin?

A. Addison's disease
B. Glucagonoma
C. Hyperparathyroidism
D. Cushing's syndrome

Answer: Option C. Hyperparathyroidism

Explanation:

Calcitonin secretion is stimulated by increases in the serum calcium concentration as seen in hyperparathyroidism.

Hypercalcitoninemia

Physiologic conditions	Sex
	Age
	Physical activity
Drugs	Omeprazole and similar drugs (interfere with the H^+ pump)
	Glucocorticoids
	Beta-blockers
	Glucagon
	CGRP
	Enteroglucagon
	Pancreozimine
Non-thyroid pathologies	Hypergastrinemias
	Hypercalcemias (hyperparathyroidism)
	Renal insufficiency
	Neuroendocrine tumors:
	• Pheochromocytoma
	• Paraganglioma
	• Enteropancreatic endocrine tumors
	• VIPoma
	• Insulinoma carcinoids
	• Small cell pulmonary tumor
Thyroid pathologies	Medullary carcinoma
	Chronic autoimmune thyroiditis

16. Which of the following is false regarding Glass Gow trauma score?

A. The lowest score is 3

B. The highest score is 15

C. Decerebrate posture is motor grade 3

D. In a patient with tracheal intubation the score is given as 1 with a modifier attached

Answer: Option C. Decerebrate posture is motor grade 3

Explanation:

Decerebrate posture is motor grade 2.

Motor grade 3 is decorticate posture.

The lowest possible GCS (the sum) is 3 (deep coma or death), while the highest is 15 (fully awake person).

Eye Response (E)

There are four grades starting with the most severe:

1. No opening of the eye.
2. Eye opening in response to pain stimulus. (A peripheral pain stimulus, such as squeezing the lunula area of the person's fingernail is more effective than a central stimulus such as a trapezius squeeze, due to a grimacing effect).
3. Eye opening to speech. (Not to be confused with the awakening of a sleeping person; such people receive a score of 4, not 3.)
4. Eyes opening spontaneously.

Verbal Response (V)

There are five grades starting with the most severe:

1. No verbal response.
2. Incomprehensible sounds. (Moaning but no words.)
3. Inappropriate words. (Random or exclamatory articulated speech, but no conversational exchange. Speaks words but no sentences.)
4. Confused. (The person responds to questions coherently but there is some disorientation and confusion.)
5. Oriented. (Person responds coherently and appropriately to questions such as the person's name and age, where they are and why, the year, month, etc.)

Motor Response (M)

There are six grades:

1. No motor response.
2. **Decerebrate posturing** accentuated by pain (extensor response: adduction of arm, internal rotation of shoulder, pronation of forearm and extension at elbow, flexion of wrist and fingers, leg extension, plantarflexion of foot).

3. **Decorticate posturing** accentuated by pain (flexor response: internal rotation of shoulder, flexion of forearm and wrist with clenched fist, leg extension, plantarflexion of foot).
4. Withdrawal from pain (absence of abnormal posturing; unable to lift hand past chin with supraorbital pain but does pull away when nailbed is pinched).
5. Localizes to pain (purposeful movements towards painful stimuli; e.g., brings hand up beyond chin when supraorbital pressure applied).
6. Obeys commands (the person does simple things as asked).

Generally, brain injury is classified as:

- Severe, GCS < 8–9
- Moderate, GCS 8 or 9–12 (controversial)
- Minor, GCS ≥ 13.

Tracheal intubation and severe facial/eye swelling or damage make it impossible to test the verbal and eye responses. In these circumstances, the score is given as 1 with a modifier attached (e.g. "E1c", where "c" = closed, or "V1t" where t = tube). Often the 1 is left out, so the scale reads Ec or Vt. A composite might be "GCS 5tc". This would mean, for example, eyes closed because of swelling = 1, intubated = 1, leaving a motor score of 3 for "abnormal flexion".

The GCS has limited applicability to children, especially below the age of 36 months (where the verbal performance of even a healthy child would be expected to be poor). Consequently, the Pediatric Glasgow Coma Scale was developed for assessing younger children.

17. Which of the following statement is false regarding tamoxifen?

A. It has a risk of endometrial carcinoma

B. Hormonal treatment is effective in estrogen receptor positive breast cancer

C. Tamoxifen is drug of choice for post menopausal women breast cancer and aromatase inhibitors are used for premenopausal women

D. It is given as 20 mg once a day for 5 days

Answer: Option C. Tamoxifen is drug of choice for post menopausal women breast cancer and aromatase inhibitors are used for premenopausal women

Explanation:

Tamoxifen is drug of choice for pre menopausal women breast cancer and aromatase inhibitors are used for postmenopausal women.

Hormonal therapy is administered to patient in whom the tumour expressed steroid hormone receptors, i.e., ER/PR. Those who are negative for ER/PR, will not benefit from these drugs.

The 1st line-anti-oestrogens-tamoxifen.

Commonly, tamoxifen in a dose of 20 mg is used for 5 years, to be started only after completion of chemotherapy.

It is given in premenopausal patients.

Raloxifene is an oral selective oestrogen receptor modulator (SERM) that has oestrogenic actions on bone and antioestrogen actions on the uterus and breast. It is used in the prevention of osteoporosis in postmenopausal women. Studies have proved that no specific advantage of raloxifene in the adjuvant treatment of breast cancer rather than established drugs such as tamoxifen.

Side effects and health risks of tamoxifen in women	
Common	Hot flashes and night sweats Irregular periods or spotting (uterine bleeding) Loss of sex drive Vaginal discharge Vaginal dryness or itching
Rare	Blood clots in the large veins (deep venous thrombosis) Blood clots in the lungs (pulmonary emboli) Bone loss (premenopausal women only) ***Uterine or endometrial cancer*** Cataracts Stroke

AROMATASE INHIBITORS

Aromatase is an enzyme which synthesises oestrogen.

- It converts androgens into oestrogen by process of aromatisation.
- Aromatase inhibitors inhibit this process.
- **In postmenopausal woman-oestrogen is produced in peripheral tissues such as fat, liver and muscle.**
- **Hence, drug of choice in postmenopausal patients is an aromatase inhibitor.**
- Anastrazole, letrozole, exemextane are the drugs.
- Cardiac problems, osteoporosis are side-effects.

18. Which of the following is statement is not true about chronic liver disease?

A. MELD score is used to find out whom needs liver transplantation early

B. Child Pugh has been classified into A, B and C

C. MELD score includes creatinine, ascites and bilirubin

D. PELD score includes creatinine, INR and Albumin

Answer: Option C. MELD score includes creatinine, ascites and bilirubin

Explanation:

MELD score include 3 variables (CBI): S. Creatinine, S. Bilirubin, INR.

MELD (Model for End-Stage Liver Disease) Score

MELD score is used to assess the severity of chronic liver disease.

It was initially developed to predict death within 3 months of surgery in patients that had undergone TIPS.

MELD score is currently used by United Network for Organ Sharing (UNOS) for prioritizing allocation of liver transplant.

It is 6–40 point scale.

The relative risk of mortality increases by 14% for each 1 point increase in need sure MELD score = 3.8 log(e) (S. bilirubin mg/dL) + 11.2 Log(e) (INR) + 9.6 Log(e) (S. creatinine mg/dL).

MELD score (CBI)	Creatinine, Bilirubin, INR
PELD (**P**ediatric **E**nd-stage **L**iver **D**isease) **score (BINAA)**	**B**ilirubin, **I**NR **N**utritional status, **A**ge, **A**lbumin

Child-Turcotte-Pugh Classification for Severity of Cirrhosis			
Clinical and Lab Criteria	**Points***		
	1	**2**	**3**
Encephalopathy	None	Grade 1 or 2	Grade 3 or 4
Ascites	None	Mild to moderate (diuretic responsive)	Severe (diuretic refractory)
Bilirubin (mg/dL)	<2	2-3	>3
Albumin (g/dL)	>3.5	2.8-3.5	<2.8
Prothrombin time			
Seconds prolonged or	<4	4-6	>6
International normalized ratio	<1.7	1.7-2.3	>2.3
***Child-Turcotte-Pugh Class obtained by adding score for each parameter (total points)**			
Class A = 5 to 6 points			
Class B = 7 to 9 points			
Class C = 10 to 15 points			

19. Which of the following condition shows small punched out lesions on endoscopy in lower esophagus in the immune-compromised patients?

A. Herpes simplex esophagitis
B. Corrosive esophagitis
C. CMV esophagitis
D. Candida esophagitis

Answer: Option A. Herpes simplex esophagitis

Explanation:

Characteristic endoscopic findings of HSV esophagitis are small, oval, punched out ulcers with shallow geographic coverage.

20. Which of the following condition shows serpiginous ulcers in distal esophagus with otherwise normal mucosa?

A. Herpes simplex esophagitis

B. Corrosive esophagitis

C. CMV esophagitis

D. Candida esophagitis

Answer: Option C. CMV esophagitis

Explanation:

Large, solitary, shallow, serpiginous ulcers or multiple discrete lesions appear in cytomegalovirus (CMV) esophagitis, especially in the distal esophagus. However, ulceration may not be present. For example, esophageal necrosis has also been reported in a kidney transplant patient, and shallow erosions have been found in a liver transplant patient.

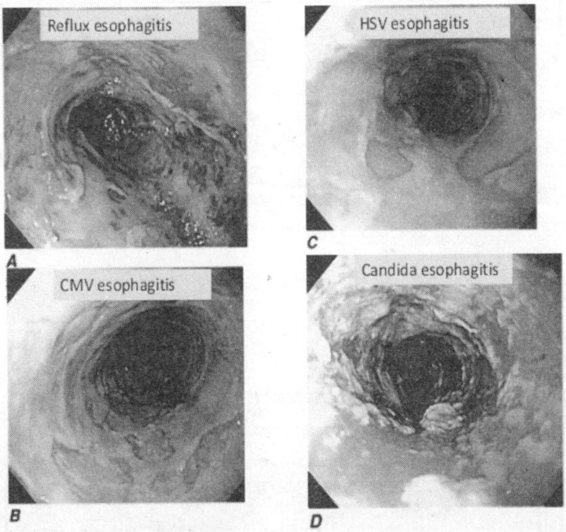

Esophagitis	Appearance
CMV	Serpiginous ulcers at distal esophagus
HSV	Volcano ulcer, punched out, small, vesicle type, lower esophagus
Eosinophilic	Circular rings, linear furrows, whitish papules and plaques (Feline esophagus)

Contd.

Contd.

Infectious	Involves proximal and diffuse ulceration
Peptic	Single and Distal esophagus
Candida	White-yellow friable plaques giving cottage-cheese appearance
Pill	Spare distal esophagus, singular and deep at point of luminal narrowing

21. A 15 weeks postnatal woman presents with fluctuant swelling in left breast with mild pain at this site, which of the following will be the treatment of this patient?

A. Incision and drainage

B. Analgesics

C. Repeated aspiration under antibiotic cover

D. Continue breastfeeding with antibiotics

Answer: Option C. Repeated aspiration under antibiotic cover

Explanation:

Here, 15 weeks postnatal woman presents with fluctuant swelling in left breast with mild pain at this site, that suggest patient has developed breast abscess. **Needle aspiration with concurrent antibiotic therapy** is currently recommended as the first line therapy for the treatment of lactational breast abscesses.

Incision and drainage is indicated only in large breast abscesses (>5 cm), abscesses with thinning or necrosis of overlying skin, failure of needle aspiration therapy and recurrent abscesses.

Lactational infections are thought to arise from entry of bacteria through the nipple into the duct system and are characterized by fever, leukocytosis, erythema and tenderness. Infections are most often caused by *Staphylococcus aureus* and may be manifested as cellulitis with breast parenchymal inflammation and swelling, termed *mastitis,* or as abscesses.

Breast Abscess

Typically seen in staphylococcal infections.

Infection starts in one segment of the breast and presents with a painful, erythematous, tender and fluctuant swelling of the breast.

Present with point tenderness, erythema and hyperthermia.

Related to lactation and occur within the first few weeks of breastfeeding.

S. aureus are transmitted via suckling neonate.

This may be associated with systemic symptoms including fever and malaise.

Staphylococcal infections **(MC)**	**Localized** and situated **deep** in the breast tissues
Streptococcal infections	**Diffuse superficial involvement**

Diagnosis

Preoperative ultrasonography is effective in delineating the required extent of the drainage procedure.

Treatment

- Management of lactational breast abscess includes general supportive measures and specific measures. The two fundamental cornerstones of specific measures include infection control and breast emptying.
- Surgical options include incision and drainage, needle aspiration and vacuum assisted biopsy. Needle aspiration with concurrent antibiotic therapy is currently recommended as the first line therapy for the treatment of lactational breast abscesses. Incision and drainage is indicated only in large breast abscesses (>5 cm), abscesses with thinning or necrosis of overlying skin, failure of needle aspiration therapy and recurrent abscesses.

22. Which of the following statement is false regarding Frey's syndrome?

A. There is aberrant misdirection of parasympathetic fibers of auriculotemporal nerve

B. There is less chances with enucleation than parotidectomy

C. Botulinum toxin is one of the treatment option

D. It is called as Gustatory sweating

Answer: Option A. There is aberrant misdirection of parasympathetic fibers of auriculotemporal nerve

Explanation:

Cross innervation between **somatic sensory supply (greater auricular)** and **parasympathetic secretomotor fibers to the parotid** is considered to be part of the anatomical basis for the phenomenon of gustatory sweating (Frey's syndrome) seen after parotid surgery, when the nerve is at risk of injury.

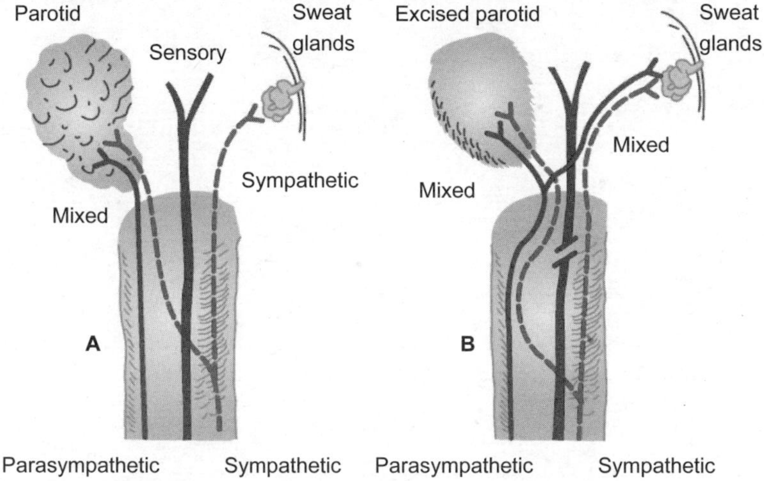

Frey's Syndrome or Auriculotemporal Syndrome (Gustatory Sweating)

It results from damage of the auriculotemporal nerve during dissection in parotidectomy.

Aberrant cross innervations between secretomotor parasympathetic fibers of the parotid gland and sympathetic fibers supplying the sweat gland.

Clinical Features

- Sweating and erythema over the region of the parotid glands as a consequence of autonomic stimulation of salivation by smell or taste of food.

Diagnosis

- Minor's starch iodine test.

Treatment

Antiperspirant (aluminium chloride) application.

Botulinum toxin treatment is used for symptomatic Frey's syndrome.

Surgical interruption of secretary fibers by tympanic neurectomy, in non-responding ca.

There is less chances of Frey's syndrome with enucleation, partial superficial parotidectomy and extracapsular dissection of parotid tumour than total parotidectomy.

23. Frey's syndrome occurs due to injury to which of the following nerve?

Or

Frey's syndrome occurs due to aberrant misdirection of fibers from salivary glands to sweat gland. Which of the following nerve is involved in this condition?

A. Glossopharyngeal nerve
B. Auriculotemporal nerve
C. Trigeminal nerve
D. Great auricular nerve

Answer: Option B. Auriculotemporal nerve

Explanation:

AURICULOTEMPORAL SYNDROME (SYN. FREY'S SYNDROME)

Partial injury to the auriculotemporal nerve gives rise to such syndrome.

This type of injury:

- May be congenital, possibly due to birth trauma.
- May be accidental injury.
- May be caused by inadvertent incision for drainage of parotid abscess.
- May occasionally follow superficial parotidectomy.

Clinical Features

There is flushing and sweating of the skin innervated by the auriculotemporal nerve particularly during meal and presence of cutaneous hyperaesthesia in front and above (the ear the area supplied by the auriculotemporal nerve). The Explanation of this syndrome is:

The postganglionic parasympathetic fibres become united to the sympathetic nerves from the superior cervical ganglion which are concerned to supply vessels and sweat glands of that region. This causes flushing and sweating of the skin.

Following injury to the auriculotemporal nerve, postganglionic parasympathetic fibres from the otic ganglion grow down the sheaths of the cutaneous filaments, so hyperaesthesia follows stimulation of the secretomotor nerves.

Treatment: If the symptoms persist, the treatment is avulsion of the auriculotemporal nerve in front of the auricle where it lies just posterior to the superficial temporal vessels.

24. A 25 years traumatic patient presets with acute breathlessness. Breath sounds are absent on one side with resonant percussion note. Which of the following statement is false regarding procedure performed in this condition?

A. Treatment consists of insertion of needle into 2nd intercostal space in the mid-clavicular line

B. Needle is inserted in lower border of upper rib to avoid injury

C. 28 french ICD tube is generally used, direction of tube insertion is superior and anterior

D. To verify that the pleural space, an index finger inserted

Answer: Option B. Needle is inserted in lower border of upper rib to avoid injury

Explanation:

Insert the large bore needle (3.25 inch, 14 gauge) into the second intercostal space in mid clavicular line at a 90-degree angle to the chest, just over the third rib. There are blood vessels running along the bottom of the ribs. **Ensure the needle is closer to the top margin upper border of the lower rib in the intercostal space**. This will prevent these vessels from being damaged.

Tension Pneumothorax

Etiology	Management
Penetrating chest trauma **Blunt chest trauma (with parenchymal injury and air leak that did not spontaneously close)**	• **Iatrogenic lung punctures** (e.g. due to **subclavian central venepuncture**) • Mechanical **positive pressure ventilation**

A tension pneumothorax develops when a 'one-way valve' air leak occurs either from the lung or through the chest wall.

Air is forced into thoracic cavity without any means of escape, completely collapsing the affected lung.

Clinical Features

The patient is panicky with tachypnoea, dyspnoea and distended neck veins (similar to pericardial tamponade).

Clinical examination can reveal tracheal deviation (a late finding – not necessary to clinically confirm diagnosis), hyperresonance and absent breath sounds over the affected hemithorax.

Diagnosis

Tension pneumothorax is a clinical diagnosis and treatment should not be delayed by waiting for radiological confirmation.

Treatment

Treatment consists of immediate decompression by rapid insertion of a large-bore needle into the 2nd intercostal space in the mid-clavicular line of the affected hemithorax.

This is immediately followed by insertion of a chest tube through the 5th intercostal space in the anterior axillary line.

If the tension in the pleural space is not relieved, the patient is likely to die from inadequate cardiac output or marked hypoxemia.

CHEST TUBE INSERTION – STANDARD METHOD

Sterile thoracotomy tube, Available sizes are 28 F, 32 F, or 36 F. Choose the tube best suited for the patient is indicated.

1. Identify the insertion site, which is usually the fourth or fifth intercostal space in the mid-to-anterior axillary line (just lateral to the nipple in males), immediately behind the lateral edge of the pectoralis major muscle. **Direct the tube as high and anteriorly as possible for a pneumothorax**. For a hemothorax, the tube is usually inserted at the level of the nipple and directed posteriorly and laterally. Elevate the head of the bed 30 to 60 degrees, and place (and restrain) the arm on the affected side over the patient's head. Do not direct the tube toward the mediastinum because contralateral pneumothorax may result. The diaphragm, liver, or spleen can be lacerated if the patient is not properly positioned or the tube is inserted too low.

2. Assemble the suction-drain system according to manufacturer's recommendations. Connect the suction system to a wall suction outlet. Adjust the suction as needed until a small, steady stream of bubbles is produced in the water column.
3. Prep the skin with povidone-iodine or Chlorhexidine solution and allow to dry. Drape the site with fenestrated sheet. Using the 10 ml syringe and 25 gauge needle, raise a skin wheal at the incision area (in the interspace one rib below the interspace chosen for the pleural insertion) with 1% solution of Lidocaine with Epinephrine.
4. Liberally infiltrate the subcutaneous tissue and intercostal muscles, including the tissue above the middle aspect of the inferior rib to the interspace where pleural entry will occur and down to the parietal pleura. Using the anesthetic needle and syringe, aspirate the pleural cavity, and check for the presence of fluid or air. If none is obtained, change the insertion site. Be careful to keep away from the inferior border of the rib to avoid the intercostal vessels.
5. Make a 2 to 3 cm transverse incision through the skin and the subcutaneous tissues overlying the interspace. Extend the incision by blunt dissection with a Kelly clamp through the fascia toward the superior aspect of the rib above. After the superior border of the rib is reached, close and turn the Kelly clamp, and push it through the parietal pleura with steady, firm, and even pressure. Open the clamp widely, close it, and then withdraw it. Be careful to prevent the tip of the clamp from penetrating the lung, especially if no chest radiograph was obtained or if the X-ray film does not clearly show that the lung is retracted from the chest wall.
6. **Insert an index finger to verify that the pleural space, not the potential space between the pleura and chest wall, has been entered.** Check for unanticipated findings, such as pleural adhesions, masses, or the diaphragm.
7. Grasp the chest tube so that the tip of the tube protrudes beyond the jaws of the clamp, and advance it through the hole into the pleural space using your finger as a guide. Direct the tip of the tube posteriorly for fluid drainage or anteriorly and superiorly for pneumothorax evacuation. Advance it until the last side hole is 2.5 to 5 cm (1 to 2 inches) inside the chest wall. Attach the tube to the previously assembled suction-drainage system. The chest tube should be inserted with the proximal hole at least 2 cm beyond the rib margin. Position of the chest tube

with all drainage holes in the pleural space should be assessed by palpation. Confirm the correct location of the chest tube by the visualization of condensation within the tube with respiration or by drained pleural fluid seen within the tube. Ask the patient to cough, and observe whether bubbles form at the water-seal level. If the tube has not been properly inserted in the pleural space, no fluid will drain, and the level in the water column will not vary with respiration.

8. Suture the tube in place with 1-0 or 2-0 silk or other nonabsorbent sutures. The two sutures are tied so as to pull the soft tissues snugly around the tube and provide an airtight seal. Tie the first suture across the incision and second suture in a horizontal mattress or purse-string stitch around the tube at the skin incision site.

25. Which of the following statement is false regarding mixed venous oxygen saturation (SvO2)?

A. SvO2 is a measure of percentage of oxygen consumption by peripheral tissue

B. Its normal value is 50-70%

C. In a patient of septic shock, SvO2 is > 70%

D. In a patient with cardiogenic shock, SvO2 is 100%

Answer: Option D. In a patient with cardiogenic shock, SvO2 is 100%

Explanation:

SvO2 are usually below normal in patients with hypovolemia (including GI hemorrhage) and cardiogenic shock, or low-flow states; they are usually high in people with distributive shock (e.g., septic shock). So **in a patient with cardiogenic shock, SvO2 is < 50%**.

Mixed venous saturation can help assess tissue oxygen delivery.

By using the derivation of the Fick equation, the mixed venous saturation (SvO2) can be determined by:

$SvO2 = SaO2 - [(VO2) / (Hb \times 1.36 \times Q)]$

SvO2: Mixed venous saturation SaO2: arterial oxygen saturation VO2: oxygen consumption Hg: hemoglobin.

The normal SvO_2 is 65-75%, which denotes tissue oxygen extraction to be 25-35%. Normal PvO_2 is 35-45 mm Hg.

Septic Shock Management

Early fluid resuscitation and vasopressor support based on the presence of hypotension and/or elevated lactate levels, and targets a MAP higher than 65 mm Hg. If this goal is unmet, CVP is targeted to 8 mm Hg or higher or a **mixed venous oxygen saturation of 70% or higher**. In the next phase, the administration of corticosteroids for septic shock, consideration of activated protein C, glucose control, and maintenance of lower ventilatory plateau pressure are addressed. For all septic patients, it must be emphasized that identification of the cause of sepsis is crucial so that eradication or source control can be carried out; without it, the elements of this bundle stand little chance of reducing septic mortality.

High SvO_2

- Increased O_2 delivery (increased FiO_2, hyperoxia, hyperbaric oxygen).
- Decreased O_2 demand (hypothermia, anaesthesia, neuromuscular blockade).
- High flow states: **sepsis**, hyperthyroidism, severe liver disease.

Low SvO_2

- Decreased O_2 delivery:
  1. Decreased Hb (anaemia, haemorrhage, dilution)
  2. Decreased SaO_2 (hypoxaemia)
  3. Decreased Q (any form of shock except septic shock, arrhythmia)
- Increased O_2 demand (hyperthermia, shivering, pain, seizures).

Causes of High SvO_2 Despite Evidence of End-organ Hypoxia

- Microvascular shunting (e.g., sepsis).
- Histotoxic hypoxia (e.g., cyanide poisoning).
- Abnormalities in distribution of blood flow.

CHAPTER 13

PEDIATRICS

1. Scissoring gait is seen in which of the following condition?

A. Neurodegenerative disorder

B.s Spastic cerebral palsy

C. Huntington's disease

D. Progressive supra nuclear palsy

Answer: Option B. Spastic cerebral palsy

Explanation:

Scissoring gait is seen in a patient of Spastic cerebral palsy.

Spastic Cerebral Palsy

This is the most common form (65%) and is topographically classified into spastic quadriparesis, diplegia or hemiparesis. Early diagnostic features of neural damage include abnormally persistent neonatal reflexes, feeding difficulties, persistent cortical thumb after 3 months age and a firm grasp. **On vertical suspension, the infant goes into scissoring due to adductor spasm with an extensor posture and does not flex his knees or thigh.** The stretch tendon reflexes are always brisk. They have variable degrees of mental and visual handicaps, seizures and behavioral problems.

Spastic quadriparesis is more common in term babies and exhibits signs including opisthotonic posture, pseudo-bulbar palsy, feeding difficulties, restricted voluntary movements and motor deficits.

Spastic diplegia is commoner in preterm babies and is associated with periventricular leukomalacia. The lower limbs are more severely affected with extension and adduction posturing, brisk tendon jerks and contractures.

Spastic hemiplegia is usually recognized after 4-6 months age. Early hand preference, abnormal persistent fisting, abnormal posture or gait disturbance may be the presenting complaint. Vascular insults, porencephaly or cerebral anomalies may be associated.

A thorough screen for associated handicaps and developmental assessment is warranted.

2. Which of the congenital disease shows severe jaundice?

A. Gilbert syndrome

B. Crigler-Najjar syndrome 1

C. Crigler-Najjar syndrome 2

D. Dubin Johnson syndrome

Answer: Option B. Crigler-Najjar syndrome 1

Explanation:

CONGENITAL ENZYME DEFICIENCIES

Crigler-Najjar syndrome (CN) type I is an autosomal recessive disorder characterized by absence of UDP-GT activity. Thus phenobarbitone has no effect (as enzyme is absent).

Patients develop severe unconjugated hyperbilirubinemia and die by 18-24 months of age if untreated. Phototherapy, plasmapheresis and exchange transfusion are required for managing these cases in initial phases. Serum bilirubin levels should be kept below 20 mg/dl during first several months of life to prevent brain damage. Definitive treatment is possible by liver transplantation, preferably auxiliary, if available.

Crigler-Najjar syndrome type II is also known as Aria syndrome. There is marked reduction of UDP-GT. In comparison to type I, jaundice is less severe and does not result in kernicterus. The condition responds to drugs like phenobarbitone that stimulate hyperplasia of the endoplasmic reticulum. The bilirubin level significantly decreases in type II CN following administration of phenobarbitone, while no change is seen in type I patients.

Gilbert syndrome is the most common cause of unconjugated hyperbilirubinemia and affects 3-8% of the population. It results from a partial deficiency of the enzyme uridine diphosphate glucuronyl transferase (UDP-GT) and thus, impaired conjugation. Most patients are asymptomatic and exhibit chronic or recurrent jaundice (up to 6 mg/dl) precipitated by intercurrent illness, fasting or stress. Mild fatigue, nausea, anorexia or abdominal pain may be present in some patients. Other liver functions remain normal. No specific treatment is necessary for this disorder.

Dubin-Johnson syndrome is an autosomal recessive disorder resulting from impaired hepatic excretion of bilirubin and causes conjugated hyperbilirubinemia (2-6 mg/dl). The transaminases and synthetic liver functions are normal. Most patients are asymptomatic apart from jaundice. Pregnancy and oral contraceptives may worsen jaundice. Liver biopsy is often done for exclusion of other causes and shows brown-black pigmentation.

Rotor syndrome is a rare, autosomal recessive disorder manifesting as mild conjugated hyperbilirubinemia. The primary defect appears to be a deficiency in the intracellular storage capacity of the liver for binding anions. The liver histology is normal.

3. An 8 years old child presented with abdominal pain, hematuria, palpable pupura and rashes at buttock showing in below image. What is the diagnosis?

A. Henoch-Schönlein Purpura

B. SLE

C. PSGN

D. Hemolytic uremic syndrome

Answer: Option A. Henoch-Schönlein Purpura

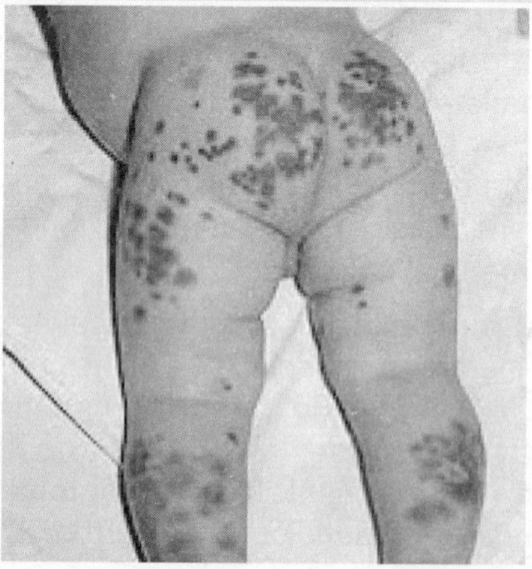

Explanation:

Here, 8 years old child presented with abdominal pain, hematuria, palpable pupura and rashes at buttock showing in above image suggest diagnosis of Henoch-Schönlein purpura.

Classification Criteria for Childhood Henoch-Schönlein Purpura

Palpable purpura in the presence of at least one of the following 4 features:

i. **Diffuse abdominal pain.**
ii. Any biopsy showing predominant IgA deposition.
iii. Arthritis or arthralgia.
iv. Renal involvement (any **hematuria** and/or proteinuria).

Henoch-Schönlein Purpura

Henoch-Schönlein purpura (HSP) is one of the most common vasculitic disorder of childhood and is characterized by the presence of a non-thrombocytopenic (and usually) palpable purpura, transient arthralgia (occasionally arthritis) and abdominal symptoms.

Henoch-Schönlein purpura is vasculitis of small vessels (capillaries, venule or arterioles) and characterized by deposition of IgA in the wall of involved vessels.

HSP is characterized by tetrad of purpura, arthritis, glomerulonephritis, and abdominal pain. Gross hematuria is seen in 2/3rd of cases. Renal manifestations usually start at the onset or within 3 months of onset of other symptoms.

The illness begins with a purpuric rash more prominent over the extensor aspects of lower extremities and buttocks. It may be macular, maculopapular or even urticaria to begin with and can be difficult to diagnose in the first few days of the illness. Glomerulonephritis is seen in approximately one-third, but only 10% patients have azotemia or nephrotic range proteinuria. Clinically, it may manifest as isolated hematuria, hypertension or a nephritic/nephrotic syndrome. This is the only long-term complication of HSP. Significant renal involvement is uncommon in children below 6 years of age.

Gastrointestinal manifestations usually occur in the first 7-10 days of the illness. Affected children may be erroneously diagnosed as having a 'surgical abdomen' and even subjected to unnecessary surgery. Abdominal pain is usually intermittent, colicky and periumbilical. Vomiting occurs in about 60% of patients but hematemesis and melena are relatively less common.

Most clinical features of HSP are self limiting and resolve in a few days. Rare manifestations include CNS vasculitis, coma, Guillain-Barré syndrome, pulmonary hemorrhage, carditis and orchitis.

Laboratory Investigations

HSP is a clinical diagnosis and none of the laboratory features are pathognomonic. There may be a nonspecific increase in total serum IgA levels. Many children may have microscopic hematuria and proteinuria. Skin biopsy from the involved sites may show the characteristic leukocytoclastic vasculitis. On indirect immunofluorescence there are deposits of IgA and C3 in skin as well as renal biopsies. Ultrasound examinations may need to be repeated at frequent intervals for evolving abdominal findings.

Treatment

Management is generally supportive with maintenance of hydration and pain relief. Prednisolone (1-1.5 mg/kg/day) is often given in children with gastrointestinal involvement and is usually continued for 2-3 weeks depending on the clinical response. There is, however, no clear evidence that steroids alter the natural course of the disease.

HSP nephritis is a serious complication and can result in chronic renal failure if not managed appropriately. There is evidence to suggest that long-term treatment with prednisolone and azathioprine can result in prolonged remissions.

Prognosis

The disease usually runs its entire course in 4 weeks and majority of the children have no permanent sequelae even when the short-term morbidity is quite significant. Children older than 6 years with significant renal involvement (especially children with rapidly progressive glomerulonephritis and fibrous crescents) need to be followed up and the long-term prognosis is guarded. Overall 1-5% of children with HSP nephritis progress to end stage renal disease.

4. Congenital infection with which virus mimics erythroblastosis fetalis?

A. Influenza B. Mumps

C. CMV D. Measles

Answer: Option C. CMV

Explanation:

Hemolytic Disease of the Newborn (HDN), also known as erythroblastosis fetalis is caused by TORCH (TORCH, which includes Toxoplasmosis, Rubella, **Cytomegalovirus (CMV)**, and Herpes infections) infection.

Hemolytic Disease of the Newborn (HDN), also known as erythroblastosis fetalis, isoimmunization, or blood group incompatibility, occurs when fetal red blood cells (RBCs), which possess an antigen that the mother lacks, cross the placenta into the maternal circulation, where they stimulate antibody production. The antibodies return to the fetal circulation and result in RBC destruction.

Differential Diagnosis of hemolytic anemia in a newborn infant:

– Isoimmunization.
– RBC enzyme disorders (e.g., G6PD, pyruvate kinase deficiency).
– Hemoglobin synthesis disorders (e.g., alpha-thalassemias).
– RBC membrane abnormalities (e.g., hereditary spherocytosis, elliptocytosis).
– Hemangiomas (Kasabach Merritt syndrome).
– **Acquired conditions, such as sepsis, infections with TORCH or Parvovirus B19 (anemia due to RBC aplasia) and hemolysis secondary to drugs.**

5. Which of the following is a stimulus for PDA closure?

A. Increase in PG E2 level

B. Increase in blood O2 level

C. Decrease in blood O2 level

D. Increase in PG E1 level

Answer: Option B. Increase in blood O2 level

Explanation:

Normal physiologic mechanisms contributing to PDA closure – increase in oxygen tension and decreased prostaglandins PGE_2 and prostacyclins (PGI_2).

The patency of the DA is primarily controlled by low fetal oxygen tension and the circulation of prostanoids produced from the metabolism of arachidonic acid by COX, with PGE_2 producing the most profound ductal relaxation among the prostanoids. Smooth muscle relaxation of the DA results from the activation of the G-coupled prostaglandin receptor EP_4 by PGE_2. Following the activation of prostaglandin receptor EP_4, a cascade of events ensues, which includes the accumulation of cyclic adenosine monophosphate, increased protein kinase A, and finally, decreased myosin light chain kinase, leading to vasodilation and ultimately DA patency. The preterm ductus is especially sensitive to the vasodilatory effects of prostaglandins, contributing to the failure of ductal closure. In term infants, as birth approaches, decreased sensitivity of the DA to prostaglandins and decreased circulating levels of PGE_2 contribute to DA closure.

Within 24–72 hours after a full-term birth, the DA closes as a result of increased oxygen tension and decreased circulating PGE_2 and prostacyclins (PGI_2). As oxygen tension increases, smooth muscle voltage-dependent potassium channels are inhibited. Through this inhibition, an influx of calcium contributes to ductal constriction. This oxygen-induced constriction fails in preterm infants potentially due to immaturity of oxygen-sensing receptors. Levels of circulating PGE_2 and PGI_2 are decreased as a result of increased metabolism in the newly functioning lung, as well as the removal of the placental source. The decreased circulating levels of these potent vasodilators allow the DA to constrict. These factors collectively contribute to smooth muscle constriction, leading to ischemic hypoxia of the inner muscle wall of the DA.

As the ductus constricts, the luminal area is diminished, resulting in a thickened vessel wall and obstructed flow through the vasa vasorum, the essential capillary network nourishing the outer cells of the vessel. This causes an increased distance of diffusion for oxygen and nutrients, including glucose, glycogen, and adenosine triphosphate (ATP), which results in nutritional deficit and oxygen starvation, leading to cell death. Ductal constriction in preterm infants is not sufficiently profound.

Consequently, preterm infants are resistant to smooth muscle hypoxia, which is paramount in triggering the cell death and remodeling required for permanent closure of the DA.Inhibition of prostaglandin and nitric oxide resulting from tissue hypoxia is not as extensive in the preterm neonate in comparison to the term infant, further contributing to resistance to DA closure in the preterm infant.

The main provider of nutrients to the DA is the lumen; however, the vasa vasorum is also a substantial provider to the outer wall of the ductus. The vasa vasorum grows toward the lumen and extends 400–500 µm from the outer wall of the ductus. The distance between the lumen and the vasa vasorum (40–500 µm) is referred to as the avascular zone and represents the maximum distance allowable for effective nutrient diffusion. In full-term infants, this avascular zone is expanded beyond the effective diffusion distance, therefore contributing to cell death. In preterm infants, the avascular zone does not sufficiently expand, resulting in cell survival and maintenance of ductal patency. If the levels of circulating PGE_2 and other prostaglandins are decreased through COX inhibition, closure is facilitated. In response to the nutritional deficit and ischemic hypoxia, vascular endothelial growth factor and transforming growth factor beta (both of which contribute to endothelial proliferation), in combination with other inflammatory mediators, contribute to the remodeling of the DA into the non-contractile ligament commonly referred to as the ligamentum arteriosum.

6. What is the best site for measurement of O_2 saturation in a patient with coarctation of aorta?

A. Right upper limb B. Right lower limb
C. Left upper limb D. Left lower limb

Answer: Option A. Right upper limb

Explanation:

Answer is by understanding that out of all four limb only right upper limb always measure true SpO_2 in a patient with coarctation of aorta (whether its pre or post ductal type). Rest of the limb measures slightly low SpO_2. Therefore SpO_2 in right upper limb will truly reflect blood oxygen circulating in brain. Therefore right upper limb is the best site for measurement of O_2 saturation in a patient with coarctation of aorta.

Coarctation of the Aorta

Coarctation of the aorta is located at the junction of the arch with the descending aorta. It is a sharp indentation involving the anterior, lateral and posterior wall of the aorta; the medial wall is spared. It may be distal or proximal to the ductus or ligamentum arteriosus and also the left subclavian artery. 40 to 80% patients have a bicuspid aortic valve.

Hemodynamics

In fetal life, the right ventricular output passes down the descending aorta through a wide ductus arteriosus.The left ventricular output empties into the innominate, left carotid and left subclavian arteries and little output reaches the descending aorta. The portion of the aorta distal to the left subclavian and before the portion where the ductus arteriosus joins is called the isthmus. At birth, the isthmus is the narrowest part of the aorta. Following closure of the ductus arteriosus, the descending aorta must receive its total supply from the left ventricle via the ascending aorta. Neonates with severe coarctation therefore become symptomatic immediately as the duct starts to close. However, a significant proportion present late.

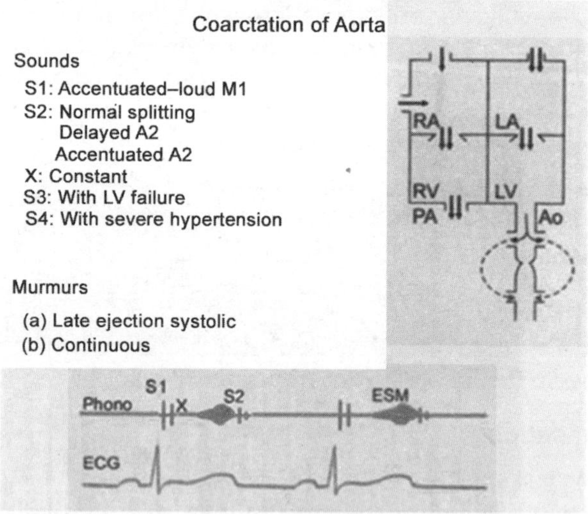

Clinical Features

Coarctation has a continuum of severity and the age at presentation is linked to severity. Newborns with severe coarctation presents as soon as the duct start to close (see duct dependent circulation). Infants with coarctation occasionally present with left ventricular dysfunction and heart failure. It is important to examine femoral pulses in newborns and infants with heart failure. Later in life, coarctation is often not associated with symptoms.

The only symptoms in uncomplicated coarctation may be intermittent claudication, pain and weakness of legs and dyspnea on running. Examination shows delayed and weak femorals compared to strong brachial arteries. The heart size remains normal with a left ventricular forcible or heaving apex. A systolic thrill may be palpable in the suprasternal notch. There are prominent arterial pulsations in the suprasternal notch and the carotid vessels. The first sound is accentuated and sometimes followed by a constant ejection click. The second sound is normally split with a loud aortic component. A variable intensity ejection systolic murmur is heard with the point of maximum intensity over the back in the interscapular area. The murmur starts late in systole after a considerable gap from the first sound and click. It may appear to go through the second sound suggesting a continuous murmur. This is because of delay in the transmission of pulse from the heart to the site of coarctation. Continuous murmurs may be audible over collaterals in the chest wall but are uncommon. An aortic ejection systolic murmur and/or an aortic regurgitation murmur may also be present because of the commonly associated bicuspid aortic valve.

Radiological Finding

(1) Abnormal aortic arch is the most common finding. Site of narrowing may be seen as an indentation. Classical, 3 Sign or 'double bulge sign' on left border of aortic shadow is formed by (above down word): pre stenotic dilatation, coarctation itself (indentation) and poststenotic dilatation.

(2) Rib notching is seen on 'inferior' border of 3'd or 4th rib downward due to enlargement of intercostals arteries (collateral vessels). Rib notching is seen in adulthood (not seen until late childhood).

Causes of Death

The causes of mortality in co-arctation of aorta are: Hypertension, Rupture of aorta, Cerebral hemorrhage (due to aneurysm rupture) Aortic dissection, Left ventricular failure, Infective endocarditis.

7. Which is the most common condition for liver transplantation in children?

A. Viral hepatitis

B. Biliary atresia

C. Choledochocele

D. Alpha -1 antitrypsin deficiency

Answer: Option B. Biliary atresia

Explanation:

Biliary atresia is most common indication for liver transplantation in pediatric age group.

"Percutaneous liver biopsy is the most valuable procedure in the evaluation of neonatal cholesteatosis."

Most common cause of neonatal cholestasis end intrahepatic neonatal cholestasis: Neonatal hepatitis.

2nd most common cause of neonatal cholestasis: Extrahepatic biliary atresia.

Most common cause of extrahepatic neonatal cholestasis; Extrahepatic biliary atresia.

3rd most common cause of neonatal cholestasis; Alpha 1 antitrypsin deficiency.

Liver Transplantation

- Liver transplantation is possible for a number of disorders. The graft is obtained either from the cadaver or can be a split graft (left lateral graft or left lobe) from a living donor. Auxiliary liver transplantation is another method where native liver is not removed and a liver graft from the donor is surgically placed in addition to the native liver. This is usually done for Crigler-Najjar type I or acute liver failure.
- **The main indications for liver transplantation are biliary atresia, fulminant hepatic failure and chronic liver disease secondary to multiple causes and hepatic tumors.** Careful selection of a blood group compatible donor is necessary, including detailed evaluation of liver functions and viral serologies. The recipient's diseased liver is removed and the new liver is transplanted, ensuring

vascular and biliary anastomoses. Patients require lifelong immunosuppression using corticosteroids, tacrolimus and mycophenolate mofetil initially and later maintenance therapy with tacrolimus. Rejection and infection are major complications following transplantation. Five-year patient survival rate exceeds 80%.

Diagnosis in Case of Biliary Atresia

Infant with pale stools, HIDA scan is not of discriminatory value as both biliary atresia and severe intrahepatic cholestasis show a nonexcretory pattern, i.e., no activity in intestine at 24 hours. Priming with UDCA or phenobarbitone for 3 days before HIDA scan improves the diagnostic efficacy of HIDA. Liver biopsy is an accurate (90-95%) test for differentiating biliary atresia from other causes of neonatal cholestasis. In biliary atresia, portal tract expansion, ductular proliferation and fibrosis is seen, whereas in neonatal hepatitis, there is alteration in lobular architecture, focal hepatocellular necrosis and giant cells formation. Laparotomy and peroperative cholangiography may be required in an infant with equivocal biopsy findings and no excretion on HIDA scan, to confirm the diagnosis of biliary atresia.

Biliary atresia is managed by Kasai procedure (hepatoportoenterostomy). The best results are obtained if it is done early (<60 days of age) and at centers with expertise. Liver transplantation is indicated in children who fail to drain bile after Kasai procedure or have progressed to end stage cirrhosis either despite surgical treatment or due to late diagnosis.

8. When will Bidextrous grasp develop in children?

A. 10 months
B. 8 months
C. 6 months
D. 4 months

Answer: Option D. 4 months

Age	Milestone
4 months	***Bidextrous grasp (reaching out for objects with both hands)***
6 months	Unidextrous grasp (reaching out for objects with one hand); transfers objects

Contd.

Contd.

9 months	Immature pincer grasp; probes with forefinger
12 months	Pincer grasp mature
15 months	Imitates scribbling; tower of 2 blocks
18 months	Scribbles; tower of 3 blocks
2 years	Tower of 6 blocks; vertical and circular stroke
3 years	Tower of 9 blocks; copies circle
4 years	Copies cross; bridge with blocks
5 years	Copies triangle; gate with blocks

9. Which of the following is a characteristic cardiac lesion in a patient of congenital Rubella syndrome?

A. Tricuspid atresia B. TAPVC

C. Pulmonary stenosis D. TGA

Answer: Option C. Pulmonary stenosis

Explanation:

Rubella causes following congenital heart disease:

- PDA (most common)

Peripheral pulmonary stenosis (2nd most common)

VSD (3rd most common))

ASD (least common)

Prenatal Exposure that Increase Risk of Congenital Heart Disease

- Gestational diabetes (transposition, atrioventricular septal defects, hypoplastic left heart, cardiomyopathy, PDA)
- Febrile illness in first trimester (increased risk)
- Lupus (complete heart block)
- Phenylketonuria (VSD, TOF, PDA, single ventricle)
- Vitamin deficiency (increased risk of heart disease)
- Teratogens (first trimester), e.g., anticonvulsants, NSAIDs, cotrimoxazole, thalidomide, retinoic acid
- Exposure to organic solvents, herbicides, pesticides, ionizing radiation.

10. Which of the following is not true about cystic fibrosis?

A. It causes biliary cirrhosis

B. Pancreatic sufficiency

C. Sweat has low chloride

D. Autosomal recessive disease

Answer: Option C. Sweat has low chloride

Explanation:

First we see, the options, which are totally right.

A. It causes biliary cirrhosis–As it causes bile duct obstruction and biliary cirrhosis.

D. Autoşomal recessive disease–Cystic fibrosis is an autosomal recessive disorder of ion transport in epithelial cells that affect fluid secretion in exocrine glands and the epithelial lining of the respiratory, gastrointestinal and reproductive tracts.

Now about option **B. Pancreatic sufficiency**–It is not totally wrong.

Approximately 10% of CF patients manifest symptoms in only a subset of the organ systems affected in PI-CF (pancreatic insufficient). This phenotype is variable and frequently milder as the majority of these patients are pancreatic sufficient (PS-CF). Diagnosis of PS-CF can be difficult due to the incomplete clinical presentation and inconclusive results of sweat chloride testing. Testing of the *CFTR* gene for mutations can aid in diagnosis, particularly in adults who present late in life with an atypical phenotype.

Option C. Sweat has low chloride is totally wrong because cystic fibrosis diagnosis is confirmed by the demonstration of a high sweat chloride (>60 mEq/1) on at least two occasions.

Common clinicalfeatures of cytic fibrosis (%)	
Age group, symptoms	**Proportion**
0-2 years	
Meconium ileus	10–15%
Obstructive jaundice	
Hypoproteinemia or anemia	

Contd.

Contd.

Bleeding diathesis	
Heat prostration or hyponatremia	
Failure to thrive	
Steatorrhoea	85%
Rectal prolapse	20%
Bronchitis or bronchiolitis	
Staphylococcal pneumonia	
2–12 years	
Malabsorption	85%
Recurrent pneumonia	60%
Nasal polyposis	6–36%
Intussusception	1–5%
> 13 years	
Chronic pulmonary disease	70%
Clubbing	
Abnormal glucose tolerance	20–30%
Diabetes mellitus	7%
Chronic intestinal obstruction	10–20%
Focal biliary cirrhois	
Portal hypertension	25%
Gallstones	4–14 %
Azoospermia	98%

CYSTIC FIBROSIS (CF)

Etiology

Mutation in the gene encoding the chloride conductance channel, CF transmembrane conductance regulator (CFTR) is the underlying cause. The failure of chloride conductance by epithelial cells leads to dehydration of secretions that are too viscid and difficult to clear. The defective gene is located at long arm of chromosome 7; the most common mutation is delta **F508.**

Clinical Features

The features depend on age of diagnosis and treatment received. The common clinical presentation includes meconium ileus in neonatal period, recurrent bronchiolitis in infancy and early childhood, recurrent lower respiratory tract infections, chronic lung disease, bronchiectasis, steatorrhoea and with increasing age pancreatitis and azoospermia. **Pancreatic insufficiency is present in >85% of CF patients.** Most common infecting organism is Pseudomonas aeruginosa in non-mucoid strain.

Diagnosis

The diagnosis should be suspected by the presence of a typical phenotype or family history and confirmed by the demonstration of a high sweat chloride (>60 mEq/1) on at least two occasions and/or by identifying CF causing mutations. Nasal potential difference measurements can be used as an adjunct to sweat test but is not widely available.

Management

The treatment of cystic fibrosis includes respiratory management, nutritional care, anticipation and early diagnosis of liver disease, diabetes and other organ dysfunction. The principles of respiratory management include airway clearance techniques, antibiotics and anti-inflammatory agents. The aim of nutrition management is to achieve normal growth and development. Nutritional management of CF includes the following measures:

- Increasing caloric intake by encouraging parents to feed the child more frequently. If appetite is poor due to persistent infection; feeding may be given by nasogastric route or by gastrostomy.
- Supplement fat soluble vitamins at twice the recommended doses. These should be given along with food and enzymes.
- Enteric coated tablets or spherules of pancreatic enzymes are given with each feed. Enzymes are started at doses of 12000 IU of lipase/kg in divided doses and increased by observing improvement in malabsorption by noting weight gain, nature of stool and abdominal symptoms.

11. Which of the following metabolic abnormalities occur in child with necrotizing enterocolitis?

A. Respiratory alkalosis, thrombocytosis, normal CRP

B. Metabolic alkalosis, thrombocytopenia, normal CRP

C. Respiratory acidosis, thrombocytosis, elevated CRP

D. Metabolic acidosis, thrombocytopenia, elevated CRP

Answer: Option D. Metabolic acidosis, thrombocytopenia, elevated CRP

Explanation:

Laboratory derangements in necrotizing enterocolitis is characterized by neutropenia, thrombocytopenia, metabolic acidosis and high C-reactive protein levels.

Signs of necrotizing enterocolitis	
Systemic	**Gastrointestinal**
Temperature instability	Abdominal distension
Lethargy	Abdominal wall discoloration
Apnea/bradycardia	Fewer stools with increased feeds
Hypotension-shock	Feeding intolerance (residuals)
Metabolic acidosis-mixed	Emesis (bilious)
Glucose instability	Carbohydrate intolerance
Left-shifted WBC differential	Positive stool clinitest
Neutropenia	Breath hydrogen elevated
Thrombocytopenia	Bloody stool
Eosinophilia	Gross blood 25%
Coagulopathy	Occult blood 25–60%
Positive blood culture	
Elevated C-reactive protein	

Necrotizing Enterocolitis

Necrotizing enterocolitis (NEC) occurs among smaller premature infants, often those less than 32 weeks. The clinical picture mimicks neonatal septicemia because of the presence of abdominal distension, apnea, bradycardia, instability of temperature, cyanosis and lethargy.

NEC is believed to result from interaction of several factors such as gut immaturity, mucosal injury due to hypoxia-ischemia, milk feeding and infection. Antenatal steroids and breastfeeding protect against NEC. Delaying enteral feeding does not prevent NEC.

Risk factors include congenital heart disease, birth asphyxia, exchange transfusion, and prolonged rupture of membranes. The underlying mechanism is believed to involve a combination of poor blood flow and infection of the intestines. Diagnosis is based on symptoms and confirmed with medical imaging.

Prevention includes the use of breast milk and probiotics. Treatment includes bowel rest, orogastric tube, intravenous fluids, and intravenous antibiotics. Surgery is required in those who have free air in the abdomen. A number of other supportive measures may also be required. Complications may include short-gut syndrome, intestinal strictures, or developmental delay.

About 7% of those that are born premature develop necrotizing enterocolitis. Onset is typically in the first four weeks of life. Among those affected, about 25% die. The sexes are affected equally frequently.

The diagnosis is usually suspected clinically but often requires the aid of diagnostic imaging modalities, most commonly radiography. Specific radiographic signs of NEC are associated with specific Bell's stages of the disease:

- **Bell's stage 1 (suspected disease):**
  - Mild systemic disease (apnea, lethargy, slowed heart rate, temperature instability)
  - Mild intestinal signs (abdominal distension, increased gastric residuals, bloody stools)
  - Non-specific or normal radiological signs
- **Bell's stage 2 (definite disease):**
  - Mild to moderate systemic signs
  - Additional intestinal signs (absent bowel sounds, abdominal tenderness)
  - Specific radiologic signs (pneumatosis intestinalis or portal venous air)

- Laboratory changes (metabolic acidosis, thrombocytopenia)

- **Bell's stage 3 (advanced disease):**
  - Severe systemic illness (low blood pressure)
  - Additional intestinal signs (striking abdominal distension, peritonitis)
  - Severe radiologic signs (pneumoperitoneum)
  - Additional laboratory changes (metabolic and respiratory acidosis, disseminated intravascular coagulation)

More recently, ultrasonography has proven to be useful as it may detect signs and complications of NEC before they are evident on radiographs, specifically in cases that involve a paucity of bowel gas, a gasless abdomen, or a sentinel loop. Diagnosis is ultimately made in 5–10% of very low-birth-weight infants (<1,500 g).

Management

Oral feeding should be withheld. A nasogastric tube is inserted to relieve distension and to aspirate stomach contents. Fluids and electrolytes in adequate quantities should be administered. Parenteral nutrition may be administered.

12. Which of the following drug Apgar score is regarded as severe?

A. 10 B. 7

C. 5 D. 3

Answer: Option D. 3

Explanation:

National Neonatology Forum of India (NNF) and WHO use an Apgar of 0-3 and 4-7, at 1 min, to define severe and moderate birth asphyxia respectively. For the community settings NNF defines asphyxia as absence of cry at 1 min and severe asphyxia as absent or inadequate breathing at five minutes.

Essential Criteria for Perinatal Asphyxia

Prolonged metabolic or mixed acidemia (pH <7.0) on an umbilical arterial blood sample.

Persistence of Apgar score of 0-3 for >5 min

Neurological manifestations, e.g., seizures, coma, hypotonia or hypoxic ischemic encephalopathy (HIE) in the immediate neonatal period.

Evidence of multiorgan dysfunction in the immediate neonatal period.

Perinatal asphyxia: Apgar score: 3 at 5 min and/or hypoxic ischemic encephalopathy.

Immediately after birth, the Apgar scores are assigned at 1 and 5 minutes. If the score is less than 7, it is assigned every 5 minutes until 20 minutes or till two successive score are 7 or greater. These scores rapidly assess the cardiopulmonary status. Apgar scores may be falsely low in infants born very preterm and those with maternal drug intake, sepsis, congenital heart disease and central nervous system malformations. Low Apgar scores are poor predictor of long-term neurodevelopmental outcome.

Role of Apgar Scores in Resuscitation

The Apgar score is an objective method of evaluating the newborn's condition. It is generally performed at 1 minute and again at 5 minutes after birth. However, resuscitation must be initiated before the 1-minute score is assigned. Therefore, the Apgar score is not used to guide the resuscitation.

While the Apgar score is not useful for decision making at the beginning of resuscitation, the change of score at sequential time points following birth can reflect how well the baby is responding to resuscitative efforts. Hence, Apgar scores should be obtained every 5 minutes for up to 20 minutes, if the 5-minute Apgar score is less than 7.

Apgar score			
Sign	**0**	**1**	**2**
Heart rate	Absent	Slow (<100 beats/min)	Normal (>100 beats/min)
Respiration	Absent	Weak cry	Good strong cry
Muscle tone	Limp	Some flexion	Active movements
Reflex irritability	No reponse	Grimace	Cough or sneeze
Color	Blue or pale	Body pink, extremities blue	Completely pink

13. Which of the following statement defines severe acute malnutrition?

A. Weight for height is less than 3 standard deviation

B. Weight for age is less than 3 standard deviation

C. Weight for height is less than 2 standard deviation

D. Weight for age is less than 2 standard deviation

Answer: Option A. Weight for height is less than 3 standard deviation

Explanation:

Severe Acute Malnutrition

Severe acute malnutrition (SAM) among children 6-59 months of age is defined by World Health Organization (WHO) and UNICEF as any of the following:

(i) **Weight-for-height below–3 standard deviation (SD or Z scores) of the median WHO growth reference.**

(ii) Visible severe wasting.

(iii) Presence of bipedal edema.

(iv) Mid upper arm circumference below 11.5 cm. This classification is used to identify children at high-risk of death.

Children having SAM require urgent attention and management in the hospital. In a child below 6 months of age, the MUAC cannot be used, and SAM should be diagnosed in the presence of (i), (ii) or (iii).

14. In a patient of 6 months old child, fast breathing is defined when respiratory rate is more than:

A. 40 B. 50

C. 60 D. 30

Answer: Option B. 50

Explanation:

According to IMNCI respiratory rate of more than 50 is considered as fast breathing in a child of 6 months age.

- Cough
- Increased respiratory rate
  - ≥ 60 if age < 2 months
  - ≥ 50 if age 2-12 months
  - ≥ 40 if age 12 months to 5 years
- Lower chest retractions
- Fever

} = Pneumonia

Following 'danger signs' in newborn when need to bring the baby to the hospital:

- Difficulty in feeding
- Convulsion
- Lethargy (movement only when stimulated)
- Fast breathing (RR >60/min)
- Severe chest indrawing
- Temperature of more than 37.5°C or below 35.5°C.

15. Which of the following is true regarding congenital rubella syndrome?

A. Associated with hydrocephalus, deafness and cerebral calcification

B. Associated with hydrocephalus, cerebral hemorrhage and chorioretinitis

C. Associated with cataract, VSD and mental retardation

D. Associated with hydrocephalus, cerebral calcification and chorioretinitis

Answer: Option C. Associated with cataract, VSD and mental retardation

Explanation:

CLINICAL FEATURES OF CONGENITAL RUBELLA SYDROME

Ear: Organ of corti– Sensorineural hearing loss most comman finding at congenital ruhella.

Heart: PDA (most common), peripheral pulmonary stenosis (2nd most common), ***VSD* (3rd most common)** ASD (least common, TOF, pulmonary artery hypoplasia.

Eye: Cataract retinopathy, microphthalmia, myopia, glaucoma.

CNS: Mental retardation spastic diplegia, microcephaly, seizures, behavioral disorders.

The skin lesion: Thrombocytopenic purpura; Blueberry muffin.

Other: IDDM, thyroid disorders, inguinal hernia, cryptorchidism, interstitial pneumonia.

Rubella or German measles (RNA virus) is transmitted by respiratory droplet exposure. Maternal Rubella infection is manifested by rash, malaise, fever, lymphadenopathy and polyarthritis. Fetal infection is by transplacental route throughout pregnancy. Risk of major anomalies when this infection occurs in first, second and third month is approximately 60%, 25% and 10%, respectively. Multisystem abnormalities are seen following congenital rubella infection. Congenital rubella syndrome (CRS) predominantly include cochlear (sensorineural deafness), cardiac (septal defects, PDA), hematologic (anemia, thrombocytopenia), liver and spleen (enlargement, jaundice), ophthalmic (cataracts, retinopathy, cloudy cornea), bone (osteopathy) and chromosomal abnormalities. **The virus predominantly affects** the fetus and is extremely teratogenic if contracted within the first trimester. **There is increased chance** of abortion, stillbirth and congenitally malformed baby. Infants born with congenital rubella shed the virus for many months and is a source of infection to others. Test for rubella specific antibody (IgM) should be done within 10 days of the exposure to know whether the patient is immune or not. Rubella specific IgG antibodies are present for life after natural infection or vaccination. **If the patient is not immune, question of therapeutic termination should be seriously considered.** Detection of viral RNA by PCR is possible. Prenatal diagnosis of rubella virus infection using PCR can be done from chorionic villi, fetal blood and amniotic fluid samples.

Active immunity can be conferred in non-immune subjects by giving live attenuated rubella virus vaccine (MMR) preferably during 11–13 years. **It is not recommended in pregnant women. When given during the child-bearing period, pregnancy should be prevented within three months by contraceptive measure.** However, if pregnancy occurs during the period, termination of pregnancy is not recommended.

Congenital Rubella

- Transmissibility is highest in the first trimester and so is the rate of fetal disease (90% at <11 weeks). The fetus is completely spared if infection occurs beyond 16 weeks. Clinical manifestations are as mentioned earlier; the classical triad of congenital rubella syndrome consists of deafness, cataract and congenital heart disease. Delayed manifestations such as diabetes mellitus and renal disease have also been described. Diagnosis is by demonstration of positive rubella IgM in cord or neonatal blood. No treatment exists. A unequivocal diagnosis of rubella in the first trimester of pregnancy is an indication for maternal termination of pregnancy. Vaccinating all children and particularly all adolescent girls against rubella is strongly recommended to reduce the burden of congenital rubella.

16. Triad of congenital toxoplasmosis:

A. Hydrocephalus, cerebral hemorrhage and chorioretinitis

B. Hydrocephalus, cerebral calcification and chorioretinitis

C. Hydrocephalus, cerebral calcification and cataract

D. Infarction, cerebral calcification and chorioretinitis

Answer: Option B. Hydrocephalus, cerebral calcification and chorioretinitis

Explanation:

In toxoplasmosis, affected baby may develop hydrocephalus, chorioretinitis, cerebral calcification, microcephaly, seizures and mental retardation.

	Toxoplasmosis	CMV	HSV	Rubella
Hydrocephalus	++	+	+	Rare
Microcephaly	++	++	+	+
Intracranial calcification	++	++	+	+/-

Toxoplasmosis

Toxoplasmosis is a protozoan infestation caused by *Toxoplasma gondii*.

Infection is transmitted through encysted organism by eating infected raw or uncooked meat or through contact with infected cat feces. It can also be acquired across the placenta. **The fetal risk of infection increases** with duration of pregnancy and is approximately 15%, 30% and 60% in the first, second and third trimesters respectively. The fetus is only at risk if the mother is seronegative. **Risk of fetal damage decreases** from 60% in first trimester to almost zero percent at the end of pregnancy. There is increased rate of abortion, IUGR and stillbirth. **During parasitemia, transplacental infection to the fetus occurs.** The presence of IgM antibody in the neonates indicates congenital infection. IgG transmitted from the mother persists for many years.

Maternal infection is mostly asymptomatic when she is immunocompetent.

Acute infection is diagnosed by detecting IgM specific antibody, high level of IgG antibody titer and detection of seroconversion for IgG from negative to positive. Neonatal infection is common (40%) when mother suffers with acute toxoplasmosis. Routine screening is usually not done. Chronic maternal toxoplasmosis is not considered to be a significant cause of recurrent abortion as parasitemia will not be repeated in subsequent pregnancies.

If current infection is confirmed the following tests are carried out: (1) Amniocentesis and cordocentesis for detection of IgM antibody in the amniotic fluid and fetal blood. PCR for T. gondii gene is also done (2) Ultrasonography findings suggestive of fetal infection are: ventriculomegaly, intracranial calcification, microcephaly, hepatosplenomegaly, ascites and IUGR at 20–22 weeks. If the fetus is infected and hydrocephalus is present, counseling for termination is to be done.

Treatment: Toxoplasmosis is a self-limited illness in an immunocompetent adult and does not require any treatment. Pyrimethamine 25 mg orally daily and oral sulfadiazine 1 gm four times a day is effective. Leucovorin is added to minimize toxicity. Four to six weeks course is usually given. Pyrimethamine is not given in the first trimester. Spiramycin (3 gm orally daily) has also been used as an alternative. Acute toxoplasmosis during pregnancy is treated with spiramycin. Extended courses may be needed in an immunocompromised patient to cure infection. Treatment to the mother reduces the risk of congenital infection and the late sequelae.

Prevention: Uncooked meat, unpasteurized milk and contact with stray cat or cat litter are to be avoided.

17. Which of the following is a true regarding Fragile X syndrome?

A Trinucleotide repeat sequence is CAG

B Females are affected in 10-20% cases

C Affected males have average IQ of 20-60

D It occurs due to gain of function mutation

Answer: Option C. Affected males have average IQ of 20-60

Explanation:

Fragile X syndrome (FXS) is a genetic disorder, symptoms often include **mild to moderate intellectual disability.**

The average IQ in males is under 60. Males are usually more affected than females. Females have a milder phenotype than males due to variability in X-inactivation.

Fragile X syndrome is estimated to occur in 1.4 in 10,000 males and **0.9 in 10,000 females (9-10%), so Females are affected in less than 10% cases**.

FXS is seen as a **loss of function disorder.**

Physical features may include a long and narrow face, large ears, flexible fingers, and large testicles. About a third of those affected have features of autism such as problems with social interactions and delayed speech. Hyperactivity is common and seizures occur in about 10%.

Fragile X syndrome is inherited in an X-linked dominant pattern.

Women with a premutation have an increased risk of having an affected child.

It is typically due to an expansion of **the CGG triplet repeat within the Fragile X mental retardation 1 (FMR1) gene on the X chromosome.** This results in not enough fragile X mental retardation protein (FMRP), which is required for the normal development of connections between neurons.

Diagnosis is by genetic testing to determine the number of CGG repeats in the FMR1 gene. Normal is between 5 and 40 repeats, fragile X syndrome occurs with more than 200, and a premutation is said to be present when a middle number of repeats occurs.

Testing for permutation carriers may allow for genetic counseling.

Inheritance

Fragile X syndrome has traditionally been considered an X-linked dominant condition with variable expressivity and possibly reduced penetrance. However, due to genetic anticipation and X-inactivation in females, the inheritance of Fragile X syndrome does not follow the usual pattern of X-linked dominant inheritance.

Before the FMR1 gene was discovered, analysis of pedigrees showed the presence of male carriers who were asymptomatic, with their grandchildren affected by the condition at a higher rate than their siblings suggesting that genetic anticipation was occurring.This tendency for future generations to be affected at a higher frequency became known as the Sherman paradox after its description in 1985. Due to this, male children often have a greater degree of symptoms than their mothers.

The explanation for this phenomenon is that male carriers pass on their premutation to all of their daughters, with the length of the FMR1 CGG repeat typically not increasing during meiosis, the cell division that is required to produce sperm.

Incidentally, males with a full mutation only pass on premutations to their daughters. However, females with a full mutation are able to pass this full mutation on, so theoretically there is a 50% chance that a child will be affected.

In addition, the length of the CGG repeat frequently does increase during meiosis in female premutation carriers due to instability and so, depending on the length of their premutation, they may pass on a full mutation to their children who will then be affected.

Repeat expansion is considered to be a consequence of strand slippage either during DNA replication or DNA repair synthesis.

Down's syndrome is the most common genetic cause of mental retardation, and fragile-X is second to Down's syndrome.

- **Most common inherited cause of mental retardation is fragile-X syndrome (because Down's syndrome is congenital cause but not inherited).**

18. Which of the following drug causes apnoea with ocular hypotension in children?

A. Timolol
B. Acetazolamide
C. Brimonidine
D. Apraclonidine

Answer: Option C. Brimonidine

Explanation:

Brimonidine can cause CNS depression and apnea in neonates and are contraindicated in children <2 years of age. It lowers intraocular pressure.

Brimonidine

Brimonidine (ALPHAGAN, others), is another clonidine derivative that is administered ocularly to lower intraocular pressure in patients with ocular hypertension or open-angle glaucoma. Brimonidine is a alpha$_2$-selective agonist that reduces intraocular pressure both by decreasing aqueous humor production and by increasing outflow. The efficacy of brimonidine in reducing intraocular pressure is similar to that of the timolol. **Unlike apraclonidine, brimonidine can cross the blood-brain barrier and can produce hypotension and sedation**, although these CNS effects are slight compared to those of clonidine. As with all alpha $_2$ agonists, this drug should be used with caution in patients with cardiovascular disease.

Ocular and skin allergies from topical epinephrine, related prodrug formulations, apraclonidine, and brimonidine are common. Brimonidine is less likely to cause ocular allergy and therefore is more commonly used.

19. Which of the following is a target SpO_2 in neonate at 3 minutes after birth?

A. 60-65%
B. 65-70%
C. 70-75%
D. 75-80%

Answer: Option C. 70-75%

Explanation:

70-75% is a target SpO_2 in neonate at 3 minutes after birth.

Targeted pre ductal SpO_2 after birth	
1 Min	60-65%
2 Min	65-70%
3 Min	**70-75%**
4 Min	**75-80%**
5 Min	80-85%
10 Min	85-95%

CHAPTER 14

OBSTETRICS AND GYNECOLOGY

1. Which is the engaging diameter of a well flexed fetus with vertex presentation?

A. Occipitofrontal
B. Suboccipitobregmatic
C. Submentovertical
D. Mentovertical

Answer: Option B. Suboccipitobregmatic

Explanation:

Varieties of Cephalic Presentations in Different Attitudes

Diameters	Attitude of Head	Presentation
1. Suboccipito-bregmatic	9.5 cm, extends from the nape of the neck to the center of the bregma	Complete flexion Vertex
2. Suboccipitofrontal	10 cm, extends from the nape of the neck to the anterior end of the anterior fontanelle or center of the sinciput	Incomplete flexion Vertex
3. Occipitofrontal	11.5 cm, extends from the occipital eminence to the root of the nose (glabella)	Marked deflexion Vertex
4. Mentovertical	14 cm, extends from the midpoint of the chin to the highest point on the sagittal suture	Partial extension Brow
5. Submentovertical	11.5 cm, extends from junction of floor of the mouth and neck to the highest point on sagittal suture	Incomplete extension Face
6. Submentobregmatic	9.5 cm, extends from junction of floor of the mouth and neck to the center of the bregma	Complete extension Face

2. Which of the following is treatment of choice in pruritus vulva with atrophic vaginitis?

A. Antibiotics

B. Local estrogen application

C. Local progesterone application

D. Local steroid application

Answer: Option B. Local estrogen application

Explanation:

Indications of estrogen therapy in menopause are:

Presence of vasomotor symptoms, prevention of **atrophic vaginitis,** urethritis and osteoporosis. Estrogen increases calcium absorption and reduces bone reabsorption.

Atrophic Vaginitis (Senile Vaginitis)

- **Vaginitis in postmenopausal women is called atrophic vaginitis**. The term is preferable to senile vaginitis.
- There is atrophy of the vulvovaginal structures due to estrogen deficiency. The vaginal defence is lost. Vaginal mucosa is thin and is more susceptible to infection and trauma. There may be desquamation of the vaginal epithelium which may lead to formation of adhesions and bands between the walls.

Clinical Features

(a) Yellowish or blood stained vaginal discharge.

(b) Discomfort, dryness, soreness in the vulva.

(c) Dyspareunia.

On Examination

(a) Evidences of pruritus vulvae.

(b) Vaginal examination is often painful and the walls are found inflamed.

Diagnosis: Senile endometritis may co-exist and **carcinoma body or the cervix should be excluded prior to therapy.**

Treatment

Improvement of general health and treatment of infection

if present should be done. Systemic estrogen therapy may be considered if there is no contraindication. This improves the vaginal epithelium, raises glycogen content, and lowers vaginal pH.

Intravaginal application of estrogen cream by an applicator is also effective. About one-third of the vaginal estrogen is systemically absorbed.

3. Best time for measurement of Nuchal translucency during antenatal period:

A. 11-14 weeks B. 22-24 weeks

C. 16-18 weeks D. 8-10 weeks

Answer: Option A. 11-14 weeks

Explanation:

Nuchal translucency—Increased fetal nuchal skin thickness (in the first trimester **11-14 weeks**) >3 mm by TVS is a strong marker for chromosomal anomalies (trisomy 21, 18, 13, triploidy and Turner's syndrome.

(See Table on the Next Page)

4. What is the value of anti-mullerian hormone in case of poor ovarian reserve?

A. 1000 ng/ml B. 100 ng/ml

C. < 1 ng/ml D. 10 ng/ml

Answer: Option C. < 1 ng/ml

Explanation:

DETECTION OF DIMINISHED OVARIAN RESERVE (DOR)

Tests for detection of DOR can indentify the women who are likely to have poor response with gonadotropin and lower pregnancy rate.

(i) Levels of cycle D3 serum FSH > 10–15 IU/L.

(ii) Levels of D3 serum estradiol > 60–80 pg/ml.

(iii) **Clomiphene Citrate Challenge Test:** Levels of D3 serum FSH and estradiol are measured. The women is given clomiphene citrate (100 mg daily from D5–D9). Serum

Q. No. 3

Prenatal Diagnosis: Biochemical and Biophysical Screening Test

	β-hCG+PAPP-A + NT	**MSAFP**	**MSAFP, hCG, uE, (Triple Test)**	**MSAFP, uE, hCG, Inhibin A**	**Soft Tissue Marker (Nuchal Translucency; Nasal Bone)**
Time (weeks)	11–14	15–20	15–18	15–20	11–14
Observation	β-hCG (↑), PAPP-A(↓)	MSAFP(↑)	MSAFP (↓); uE,↓; hCG(↑)	MSAFP (↓); uE, ↓; hCG (↑); Inhibin (↑)	Nuchal thickness (NT) > 3 mm, Nasal bone absent
Anomaly to detect	**Down's syndrome**	**Open neural tube defects**	**Down's syndrome**	**Down's syndrome**	**Down's syndrome, Turner's syndrome and other**
Comment	A cut off value 1 in 300 is screen positive	Cut-off level of 2.5 MOM can detect 90% of anencephaly, 80% open spina bifida	A cut-off value of 1 in 200 is screen positive	Detection rate is high	Detection rate of Down's syndrome is high (92%), when NT and NB are combined (see p. 515)
Detection rate	85–92%	85%	73%	85–92%	85–92%
False-positive rate	5%	3–5%	5%	0.9%	3–5%

levels of FSH is measured again on D10 and elevated values of serum FSH (more than 2 SD of the mean) are obtained.

(iv) **Levels of cycle D3 serum anti-Müllerian Hormone (AMH)**—Low (0.2–0.7 ng/ml).

(v) **Levels of basal serum inhibin B**—Low (< 40 pg/ml). However, it is not a reliable measure.

(vi) **Antral Follicle Count (AFC):** Total number of antral follicles (measuring 2–10 mm) in both the ovaries using TVS is proportional to the number of primordial follicles present in the ovaries. So a low AFC indicates poor ovarian reserve. A woman in her reproductive age, usually have 20–150 growing follicles in the ovaries at any time.

(vii) **Ovarian Volume Measurement (OVM):** Ovarian volume decreases with progressive follicular loss. Poor ovarian reserve indicates poor outcome with IVF.

Anti-Müllerian Hormone (AMH)

It is a peptide produced by the granulosa cells of primordial follicles (< 6 mm).

It causes Müllerian duct regression during male sexual differentiation.

AMH levels reflect the number of growing follicles in the ovary and it helps oocyte maturation and follicular development.

Low levels of AMH is observed with rise of FSH and E_2 levels and also with increasing age of the women (as the follicle number declines).

Estimation of serum AMH is used as a screening test of ovarian reserve.

5. Which of the following statement is true about Group B Streptococcal infection?

A. Antimicrobial prophylaxis 1 week after delivery

B. No prophylaxis is indicated

C. Antimicrobial prophylaxis 4-6 hours after delivery

D. Intrapartum antimicrobial prophylaxis 4-6 hours before delivery

Answer: Option D. Intrapartum antimicrobial prophylaxis 4-6 hours before delivery

Explanation:

INTRAPARTUM ANTIMICROBIAL PROPHYLAXIS

Prophylaxis administered 4 or more hours before delivery is highly effective (Fairlie, 2013).

Regardless of screening method, penicillin remains the first-line agent for prophylaxis, and ampicillin is an acceptable alternative. Women with a penicillin allergy and no history of anaphylaxis should be given cefazolin. Those at high risk for anaphylaxis should have antimicrobial susceptibility testing performed to exclude clindamycin resistance. Clindamycin-sensitive but erythromycin-resistant isolates should have a D-zone test performed to assess for inducible clindamycin resistance. If clindamycin resistance is confirmed, vancomycin should be administered. *Erythromycin is no longer used for penicillin-allergic patients*.

Vaginal and rectal GBS screening cultures at 35–37 weeks' gestation for ALL pregnant women (unless patient had GBS bacteriuria during the current pregnancy or a previous infant with invasive GBS disease)	
Intrapartum prophylaxis indicated	**Intrapartum prophylaxis not indicated**
• Previous infant with invasive GBS disease • GBS bacteriuria during current pregnancy • Positive GBS screening culture during current pregnancy (unless a planned cesarean delivery, in the absence of labor or amnionic membrane rupture, is performed) • Unknown GBS status (culture not done, incomplete, or results unknown) and any of the following: – Delivery at < 37 weeks' gestation – Amnionic membrane rupture in 18 hours – Intrapartum temperature 100.4F (38 °C) – Intrapartum nucleic acid amplification test (NAAT) positive for GBS	• Previous pregnancy with a positive GBS screening culture (unless a culture was also positive during the current pregnancy) • Planned cesarean delivery performed in the absence of labor or membrane rupture (regardless of maternal GBS culture status) • Negative vaginal and rectal GBS screening culture in late gestation during the current pregnancy, regardless of intrapartum risk factors

Group B streptococcal infection (GBS): Maternal infection with GBS is an important cause of high perinatal mortality. Vaginal and anorectal colonization of GBS is the main source of infection. Main risk factors for neonatal infection are prolonged rupture of membranes, preterm labor, prolonged labor and low birth weight. Neonatal infections include R.D.S., pneumonia, jaundice, hypotension, septicemia and meningitis. Neonatal mortality is about 30–40%.

Maternal complications include: Endometritis, UTI, PROM and preterm labor and wound infection. Diagnosis is made by culture of specimens obtained from vagina, perineum using a cotton swab. PCR can also be used.

Currently universal cultures for all patients is recommended (CDC, 2002) for prevention of GBS infection. Intrapartum therapy with ampicillin 2 gm initially, then 1 gm 6 hourly is effective.

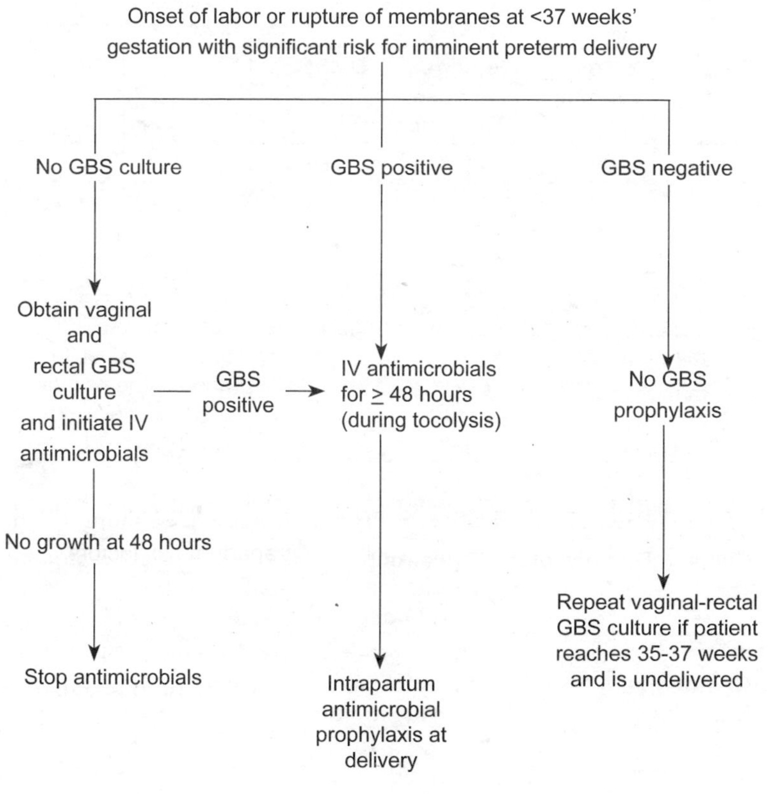

6. What is the fasting blood sugar for diagnosis of diabetes mellitus during pregnancy?

A. 200 mg B. 126 mg

C. 140 mg D. 100 mg

Answer: Option B. 126 mg

Explanation:

Fasting blood sugar for diagnosis of diabetes mellitus during pregnancy should be more than 126 mg/dl according to American Diabetes Association.

Criteria for Diagnosis of Impaired Glucose Tolerance and Diabetes with 75 gm Oral Glucose (American Diabetic Assocation)				**International Association of Diabetes and Pregnancy Study Groups (IADPSG) (75 gm Oral Glucose) (mg/dL)**	
Time	**Normal Tolerance**	**Impaired Glucose Tolerance**	**Diabetes**	**Time**	**Value**
				Fasting	92
Fasting	<100	≥ 100 and <126	≥ 126	1-hour	180
2-hour post glucose	<140	≥ 140 and <200	≥ 200	2-hour	153
• Venous whole blood values are 15% less than the plasma • m mol/1=mg% × 0.0555				Based on IADPSG, diagnosis of GDM is made if one or more thresholds are met or exceeded.	

White's Classification of Pregnant Diabetic Women				
Class	**Onset**	**Fasting plasma glucose**	**2-hour post prandial**	**Treatment**
A Gestational Diabetes	**Any Age**	**A1: Glucose <105 mg/dl** **A2: > 105 mg/dl**	**< 120 mg/dl** **> 120 mg/dl**	**Diet** **Insulin**

Class	Age of Onset	Duration (years)	Vascular Disease	Treatment
B	>20 years	<10 years	None	Insulin
C	10–19 years	10–19 years	None	Insulin
D	<10 years	>20 years	Benign retinopathy	Insulin
F	Any	Any	Nephropathy	Insulin
H	Any	Any	Coronary artery diseae	Insulin
R	Any	Any	Proliferative retinopathy	Insulin
T	Any	Any	Renal transplant	Insulin

7. Maximum contribution of amniotic fluid after 20 weeks:

A. Secretion from amniotic epithelium

B. Transudation of fetal plasma

C. Fetal urine

D. Transudation of maternal serum

Answer: Option C. Fetal urine

Explanation:

Maximum contribution of amniotic fluid after 20 weeks is by fetal urine.

<table>
<tr><th>Contribution of amniotic fluid</th><th></th></tr>
<tr><td>Transudation of maternal serum across the placental membranes</td><td rowspan="6">Fetus swallows about 500–1,000 mL of liquor every day.
Intramembranous absorption of water and solutes (200–500 mL/day) from the amniotic compartment to fetal circulation through the fetal surface of the placenta.</td></tr>
<tr><td>Transudation from fetal circulation across the umbilical cord or placental membranes</td></tr>
<tr><td>Secretion from amniotic epithelium</td></tr>
<tr><td>Transudation of fetal plasma through the highly permeable fetal skin before it is keratinized at 20th week</td></tr>
<tr><td>Fetal urine — Daily output at term is about 400–1,200 mL after 20 weeks of gestation</td></tr>
<tr><td>Fetal lung that enters the amniotic cavity add to its volume.</td></tr>
</table>

AMNIOTIC FLUID

Circulation: The water in the amniotic fluid is completely changed and **replaced in every 3 hours** as shown by the clearance of radioactive sodium injected directly into the amniotic cavity. The presence of lanugo and epithelial scales in the meconium shows that the fluid is swallowed by the fetus and some of it passes from the gut into the fetal plasma.

Volume: Amniotic fluid volume is related to gestational age. It measures about 50 mL at 12 weeks, 400 mL at 20 weeks and reaches its peak of 1 liter at 36–38 weeks. Thereafter the amount diminishes, till **at term it measures about 600–800 mL**. As the pregnancy continues post term, further reduction occurs to the extent of about 200 mL at 43 weeks.

Physical Features: The fluid is faintly alkaline with low specific gravity of 1.010. It becomes highly hypotonic to maternal serum at term pregnancy. **An osmolarity of 250 mOsmol/L is suggestive of fetal maturity**. The amniotic fluid's osmolality falls with advancing gestation.

Abnormal color: Deviation of the normal color of the liquor has got clinical significance.

Meconium stained (green) is suggestive of fetal distress in presentations other than the breech or transverse. Depending upon the degree and duration of the distress, it may be thin or thick or pea soup (thick with flakes). Thick with presence of flakes suggests chronic fetal distress.

Golden color in Rh incompatibility is due to excessive hemolysis of the fetal RBC and production of excess bilirubin.

Greenish yellow (saffron) in post maturity.

Dark colored in concealed accidental hemorrhage is due to contamination of blood.

Dark brown (tobacco juice) amniotic fluid is found in IUD. The dark color is due to frequent presence of old HbA.

8. All of the following are physiological changes in pregnancy except:

A. Decreased residual volume (RV)

B. No change in total lung capacity (TLC)

C. Increase inspiratory capacity (IC)

D. Increased FRC

Answer: Option D. Increased FRC

Explanation:

- Decreased functional residual capacity is seen, typically falling from 1.7 to 1.35 litres, due to the compression of the diaphragm by the uterus.
- The compression also causes a decreased total lung capacity (TLC) by 5% and decreased expiratory reserve volume.
- Tidal volume increases with 30-40%, from 0.45 to 0.65 litres, and minute ventilation by 30-40% giving an increase in pulmonary ventilation.
- This is necessary to meet the increased oxygen requirement of the body, which reaches 50 mL/min, 20 mL of which goes to reproductive tissues. Overall, the net change in maximum breathing capacity is zero.

Lung volume changes associated with pregnancy:

- Decreases : FRC (10-25%)
  ERV (8-40%)
  RV (7-22%)
- Increases : IC
- No change : TLC
  VC

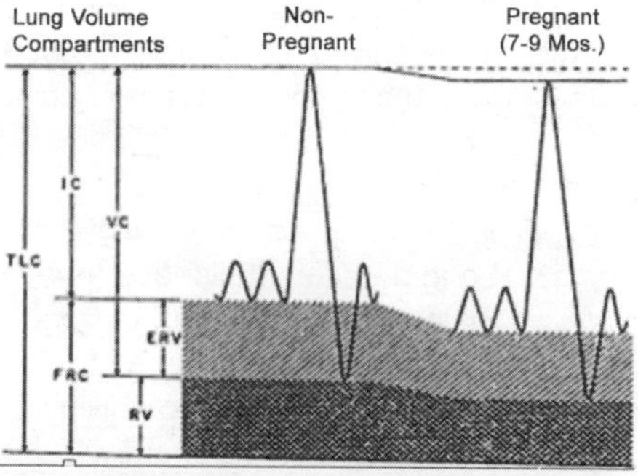

9. Which of the following is not a gestational trophoblastic disease?

A. Placental site trophoblastic tumor

B. Primary choriocarcinoma of ovary

C. Invasive mole

D. Partial mole

Answer: Option B. Primary choriocarcinoma of ovary

Explanation:

Non-gestational trophoblastic disease occurs as a primary choriocarcinoma of the ovary and is probably a teratomatous tumor.

Definition: Gestational trophoblastic disease (GTD) encompasses a spectrum of proliferative abnormalities of trophoblasts associated with pregnancy. Persistent GTD (persistently raised β-hCG) is referred as gestational trophoblastic neoplasia (GTN).

Classification of GTD
Hydatidiform mole: – Complete – Partial **Invasive mole** **Placental site trophoblastic tumor** **Choriocarcinoma** **Non metastatic disease (confined to the uterus)** **Metastatic disease** **A.** *Low risk (good prognosis)* Disease is present < 4 months duration Initial serum hCG level < 40,000 mIU/mL Metastasis limited to lung and vagina No prior chemotherapy No preceding term delivery **B.** *High risk (poor prognosis)* Long duration of disease (> 4 months) Initial serum hCG > 40,000 mIU/mL Brain or liver metastasis Failure of prior chemotherapy Following term pregnancy WHO score > 7

10. OC pill can prevent all of the following except:

A. Endometrial cancer

B. Ectopic pregnancy

C. Thromboembolic event

D. Osteoporosis

Answer: Option C. Thromboembolic event

Explanation:

Thromboembolic event is an absolute contraindications for combined OC pills according to WHO category IV.

Benefits of combined oral contraceptives

(a) ***Contraceptive benefits:***

(i) Protection against unwanted pregnancy (failure rate – 0.1 per 100 women year) (ii) Convenient to use (iii) Not intercourse related (iv) Reversibility (v) Improving maternal and child health care.

(b) ***Non-contraceptive benefits:***

Improvement of menstrual abnormalities—(1) Regulation of menstrual cycle (2) Reduction of dysmenorrhea (40%) (3) Reduction of menorrhagia (50%) (4) Reduction of premenstrual tension syndrome (PMS) (5) Reduction of Mittelschmerz's syndrome (6) Protection against iron-deficiency anemia.

Protection against health disorders— (7) Pelvic inflammatory disease (thick cervical mucus) (8) ***Ectopic pregnancy*** (9) Endometriosis (10) Fibroid uterus (11) Hirsutism and acne (12) Functional ovarian cysts (13) Benign breast disease (14) ***Osteopenia and postmenopausal osteoporotic fractures*** (15) Autoimmune disorders of thyroid (16) Rheumatoid arthritis.

Prevention of malignancies—(17) **Endometrial cancer (50%)** (18) Epithelial ovarian cancer (50%) (19) Colorectal cancer (40%).

SIDE EFFECTS AND RISKS

Breakthrough bleeding: This is slightly more common with the lower-dose pills. The women should have two pills a day for 2 or 3 days, which usually controls BTB; if not, EE 0.02 mg may be taken for 7 days along with the pills.

Oligomenorrhea happens sometimes with low-dose pills. The women should be reassured that oligomenorrhea is not harmful but rather good for health. But if they are not convinced, EE 0.02 mg may be added in the last 7 days for a few cycles.

Amenorrhea is usually temporary and not harmful. Change to triphasic pills or supplementation with EE for two to three cycles usually cures amenorrhea.

Stroke and myocardial infarction: Women who do not smoke, have their blood pressure checked, and do not have hypertension or diabetes are at no increased risk of myocardial infarction if they use low-dose COCs, irrespective of their age and duration of OC use. The risk of hemorrhagic stroke does not increase in women below 35 years of age who do not smoke and are not hypertensive. Current users of low-dose COCs have a low absolute risk of VTE mainly because incidence of VTE is very low in nonpregnant women. Nevertheless, this risk is three to six times more than nonusers. The absolute risk of VTE attributable to OC use rises with increasing age, recent surgery, and some forms of thrombophilia. Progestogens are associated with the increase of low-density lipoprotein cholesterol and a decrease of high-density cholesterol, which enhance the risk of atherosclerosis, coronary heart disease and cerebral thrombosis; but estrogens have the opposite effect, and these actions seem relatively balanced in low-dose COCs.

Breast and cervical cancer: There is a small increase in risk of current users of the pill (relative risk 1.24), and the risk reduces gradually over the 10 years after discontinuing use. Breast cancer in current or past OC users is largely localized in the breast—a condition that usually has a better prognosis. The risk of breast cancer is due to the progestogen component of the pills, as the risk is same among users of progestogen-only methods. Studies in developed and developing countries have shown a modest increase in the risk of cervical cancer (1.3–1.8-fold) among women who have used COCs for more than 5 years. However, it is not clear whether the increased risk is due to direct effect of the pill or some characteristics of the pills' users such as age at first intercourse, number of sexual partners, parity and smoking status.

Liver tumor: OCs increase the incidence of a rare benign liver tumor, namely, primary hepatocellular adenoma.

Vitamin B6 (pyridoxine) may help curing depression after OC use.

WHO Category 4: Absolute contraindications for combined OC pills	
• Active liver disease (hepatitis/ tumor) • Postpartum: breastfeeding women <6 week • Postpartum • ***Thrombophilias*** • Ischemic heart disease • Complicated migraine • Pregnancy • Complicated valvular heart disease	• Breast cancer (current or past history) • Severe hypertension (systolic >160 or diastolic >100) • DM with vascular complications • Current history of thrombo-embolism/stroke/deep vein thrombosis

11. A 25 years sexually active female presented with frothy discharge, her vaginal fluid pH is 5.4, now microscopy shows which organism?

A. Bacterial vaginosis

B. Chlamydia

C. Trichomonas vaginalis

D. Candidiasis

Answer: Option C. Trichomonas vaginalis

Explanation:

(See Table on the next page)

Vaginal trichomoniasis is the most common and important cause of vaginitis in the childbearing period.

Causative Organism: It is caused by Trichomonas vaginalis

Clinical Features

(a) There is sudden profuse and offensive vaginal discharge often dating from the last menstruation.

(b) Irritation and itching of varying degrees within and around the introitus are common.

(c) There is presence of urinary symptoms such as dysuria and frequency of micturition.

Q. No. 11

Differential Diagnosis of Vaginal Discharge

Characteristics	Trichomoniasis	Candidiasis	Bacterial vaginosis	Chlamydia	Normal vaginal discharge
Color	Greenish yellow	Curdy white	Gray white to green yellow white	Mucopurulent	White
Consistency	Thin, frothy	Thick	Thin	Thick	Thin
Whiff test (see p. 148)	Negative	Negative	Positive (Fishy amine)	Negative	Negative
pH	≥ 5	< 4.5	≥ 5	< 4.5	< 4.5
Pruritus	+++	++	Non-irritating	–	–
Diagnosis (Wet mount microscopy)	Motile Trichomonas (see p. 164)	Hyphae or spores (see p. 165)	Clue cells (> 20%) (see p. 152)	Chlamydia NAAT (see p. 150)	–
Treatment	Metronidazole 2 gm single dose or 200 mg. TID × 7 days (see p. 164)	Imidazole Fluconazole 150 mg P.O. weekly for 6 weeks	Metronidazole 200 mg. TID × 7 days (see p. 152)	Azithromycin 1 gm orally single dose (see p. 150)	–

(d) There may be history of previous similar attacks. Women with trichomoniasis should be evaluated for other STDs including *N. gonorrheae, C. trachomatis* and HIV.

On Examination

(a) There is thin, greenish-yellow and frothy offensive discharge per vaginum.

(b) The vulva is inflamed with evidences of pruritus.

(c) Vaginal examination may be painful. The vaginal walls become red and inflamed with multiple punctate hemorrhagic spots. Similar spots are also found over the mucosa of the portio vaginalis part of the cervix on speculum examination giving the appearance of 'strawberry'.

Diagnosis

(a) Identification of the trichomonas is done by hanging drop preparation. If found negative even on repeat examination, the confirmation may be done by culture.

(b) Culture of the discharge collected by swabs in Diamond's TYM or Feinberg Whittington medium.

12. Which of the following drug is a true statement regarding acute fatty liver in pregnancy?

A. It occurs late in pregnancy

B. Hyperbilirubinemia is more than 10 mg/dL

C. Abnormal carbohydrate metabolism

D. It causes hyperglycemia as complication

Answer: Option A. It occurs late in pregnancy

Explanation:

Acute Fatty Liver of Pregnancy = Acute Metamorphosis = Acute Yellow Atrophy

It occurs late in pregnancy in the third trimester or early postpartum period.

- ***Abnormal fatty acid oxidation.***
- LCHAD deficiency (long-chain hydroxyl acyl coenzyme A dehydrogenase) Microvascular steatosis with periportal sparing.

- Greasy soft yellow liver.
- ***Hyperbilirubinemia is less than 10 mg/dL.***
- Complications—Hypoglycemia, hepatic encephalopathy, coagulopathy, renal failure, mortality (10–75%), and increased risk of PIH.
- Decrease in fibrinogen and increase in ammonia and SGOT.
- Treatment—Fresh frozen plasma, cryoprecipitate, platelets and blood. Treat hepatic encephalopathy, deliver the patient.
- **Transient diabetes insipidus occurs during the period of recovery (due to elevated vasopressinase concentration).**

(See Table on the next page)

13. What is the maximum dose of 15-methyl PGF2 alpha?

A. 20 microgram
B. 200 microgram
C. 2000 microgram
D. 20 mg

Answer: Option C. 2000 microgram

Explanation:

Midtrimester termination of pregnancy

Prostaglandin $F_{2\alpha}$($PGF_{2\alpha}$), carboprost tromethamine—250 microgram IM every 3 hours for a ***maximum ten doses (2500 microgram)*** can be used. The success rate is about 90% in 36 hours. Side effects of $PGF_{2\alpha}$(nausea, vomiting, diarrhea and pain at injection site) are more. It is contraindicated in cases with bronchial asthma.

Atonic uterus: Coexistent bleeding sites from the injured area. **In refractory cases:** Injection 15 methyl $PGF_{2\alpha}$ 250 microgram IM in the deltoid muscle every 15 minutes ***(up to maximum of 2000 microgram).***

14. In all of the following condition, magnesium sulphate is useful, except:

A. Reducing RDS in newborn
B. As a tocolytic
C. It is a neuroprotector for fetus
D. Maternal eclampsia

Q. No. 12

Clinical and Laboratory Findings with Acute Liver Diseases in Pregnancy

Disorder	Onset in Pregnancy	Clinical Findings	Hepatic		Renal	Hematological and Coagulation					
			AST (U/L)	Bili (mg/dL)	Cr (mg/dL)	Hct	Plat	Fib	DD	Pt	Hemolysis
Hyperemesis	Early	Severe N & V	NL-300	NL-4	↑	↑↑	NL	NL	NL	NL	No
Choletasis	Late	Pruritus, Jaundice	NL-200	1-5	NL	NL	NL	NL	NL	NL	No
Fatty liver	**Late**	**Moderate N & V, + HTN, Liver failure**	**200-800**	**4-10**	↑↑↑	↑↑↑	↓↓	↓↓↓	↑	↑↑	↑↑↑
Preeclampsia	Mid to late	HA, HTN	NL-300	1-4	↑	↑	↓↓	NL	↑	NL	↑↑↑
Hepatitis	Variable	Jaundice	2000+	5-20	NL	↑	↓	NL	NL	↑	No

↑= increased levels; ↓= decreased levels; AST = aspartate aminotransferase; Bili = bilirubin; Cr= creatinine; DD=D-dimers; Fib=fibrinogen; HA=headache; Hct=hematocrit; HTN=hypertension; N&V=nausea and vomiting; NL=normal; Plat=platelets; PT=prothrombin time.

Answer: Option A. Reducing RDS in newborn

Explanation:

Magnesium sulfate is the drug of choice in eclampsia. It acts as a membrane stabilizer and neuroprotector. It reduces motor endplate sensitivity to acetylcholine. Magnesium also blocks neuronal calcium influx. It induces cerebral vasodilatation, dilates uterine arteries, increases production of endothelial prostacyclin and inhibits platelet activation (see p. 583). It has no detrimental effects on the neonate within therapeutic level. It has got excellent result with maternal mortality of 3%. It does not control hypertension.

Compared to other regimes, magnesium sulfate has got the following benefits: (i) it controls fits effectively without any depression effect to the mother or the infant (ii) reduced risk of recurrent convulsions (9%) (iii) significantly reduced maternal death rate (3%) and (iv) reduced perinatal mortality rate.

Magnesium sulfate (neuroprotector) to the mother to reduce neonatal cerebral palsy when pregnancy is <34 weeks. When delivery is to be done **before 32 weeks, magnesium sulfate** should be given to the mother for fetal and neonatal neuroprotection.

Use as tocolysis – Magnesium sulfate can be used if vaginal bleeding is associated with uterine contractions.

15. Which of the following is true about Gemeprost?

A. It is used in 1st trimester

B. It's a PG E1 analogue

C. It has more selective action on endometrium

D. Only act on uterus

Answer: Option B. It's a PG E1 analogue

Explanation:

Gemeprost (PGE_1 analog): 1 mg vaginal pessary every 3–6 hours for five doses in 24 hours has got about 90% success. The mean induction-abortion interval was 14–18 hours.

Prostaglandins and their analogs are very much effective. They are used extensively, specially in the second

trimester. They act on the cervix and the uterus. The PGE (dinoprostone, sulprostone, gemeprost, misoprostol) and PGF (carboprost) analogs are commonly used. PGEs are preferred as they have more selective action on the myometrium and less side effects.

16. Which of the following is diagnosis based on given below image of uterus cut section with pelvic tenderness in a 40 years old female?

A. Uterine carcinoma
B. Fibroid
C. Adenomyosis
D. Uterine polyp

Answer: Option C. Adenomyosis

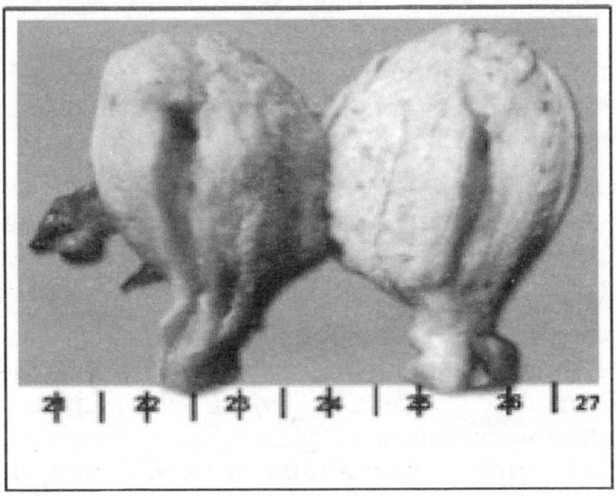

Explanation:

Here the uterus is enlarged asymmetrically, and the rounded dark areas consist of spaces full of blood. The enlargement is caused by hyperplasia of muscle cells surrounding areas of endometrium and there is thickening of the uterine wall. The cut surface presents characteristic trabeculated appearances with pelvic tenderness (due to tender uterine enlargement). **These findings are in favor of Adenomyosis**.

Leiomyoma is the most common pelvic tumor, but the majority are asymptomatic and the uterus is irregular in shape.

Uterine carcinoma presents in older women with postmenopausal bleeding and nontender uterine enlargement.

Adenomyosis is a condition in which normal endometrial glands grow into the myometrium. Symptomatic disease primarily occurs in multiparous women over the age of 35 years, compared to endometriosis, in which onset is considerably younger. Patients with adenomyosis complain of dysmenorrhea and menorrhagia, and the classical examination findings include a tender, symmetrically enlarged uterus without adnexal tenderness. Adenomyosis on USG has a Swiss cheese appearance.

Benson and Sneden's Criteria for Adenomyosis (On Histology):

Presence of endometrium within the myometrium at least two low-power field or 8 mm from basal endometrium.

Adenomyosis

Definition: Adenomyosis is a condition where there is ingrowth of the endometrium, both the glandular and stromal components, directly into the myometrium.

Causes: The cause of such ingrowth is not known. It may be related to repeated childbirths, vigorous curettage or excess of estrogen effect. Pelvic endometriosis coexists in about 40 percent.

Pathogenesis: Histologically, it is characterized by the extension of endometrial glands and stroma beneath the endometrial—myometrial interface (EMI). As the submucosa is absent, endometrial glands lie in direct contact with the underlying myometrium. It forms nests, deep within myometrium. Subsequently, threre is myometrial hyperplasia around the endometriotic foci. Myometrial zone anatomy was observed by MRI. A junctional zone (with low signal intensity on T2 weighted images) is defined at the innermost layer of myometrium. It is thought that the disturbance of normal junctional zone (JZ) predisposes to secondary infiltration of endometrial glands and stroma to inner myometrial zone. The disturbance of junctional zone (JZ) may be due to the endometrial factors, genetic predisposition or altered immune response. Trauma to the deeper endometrium (repeated curettage), causing breakdown of EMI is also taken as an important etiologic factor.

Pathology: The growth and tissue reaction in the endometrium depend on the response of the ectopic endometrial tissues to the ovarian steroids. If the basal layer is only present, the tissue reaction is much less, as it is unresponsive to hormones. But, if the functional zone is present which is responsive to hormones, the tissue reaction surrounding the endometrium is marked. There is hyperplasia of the myometrium producing diffuse enlargement of the uterus, sometimes symmetrically but at times, more on the posterior wall. The growth may be localized or may invade a polyp (adenomyomatous).

Naked Eye Appearance: There is diffuse symmetrical enlargement of the uterus; the posterior wall is often more thickened than the anterior one. The size usually does not increase more than a large orange (12–14 weeks pregnant uterus). On cut section, there is thickening of the uterine wall. The cut surface presents characteristic trabeculated appearances. **Unlike fibroid, there is no capsule surrounding the growth**. There may be visible blood spots at places.

Patient profile: The patients are usually parous with age usually above 40.

Symptoms: Menorrhagia (70%), Dysmenorrhea (30%), Dyspareunia or frequency of urination, Infertility.

Histological Examination: Histological examination reveals glandular tissue like that of endometrium surrounded by stromal cells in the myometrium. The response of the ectopic endometrial tissue to ovarian hormones is minimal as the invasion is predominantly in the basal layer.

Ultrasound and Color Doppler Characteristics are: Myometrium normally has three distinct zones of different echogenecity. The inner layer is hypoechoic relative to the middle and outer layer. This subendometrial halo is characteristic in adenomyosis. Other features are: (i) heterogenous echogenecity, (ii) hypoecoic myometrium with multiple small cysts in the myometrium (honeycomb appearance), (iii) increased vascularity within the myometrium.

Magnetic Resonance Imaging (MRI): It is more specific to the diagnosis. Low signal intensity JZ < 8 mm excludes the disease. Whereas JZ thickness > 12 mm is suggestive of adenomyosis.

Treatment: The treatment is surgical. There is little place of hormone therapy. Treatment with progestins or cyclic estrogen and progestin have got little benefit. **Levonorgestrel-releasing-IUS** (p.479) is found to improve the menorrhagia and dysmenorrhea. **Danazol**—loaded (300–400 mg) intrauterine device (IUD) is also found to improve the symptoms of menorrhagia and dysmenorrhea. Serum danozol levels were not detectable and the side effects were minimal.

Surgical Management:

(A) *Conservative surgery:*

- Adenomyomectomy
- Uterine mass reduction (Laparotomy or laparoscopy).

(B) *Hysterectomy* (parous and aged women).

17. Find out the grade of placenta previa in given below image:

A. Placenta previa type 1

B. Placenta previa type 2

C. Placenta previa type 3

D. Placenta previa type 4

Answer: Option B. Placenta previa type 2

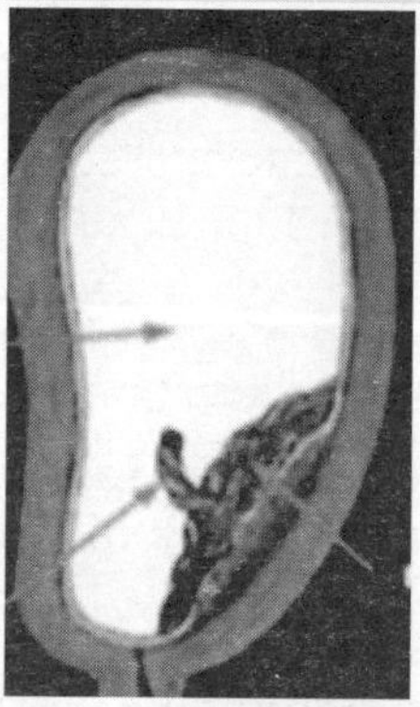

Explanation:

(2) Second degree

(Type II = P.P. marginalis):

The lower edge of the placenta reaches the margin of the internal os but does not cover it.

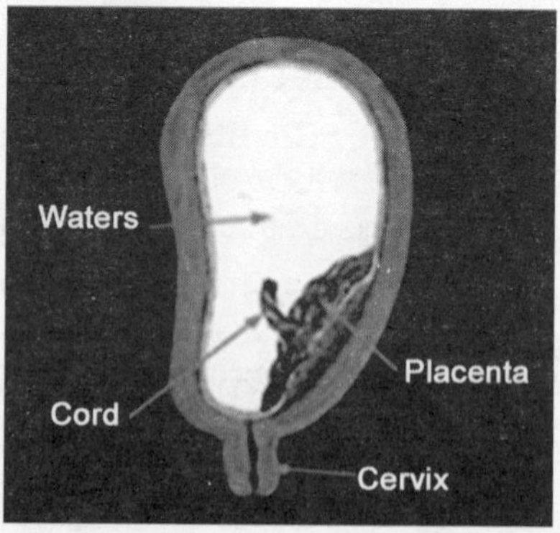

There are four types of placenta previa depending upon the degree of extension of placenta to the lower segment.

Type—I (Low-lying): The major part of the placenta is attached to the upper segment and only the lower margin encroaches onto the lower segment but not up to the os.

Type—II (Marginal): The placenta reaches the margin of the internal os but does not cover it.

Type—III (Incomplete or partial central): The placenta covers the internal os partially (covers the internal os when closed but does not entirely do so when fully dilated).

Type—IV (Central or total): The placenta completely covers the internal os even after it is fully dilated.

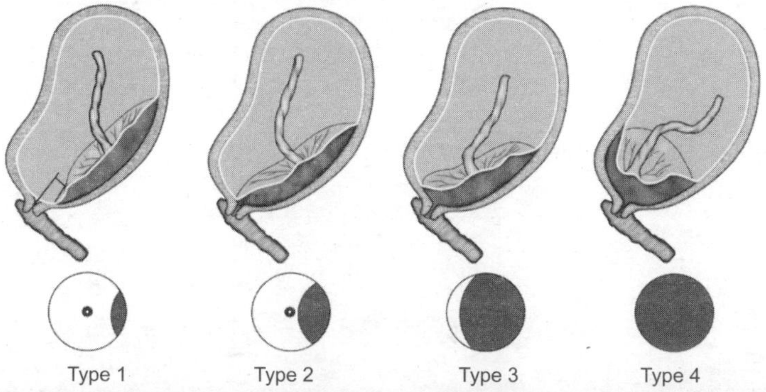

18. Which hormone is responsible for given image of uterus during menstrual cycle?

A. Estrogen
B. Progesterone
C. FSH
D. LH

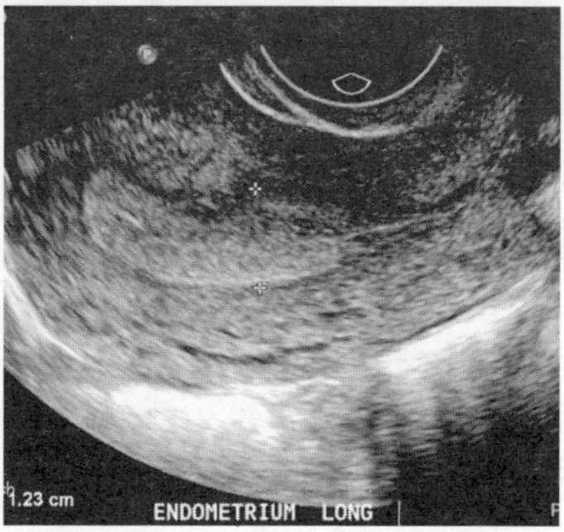

Answer: Option B. Progesterone

Explanation:

Here, above uterine USG image shows thickened (thickness is 12.3 mm), homogenous and hyperechoic endometrium which is seen during secretory phase during which progesterone is the main hormone.

Ovarian phases	Uterine (endometrial) phase	Events	Endometrium
Follicular phase (Days 1–14)	Menstrual phase (Days 1–5)	Withdrawal of the hormonal support of the endometrium at this time causes necrosis and menstruation. Low estrogens and progesterone	Hyperechoic line measuring 1 to 4 mm
	Proliferative phase (Days 6–14)	This phase is dominated by the effects of estrogen, which include the replacement of the endometrial cells lost during menses	Hyperechoic line measuring 5 to 7 mm
Ovulation (Day 14)		Characterized by the LH surge, which actually induces ovulation	Multilayered appearance with hypoechoic functional layer and hyperechoic basal layer, as well as a thin central hyperechoic layer representing overlapped or interfacing opposed layers; typically less than 11 mm
Luteal phase (Days 15–28)	**Secretory phase (Days 15–28)**	**Dominated by the elevated plasma levels of progesterone, which, along with the secreted estrogen, prepares the uterus for implantation**	**Thickened hyperechoic endometrium measuring up to 16 mm**

The normal endometrium changes in appearance as well as in thickness throughout the menstrual cycle:

- In the menstrual and early proliferative phase it is a thin, brightly echogenic stripe comprising the basal layer; minimal fluid can be appreciated endovaginally within the endometrium in the menstrual phase.
- In the late proliferative phase it develops a trilaminar appearance: outer echogenic basal layer, middle hypoechoic functional layer, and an inner echogenic stripe at the central interface.
- In the secretory phase it is at its thickest, up to 16 mm , and becomes uniformly echogenic, as the functional layer becomes oedematous and isoechoic to the basal layer; there is through transmission and posterior acoustic enhancement noted.
- The postmenopausal endometrium should be smooth and homogeneous. regular, thin hyperechoic line measuring up to 5 mm, representing the remaining basal layer of endometrium.

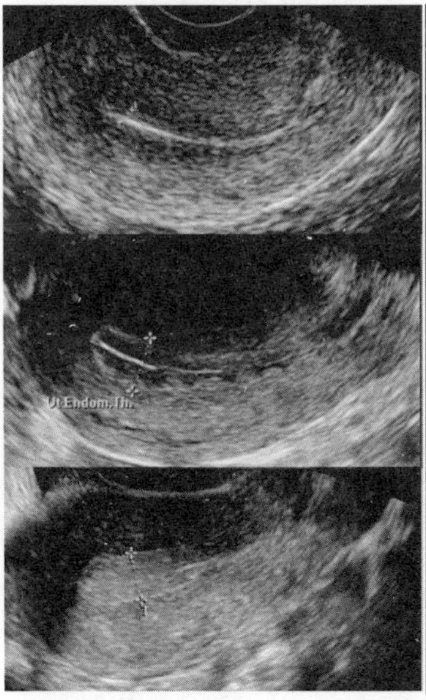

Early proliferative phase Endometrium	• Thin • Linear • Echogenic
Late proliferative phase Endometrium	• Thick • Trilaminar appearance: 1. Central thin, echogenic line 2. Darker echolucent rim in the middle 3. Surrounding echogenic basilar layer
Secretory phase Endometrium	• Thick • Hyperechoic • Homogeneous

19. Following is an image of a fetus born at 34 weeks. What disease mother may have?

A. Pre-eclampsia
B. Diabetes mellitus
C. Hypertension
D. Eclampsia

Answer: Option B. Diabetes mellitus

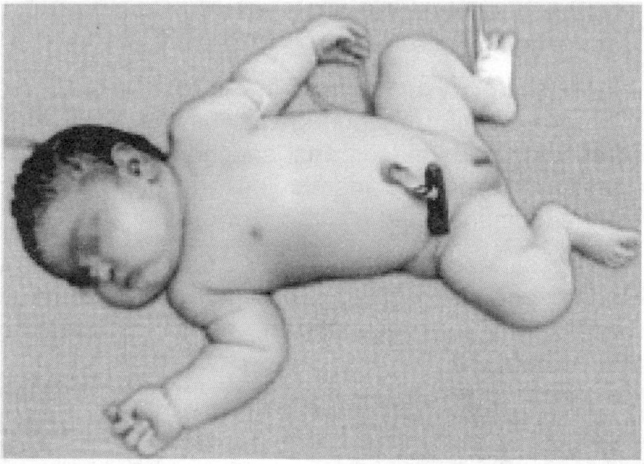

Explanation:

Above image of 34 weeks fetus is showing macrosomic baby, weighing 5.3 kg, looked plethoric (due to polycythemia), with plumpy face, buried eyes and excessive buccal fat, these features are seen in fetus of a diabetic mother.

FETAL AND NEONATAL HAZARDS:

Fetal macrosomia (40–50%) with birth weight > 4 kg (>90th percentile) probably results from:

(a) **Maternal hyperglycemia** → hypertrophy and hyperplasia of the fetal islets of langerhans → increased secretion of fetal insulin → stimulates carbohydrate utilization and accumulation of fat. Insulin like growth factors (IGF-I and II) are also involved in fetal growth and adiposity. With good diabetic control, incidence of macrosomia is markedly reduced. (b) **Elevation of maternal free fatty acid (FFA)** in diabetes leads to its increased transfer to the fetus → acceleration of triglyceride synthesis → adiposity.

Congenital malformation (6–10%) is related to these verity of diabetes affecting organogenesis, in the first trimester (both in type 1 and type 2 diabetes). **The factors associated with teratogenesis are multifactorial**: (a) Genetic susceptibility (b) Hyperglycemia (c) Arachidonic acid deficiency (d) Ketone body excess (e) Somatomedin inhibition (f) Free oxygen radical excess (superoxide dismutase, an oxygen radical scavenging enzyme can protect excess malformation). Risks of fetal chromosomal abnormalities are not increased.

Birth injuries (brachial plexus) are associated with prolonged labor and shoulder dystocia due to macrosomic baby.

Growth restriction is less commonly observed and is associated with maternal vasculopathy. Placental amino acid transporters are involved in fetal macrosomia or IUGR in women with diabetes.

Fetal death has got multifactorial pathogenesis but the final event being **hypoxia and lactic acidemia**. It is observed more in patients with poor glycemic control, vasculopathy, pre-eclampsia, ketoacidosis and fetal macrosomia. Fetal hyperglycemia and hyperinsulinemia increase fetal oxygen demand. Glycosylated hemoglobin carries less oxygen molecule. It binds O_2 more avidly and releases O_2 less. Other factors involved are fetal polycythemia and hyperviscosity.

Neonatal complications include—(a) **Hypoglycemia** (< 35 mg/dl) is due to hyperinsulinemia. It is common in macrosomic infants. (b) **Respiratory distress syndrome** is due to excess level of fetal insulin that blocks the action of cortisol. Cortisol activates type II pneumocytes for the synthesis of phospholipids (surfactant). Risk of RDS is reduced when diabetes is well controlled and delivery is done after 38 weeks of gestation (see p. 547). (c) **Hyperbilirubinemia** is high (25% to 50%) due to increased red cell production (polycythemia) and break down of red cells. (d) **Polycythemia** (e) **Hypocalcemia** (≤7 mg/dl) (f) **Hypomagnesemia** (<7 mg/dl) (g) **Cardiomyopathy** is more common when diabetes is poorly controlled. Septal hypertrophy and cardiac hypertrophy are also observed.

Long-term effects—Childhood obesity, neuropsychological effects and diabetes.

Major Birth Defects in Infants of Diabetic Mothers (6-10%)

CNS and Skeletal	Cardiovascular	Renal	Gastrointestinal	Others
• Neural tube defects	• VSD, ASD	• Renal agenesis	• Duodenal atresia	• Single umbilical artery
• Anencephaly	• Coarctation of aorta	• Hydronephrosis	• Anorectal atresia	
• Microcephaly	• Transposition of great vessels	• Double ureter	• Omphalocele	
• Caudal regression syndrome	• Situs inversus	• Polycystic kidneys	• Tracheoesophageal fistula	
• Sacral agenesis	• Fallot's tetralogy			

Good glycemic control with preconceptional counseling can reduce the incidence to 0.8-2%.

20. Testosterone is produced by which cells?

A. Granulosa cells
B. Leydig cells
C. Sertoli cells
D. Clear cells

Answer: Option B. Leydig cells

Explanation:

Leydig cells start secreting testosterone by human chorionic gonadotropin (hCG) and develop accessory organs (Wolffian duct) at eighth week.

In the male embryo, the fetal testis elaborates two substances:

(i) A Müllerian suppression substance which inhibits the development of the Müllerian ducts, Müllerian-inhibiting factor (MIF) glycoprotein secreted by the Sertoli cells of the testes.

(ii) **Testosterone derived from Leydig cells**, which is responsible for completing the development of the Wolffian structures, and fusion of the labioscrotal folds and development of the phallus, so that the external genitalia develop along the male line.

21. What is the dose of Ulipristal?

A. 300 mg
B. 3 mg
C. 30 mg
D. 0.3 mg

Answer: Option C. 30 mg

Explanation:

Ulipristal acetate as an emergency contraceptive is as effective as levonorgestrel. **A single dose 30 mg, to be taken orally as soon as possible or within 120 hours of coitus.** It acts by suppressing follicular and endometrial growth. It delays ovulation and inhibits implantation. It should not be prescribed in women with severe hepatic dysfunction nor with severe asthma.

One progesterone-receptor modulator currently available for emergency contraceptive is ulipristal acetate and is marketed as *Ella.* It is taken as a single 30 mg tablet up to 120 hours after unprotected intercourse.

The major mechanism with all hormonal regimens is inhibition or delay of ovulation. Emergency hormonal contraceptive regimens are more effective the sooner they are taken and decrease the risk of pregnancy by up to 94 percent.

22. What is the treatment of female presented with recurrent miscarriage with positive for APLA antibody?

A. Steroids
B. Aspirin only
C. Heparin only
D. Aspirin and Heparin

Answer: Option D. Aspirin and Heparin

Explanation:

Antiphospholipid antibody syndrome (APLA Syndrome): Women are treated with low-dose aspirin (50 mg/day) and heparin (5,000 units SC twice daily) up to 34 weeks. Unfractionated heparin and low molecular weight heparin (LMWH) are equally effective and safe.

In SLE antiphospholipid antibodies, e.g., lupus anticoagulant, β_2 glycoprotein, and anticardiolipin are important. These antibodies act by **dysregulation of coagulation pathways. This causes thrombosis of uteroplacental vessels and poor placental perfusion.** Obstetric complications are due to this pathology.

Antiphospholipid antibody syndrome (APAS)—is due to the presence of antiphospholipid antibodies. These are: lupus anticoagulant (LAC), anticardiolipin antibodies (ACAs) and β_2-glycoprotein 1 antibodies (Anti β_2-GP1).

Mechanisms of pregnancy loss in women with APAS are: (a) inhibition of trophoblast function and differentiation, (b) activation of complement pathway, (c) release of local inflammatory mediators (cytokines, interleukins) and (d) **thrombosis** of uteroplacental vascular bed. **Ultimate pathology is fetal hypoxia**.

Autoimmunity—Presence of **autoantibodies** causes rejection of early pregnancy (15%) in the second trimesters mainly. Antibodies responsible are: antinuclear antibodies, anti-DNA antibodies (double or single stranded) and antiphospholipid antibodies. Antiphospholipid antibody-positive women demonstrate a tendency to miscarry at progressively lower gestational ages.

23. What is the treatment of third degree of uterovaginal prolapse with cystocele and rectocele?

A Vaginal hysterectomy with pelvic floor repair

B. Fothergil's operation

C. Conservative treatment

D. Purandare sling surgery

Answer: Option A. Vaginal hysterectomy with pelvic floor repair

Explanation:

Vaginal hysterectomy with pelvic floor repair: Women above 40 years who have advanced uterine prolapse with cystorectocele, have completed their families, and are not interested in further childbearing or menstruation are fit for surgery.

SURGICAL TREATMENT FOR PROLAPSE

Age, parity status, and/type of prolapse are the factors that decide the type of surgery.

Conservative Treatment (Uterus-preserving Surgeries)

It is done for young patients desirous of further childbearing/ menstrual function.

Transvaginal

- Fothergill's operation
- Shirodkar's uterosacral ligament advancement

Abdominal (Sling Surgery/Cervicopexy)

- Purandare
- Shirodkar
- Khanna
- Virkud (composite sling)

Radical Surgery

- For old patients, family complete, postmenopausal women who are **medically fit for surgery.**
- Vaginal hysterectomy with or without anterior and posterior colporrhaphy is the best surgery.

Anterior colporrhaphy: Repair of cystocele and cystourethrocele.

Posterior colporrhaphy: Repair of rectocele and lax perineum.

1. **Fothergill's repair (Manchester operation)**: Main step is **amputation of cervix.**
   - Initially, the operation was thought to preserve the fertility status of the patient.
   - But as it is associated with many complications, it is not a preferred option nowadays.
   - Various complications include:
     a. Primary hemorrhage/secondary hemorrhage
     b. Repeated **second trimester** abortions due to **cervical incompetence**
     c. Preterm labor/PROM
     d. Cervical stenosis
     e. Cervical dystocia
     f. Infertility due to cervical factor
2. **Shirodkar's uterosacral ligament advancement surgery** (modification of Fothergill's operation): There is **no amputation of cervix,** and so the complications of Fothergill's operation are not there. It is preferred in young women desirous of further childbearing.
3. **Purandare's cervicopexy** (dynamic sling and open sling): Central part of Mersilene tape is fixed anteriorly over the exposed isthmus. The two ends of tape are attached to the **posterior rectus sheath. Good abdominal muscle tone is prerequisite for this surgery.** If the anterior abdominal tone is poor, this surgery should not be done. **Postsurgery,** the uterus becomes retroverted and the POD becomes deep. Hence, enterocele is a long-term complication of this surgery. Enterocele formation can be prevented by Moschowit's/Halban's surgery in which POD is obliterated.
4. **Shirodkar sling** (static sling): Mersilene tape is placed posteriorly on the cervix and anchored to sacral promontory (anterior longitudinal ligament). On the left side, the tape has to pass below the mesentery of sigmoid colon to reach sacral promontory. On the left side, a loop is created over the psoas muscle to avoid obstruction to the rectosigmoid.

   Complications:

   a. Injury to sigmoid colon, mesentery and ureters

b. Hemorrhage from pre-sacral/mesenteric vessels
c. Intestinal obstruction
d. Injury to genitofemoral nerve (present in psoas muscle)

5. **Khanna sling:** Mersilene tape is anchored to anterior superior iliac spine.
6. **Composite sling (Virkud):** As the complications of Shirodkar sling are mainly on the left side in this surgery, on right side the tape is attached to sacral promontory and on left side the tape is attached to rectus sheath (left-sided Purandhare + right-sided Shirodkar).
7. **Le Fort's repair (complete colpocleisis):** It is done in very elderly postmenopausal women who are unfit for major surgery (with medical complications such as heart failure, past history of myocardial infarction, severe hypertension, etc.). This procedure can be performed under local anesthesia and sedation. Prior to the procedure, PAP smear and pelvic USG should be done to rule out cervical dysplasia and pelvic pathology. Vaginal sexual activity is not possible after this surgery. If sexual function is desired, Goodell-Powel surgery (partial colpocleisis) is done (modification of Le Fort's repair).

24. Which of the following vaccine is contraindicated during pregnancy?

A. Hepatitis B. Tetanus
C. Varicella D. Rabies

Answer: Option C. Varicella

Explanation:

IMMUNIZATION

In the developing countries, immunization in pregnancy is a routine for tetanus; others are given when epidemic occurs or traveling to an endemic zone or for traveling overseas.

Live virus vaccines (rubella, measles, mumps, varicella, yellow fever) are contraindicated.

Rabies, hepatitis A and B vaccines, toxoids can be given as in nonpregnant state.

25. Which of the following is a true regarding transmission of HIV?

A. Breastfeeding is not a risk factor for transmission of HIV

B. Maternal CD4 count has no effect on transmission of HIV

C. Its transmission is directly related with maternal viral load

D. Prolonged rupture of membranes reduces transmission

Answer: Option C. Its transmission is directly related with maternal viral load

Explanation:

Risk factors for increased perinatal transmission of HIV are:

(a) ***Maternal high plasma viral load***
(b) ***Low CD4 cell count***
(c) Co-existing other STDs and opportunistic infections
(d) ***Prolonged rupture of membranes***
(e) Chorioamnionitis
(f) Invasive intrapartum procedures
(g) Preterm delivery
(h) Vaginal delivery and
(i) ***Breastfeeding.***

HUMAN IMMUNODEFICIENCY VIRUS (HIV)

Perinatal transmission of HIV: Vertical transmission to the neonates is about 14–25%. Transmission of HIV 2 is less frequent (1–4%) than for HIV 1 (15-40%). Transplacental transmission occurs: 20% before 36 weeks, over 80% of transmissions occur around the time of labor and delivery. **Vertical transmission is more in cases with preterm birth and with prolonged membrane rupture. Risks of vertical transmission is directly related to maternal viral load (measured by HIV RNA) and inversely to maternal immune status (CD^+ count).** Maternal anti-retroviral therapy reduces the risk of vertical transmission by 70%. Breastfeeding doubles the risk of MTCT transmission (14% to 28%).

Male to female transmission is about double compared to female to male transmission. Rectal intercourse is more dangerous than vaginal. Parenteral transmission is the most potent route.

Effects: Pregnancy per se has got no effect on the disease progression in HIV positive women. Increased incidence of abortion, prematurity, preeclampsia, IUGR and perinatal mortality in HIV seropositive mothers still remains inconclusive. Maternal mortality and morbidity are not increased by pregnancy.

Clinical presentation: Initial presentation of an infected patient may be fever, malaise, headache, sore throat, lymphadenopathy and maculopapular rash. Primary illness may be followed by an asymptomatic period. There may be associated constitutional symptoms like weight loss, lymphadenopathy or protracted diarrhea. CD^+ count < 200.

Diagnosis: HIV diagnosis is made by detecting HIV viral RNA in blood by PCR testing (HIV RNA PCR) or by detecting antibodies to HIV. The enzyme immunoassay (EIA) is used as a screening test for HIV antibodies. It is extremely sensitive (99.5%), inexpensive but less specific. EIA kits are commercially available. An initial positive EIA test must be confirmed with a second, more specific test Western blot or HIV RNA PCR. This is then **confirmed by Western blot, immunofluorescence assay (IFA) or HIV RNA PCR**. The western blot detects specific viral antigens P24 (Capsid), GP41 (envelope) and GP 120/160 (envelope).

Women presenting in labor; need to check her recent viral load to plan mode of delivery. Women with viral load < 400 copies/ml, neonatal infection was 1%, whereas infection rate was >30% when maternal viral load was >100,000 copies/ml.

Zidovudine (ZDV) is given IV infusion starting at the onset of labor (vaginal delivery) or 4 hours before cesarean section. loading dose 2 mg/kg/hr, maintenance dose 1 mg/kg/hr **until cord clamping is done.**

Women taking HAART can have **planned vaginal delivery** when plasma viral load is < 50 copies/ml (RCOG 2010).

Elective cesarean delivery is recommended (RCOG-2010) at 38 weeks for women taking HAART who have plasma viral load > 50 copies/ml.

Elective cesarean delivery reduces the risk of vertical transmission by about 50%. Avoidance of breastfeeding, HAART therapy and appropriate mode of delivery has reduced MTCT rates from 25–30% to <1%. Baby should be bathed immediately.

Perioperative or peripartum broad spectrum antibiotics should be given as per hospital protocol.

Invasive procedures that might result in break in the skin or mucous membrane of the infants (procedures like attachment of scalp electrode and determination of scalp blood pH) are contraindicated. Instrumentation (ventouse) is avoided.

Amniotomy and oxytocin augmentation for vaginal delivery should be avoided whenever possible.

Place of cesarean delivery to reduce MTCT: Elective CS should be done at 38 weeks gestation. CS to be done prior to onset of labor and prior to rupture of membranes if viral load is >1000 copies/ml or when viral load is unknown. ZDV IV to be started 4 hours prior to the procedure.

Health care workers should be protected from contact with potentially infected body fluids. Estimated risk of infection after parenteral or mucous membrane exposure is 0.36%.

Post exposure prophylaxis with triple therapy for 4 weeks, reduces the risk of seroconversion by more than 80% (ZDV 200 mg TDS+ lamivudin 150 mg BD + Indinavir 800 mg TDS).

26. Which is the next step in a 42 years patient suffering from heavy menstrual bleeding for 6 months and USG showing 2 cm sized intramural fibroid?

A. Bleeding time
B. Laparoscopy
C. Endometrial sampling
D. CA-125

Answer: Option C. Endometrial sampling

Explanation:

Here 42 years patient suffering from heavy menstrual bleeding for 6 months and USG showing 2 cm sized intramural fibroid. In any patient with heavy menstrual bleeding, first test is endometrial sampling and histopathological evaluation because small fibroid is unlikely to cause heavy menstrual bleeding for chronic duration. So here is the best next step is to rule out endometrial hyperplasia or carcinoma or other etiology.

- Heavy menstrual bleeding can be an early sign of endometrial cancer. Most cases of endometrial cancer are diagnosed in women in their mid 60s who are past menopause. It often is diagnosed at an early stage when treatment is the most effective.

- **Endometrial biopsy:** A sample of the endometrium is removed and looked at under a microscope. Sometimes hysteroscopy is used to guide this test. A surgical procedure called dilation and curettage (D&C) is another way this test can be done.

Progressive menorrhagia seen in intramural and submucous myoma is due to increased vascularity, endometrial hyperplasia and enlarged uterine cavity. Further away from the cavity, lesser is the possibility of menorrhagia. For this reason, subserous and pedunculated fibroids do not cause menorrhagia.

When is menstrual bleeding considered "heavy"?

Any of the following is considered to be heavy menstrual bleeding:

- Bleeding that lasts more than 7 days.
- Bleeding that soaks through one or more tampons or pads every hour for several hours in a row.
- Needing to wear more than one pad at a time to control menstrual flow.
- Needing to change pads or tampons during the night.
- Menstrual flow with blood clots that are as big as a quarter or larger.

Some of the causes include the following:

- **Cancer**–Heavy menstrual bleeding can be an early sign of endometrial cancer. Most cases of endometrial cancer are diagnosed in women in their mid 60s who are past menopause. It often is diagnosed at an early stage when treatment is the most effective.
- Fibroids and polyps.
- Adenomyosis.
- **Irregular ovulation**–If you do not ovulate regularly, areas of the ***endometrium*** (the lining of the ***uterus***) can become too thick. This condition is common during ***puberty*** and ***perimenopause***. It also can occur in women with certain medical conditions, such as ***polycystic ovary syndrome and hypothyroidism***.

- **Bleeding disorders**—When the blood does not clot properly, it can cause heavy bleeding.
- **Medications**—Blood thinners and aspirin can cause heavy menstrual bleeding. The copper ***intrauterine device (IUD)*** can cause heavier menstrual bleeding, especially during the first year of use.
- **Other causes**—***Endometriosis*** can cause heavy menstrual bleeding. Other causes include those related to pregnancy, such as ***ectopic pregnancy and miscarriage. Pelvic inflammatory disease*** also can cause heavy menstrual bleeding. Sometimes, the cause is not known.

Following tests needed:

- **Ultrasound exam**—Sound waves are used to make a picture of the pelvic organs.
- **Hysteroscopy**—A thin, lighted scope is inserted into the uterus through the opening of the ***cervix***. It allows your ob-gyn to see the inside of the uterus.
- **Endometrial biopsy**—A sample of the endometrium is removed and looked at under a microscope. Sometimes hysteroscopy is used to guide this test. A surgical procedure called ***dilation and curettage (D&C)*** is another way this test can be done.
- **Sonohysterography**—Fluid is placed in the uterus through a thin tube while ultrasound images are made of the uterus.
- **Magnetic resonance imaging**—This imaging test uses powerful magnets to create images of the internal organs.
  - In a perimenopausal women, D&C is mandatory.
  - To rule out malignancy. If benign, either hormonal therapy, ablation technique or hysterectomy will be required.
  - **Leiomyoma (AUB-L).**
  - Many leiomyomas are co-incidental findings and are not the cause of AUB.
  - Metrorrhagia in a woman over 40 requires D&C to rule out endometrial cancer, which is associated with fibroids in 3% cases.

POSTMENOPAUSAL BLEEDING PV

Never wait and watch.

Histopathological diagnosis should always be made first.

Fractional curettage (to rule out Ca cervix and Ca endometrium) is the investigation of choice.

There is no role for hormonal manipulation to control postmenopausal bleeding.

27. A multipara at 41 weeks presented with no uterine contraction, uneffaced cervix with closed OS. Which of the following drug has no role in induction?

A. PGE_1
B. PGE_2
C. PG F_2 alpha
D. Mifepristone

Answer: Option C. PG F_2 alpha

Explanation:

$PGF_{2\alpha}$ causes myometrial contraction. $PGF_{2\alpha}$ acts predominantly on the myometrium, while PGE_2 acts mainly on the cervix due to its collagenolytic property. PGE_2 is primarily important for cervical ripening whereas $PGF_{2\alpha}$ for myometrial contraction, so $PGF_{2\alpha}$ is not useful as induction of labour.

MEDICAL INDUCTION

Drugs used: Prostaglandins PGE_2, PGE_1, Oxytocin, Mifepristone.

Prostaglandins: Act locally (autocrine and paracrine hormones) on the contiguous cells. PGE_2 and $PGF_{2\alpha}$ both cause myometrial contraction. But **PGE_2 is primarily important for cervical ripening whereas $PGF_{2\alpha}$ for myometrial contraction**. **PGE_2** has greater collagenolytic properties and also sensitizes the myometrium to oxytocin. Intracervical application of dinoprostone (PGE_2 – 0.5 mg) gel is the **gold standard** for cervical ripening. It may be repeated after 6 hours for 3 or 4 doses if required. The woman should be in bed for 30 minutes following application and is monitored for uterine activity and fetal heart rate. Side effects are few.

Misoprostol (PGE_1) is currently being used either **trans-vaginally** or **orally** for induction of labor (ACOG 2003). Oral use of misoprostol is less effective than vaginal administration. A dose of 25 μg vaginally every 4 hours is found either superior or similarly effective to that of PGE_2 for cervical ripening and labor induction. With the above dose schedule, the risk of uterine hyperstimulation, meconium stained liquor and fetal heart irregularities are reduced. Total 6–8 doses are used. Buccal and sublingual use of misoprostol can avoid the first pass hepatic circulation and can maintain the serum bioavailability similar to that of vaginal use. **Side effects are:** Tachysystole, meconium passage and possibly uterine rupture. **It is contraindicated in women with previous cesarean birth.**

Oxytocin is an endogenous uterotonic that stimulates uterine contractions. Oxytocin receptors present in the myometrium are more in the fundus than in the cervix. Receptor concentrations increase during pregnancy and in labor (cf. prostaglandins). Oxytocin acts by (a) receptor mediation; (b) voltage-mediated calcium channels and (c) prostaglandin production. Because of short half life (3–4 minutes) plasma levels fall rapidly when intravenous infusion is stopped. Oxytocin is effective for induction of labor when the cervix is ripe. It is less effective as a cervical ripening agent.

Mifepristone (progesterone receptor antagonists) blocks both progesterone and glucocorticoid receptors. RU 486,200 mg vaginally daily for 2 days has been found to ripen the cervix and to induce labor. **Onapristone** is a more selective progesterone receptor antagonists.

28. Which of the following is true regarding septic pelvic thrombophlebitis?

A. Vascular intervention is required

B. Treatment is continue antibiotics and add heparin

C. Treatment is a continue antibiotics only

D. Treatment is heparin only

Answer: Option C. Treatment is a continue antibiotics only

Explanation:

(Williams Obstetrics, 25th edition, page 673)

There is no role of heparin in the management of septic pelvic thrombophlebitis.

Women with septic thrombophlebitis usually have symptomatic improvement with antimicrobial treatment, however, they continue to have fever. Although there occasionally is pain in one or both lower quadrants, patients are usually asymptomatic except for chills. Diagnosis can be confirmed by either pelvic CT or MR imaging (Klima, 2008; Sheffield, 2001). Using either, Brown and colleagues (1999) found that 20 percent of 69 women with metritis who had fever despite 5 days of appropriate antimicrobial therapy had septic pelvic thrombophlebitis.

It has been disproven that intravenous heparin causes fever to dissipate with septic phlebitis (Brown, 1986; Witlin, 1995). And although Garcia and coworkers (2006) and Klima and Snyder (2008) advocate heparin therapy, we do not recommend anticoagulation.

- Puerperal septic thrombophlebitis is likely to involve one or both ovarian venous plexuses.
- In a fourth of women, the clot extends into the inferior vena cava, and occasionally extends to the renal vein.
- Women with septic pelvic thrombophlebitis usually display some clinical improvement of their pelvic infection following antimicrobial treatment.
- When imaging modalities were not available to confirm venous involvement, "heparin challenge test" was used. If the temperature decreases on giving IV heparin, then it is diagnostic of septic pelvic thrombophlebitis.

Septic thrombophlebitis may involve either the iliofemoral or the ovarian vein but rarely involves both sites in the same patient. Vena caval thrombosis may follow either ovarian or iliofemoral phlebitis. The clinical presentation is that of a pelvic infection with pain and fever. Following antimicrobial therapy clinical symptoms usually resolve, but fever spikes may continue. Commonly patients do not appear clinically ill. The diagnosis is made by computerized tomography (CT) or by magnetic resonance imaging (MRI). Before these diagnostic modalities were available, the heparin challenge test was advocated—lysis of fever after intravenous administration of heparin was accepted as diagnostic for pelvic thrombophlebitis. It seems, however, that the course of clinical symptoms is not changed significantly by administration of heparin.

CHAPTER 15

ORTHOPEDIC

1. Foot drop occurs because of injury to which nerve?

A. Obturator nerve

B. Common peroneal nerve

C. Tibial nerve

D. Common femoral nerve

Answer: Option B. Common peroneal nerve

Explanation:

Nerve injured	Type trauma	Effect
Sciatic nerve	Posterior dislocation of the hip	Foot drop
Common peroneal nerve	***Knee dislocation/ Fracture of neck of the fibula***	***Foot drop***
Posterior interosseous nerve	Monteggia fracture	Finger drop
Radial nerve	Fracture shaft of the humerus (lower 1/3rd)	Wrist drop
Axillary nerve	Dislocation of the shoulder (Anterior and Inferior)	Deltoid palsy
Ulnar nerve	Fracture medial epicondyle humerus	Claw hand
Anterior interosseous nerve	Supra condylar fracture humerus	Kiloh nevin sign
Median nerve	Supracondylar fracture of humerus	Pointing index

Foot drop is a gait abnormality in which the dropping of the forefoot happens due to weakness, irritation or damage to the **common peroneal nerve** including the sciatic nerve, or paralysis of the muscles in the anterior portion of the lower leg. It is usually a symptom of a greater problem, not a disease in itself. Foot drop is characterized by inability or impaired ability to raise the toes or raise the foot from the ankle (dorsiflexion). Foot drop may be temporary or permanent, depending on the extent of muscle weakness or paralysis and it can occur in one or both feet. In walking, the raised leg is slightly bent at the knee to prevent the foot from dragging along the ground.

Foot drop can be caused by nerve damage alone or by muscle or spinal cord trauma, abnormal anatomy, toxins, or disease. Toxins include organophosphate compounds which have been used as pesticides and as chemical agents in warfare. The poison can lead to further damage to the body such as a neurodegenerative disorder called organ phosphorus induced delayed polyneuropathy. This disorder causes loss of function of the motor and sensory neural pathways. In this case, foot drop could be the result of paralysis due to neurological dysfunction. Diseases that can cause foot drop include trauma to the posterolateral neck of fibula, stroke, amyotrophic lateral sclerosis, muscular dystrophy, poliomyelitis, Charcot Marie Tooth disease, multiple sclerosis, cerebral palsy, hereditary spastic paraplegia, Guillain-Barré syndrome, Welander distal myopathy and Friedreich's ataxia. It may also occur as a result of hip replacement surgery or knee ligament reconstruction surgery.

Signs and Symptoms

Foot drop is characterized by steppage gait. While walking, people suffering the condition drag their toes along the ground or bend their knees to lift their foot higher than usual to avoid the dragging. This serves to raise the foot high enough to prevent the toe from dragging and prevents the slapping. To accommodate the toe drop, the patient may use a characteristic tiptoe walk on the opposite leg, raising the thigh excessively, as if walking upstairs, while letting the toe drop. Other gaits such as a wide outward leg swing (to avoid lifting the thigh excessively or to turn corners in the opposite direction of the affected limb) may also indicate foot drop.

Patients with painful disorders of sensation (dysesthesia) of the soles of the feet may have a similar gait but do not have foot drop. Because of the extreme pain evoked by even the slightest pressure on the feet, the patient walks as if walking barefoot on hot sand.

2. In a patient with painful arc syndrome, pain occurs at which part of movement?

A. Mid adduction

B. At beginning of abduction

C. Mid abduction

D. Over abduction

Answer: Option C. Mid abduction

Explanation:

Tendinitis and partial tears in the supraspinatus tendon causes a 'painful arc' since as the person elevates his arm sideways, the tendon begins to impinge under the acromion through the middle part of the arc, and this is usually relieved as the arm reaches 180 degrees (vertical).

Painful Arc Syndrome

It is anterior shoulder pain in 60–120° of glenohumeral abduction.

Most common cause is chronic supraspinatus tendinitis.

Supraspinatus tendinitis (also known as impingement syndrome and painful arc syndrome).

The classical sign of supraspinatus tendinitis is the painful arc on resisted abduction between 60 and 120 degrees when the inflamed tendon presses against the acromium – outside of this range, abduction is painless. Abduction with the arm in full external rotation is usually without pain throughout the entire range of movement.

The painful arc may also characterise a partial tear of the tendon. Weakness of resisted abduction is usually present when the tear is 2 cm or more.

Impingement syndrome can usually be diagnosed by history and examination.

- Shoulder X-rays may reveal joint pathology including acromioclavicular arthritis, variations in the acromion, and calcification.
- Ultrasound, arthrography and MRI can be used to detect rotator cuff muscle pathology.

Treatment

- Conservative treatment includes rest, cessation of painful activity and physiotherapy
  - NSAIDs and analgesia may be of benefit.
- Corticosteroid and local anaesthetic injections may be used for persistent impingement syndrome.
- Surgical treatment
  - May be done arthroscopically or as open surgery
    - ◊ Impinging structures may be removed in surgery, and the subacromial space may be widened by resection of the distal clavicle and excision of osteophytes on the under-surface of the acromioclavicular joint.
    - ◊ If surgical treatment is undertaken then damaged rotator cuff muscles can be surgically repaired.

On physical exam, the physician may twist or elevate the patient's arm to test for reproducible pain (the Neer sign and Hawkins-Kennedy test). These tests help localize the pathology to the rotator cuff; however, they are not specific for impingement. Neer sign may also be seen with subacromial bursitis.

3. In movement of neck as 'yes-yes' which of the following joint is involved?

A. Atlanto-axial

B. Atlanto-occipital

C. Between C2 and C3

D. Between C3 and C4

Answer: Option B. Atlanto-occipital

Explanation:

- **Atlanto-occipital joint:** Joint between atlas (vertebra C1) and occipital bone; movements - flexion - extension of the neck (nodding the head in **"yes" movement**).
- **Atlanto-axial joint:** Joint between atlas (C1) and axis (C2); movement: lateral rotation of atlas on axis (shaking head in **"no" movement**).

- **Ligaments of joint:** Stabilize joints and protect medulla and spinal cord; some prevent excessive movement; some are extensions of ligaments of spinal column.
  1. **Cruciate (cross) ligament:** Composed of:
     - **Transverse ligament of atlas:** Transverse band within vertebral canal which is attached to inner side of atlas; holds dens of axis against inner aspect of anterior arch of atlas.
     - **Superior and inferior bands:** Upper and lower extensions from transverse ligament of atlas to occipital bone superiorly and to body of the axis inferiorly.

     Clinical note: Tear of cruciate ligament of atlas can allow dens to be driven into spinal cord (resulting in quadriplegia) or medulla (resulting in death).
  2. **Alar ligament:** Extends laterally from dens to occipital bone; prevents excessive rotation of head.
  3. **Tectorial Membrane:** Extension of posterior longitudinal ligament of spinal column – extends from axis to occipital bone, posterior to cruciate ligament.
  4. **Anterior atlanto-occipital membrane:** Extension of anterior longitudinal ligament–extends from atlas to occipital bone.

4. A 46 years old male patient with chronic pain at upper end of right lower leg. His X-ray right leg shows lytic lesion with sclerotic margin at upper end of tibia. What is the diagnosis of this presentation?

A. Giant cell tumor
B. Brodie's abscess
C. Aneurysmal cyst
D. Metastasis

Answer: Option B. Brodie's abscess

Explanation:

Here 46 years old male patient with chronic pain at upper end of right lower leg, so based on this history we can rule out aneurysmal bone cyst (occurs before 18 years age). Now his X-ray shows lytic lesion with sclerotic margin at upper end of tibia which itself rule out giant cell tumor and metastasis (these lesion do not show sclerotic margin). So our diagnosis is Brodie's abscess which show all above mentioned features.

Brodie's abscess is an intraosseous abscess related to a focus of subacute pyogenic osteomyelitis. Unfortunately, there is no reliable way radiographically to exclude a focus of osteomyelitis. It has a protean radiographic appearance and can occur at any location and in a patient of any age. It might or might not be expansile, have a sclerotic or nonsclerotic border, or have associated periostitis.

Epidemiology

Typically these present in children with unfused epiphyseal plates, more frequently in boys.

Etiology

S. aureus (most common); cultures often negative.

Location

It has a predilection for ends (metaphysis) of tubular bones:

- Proximal/distal tibial metaphysis (most common).
- Carpal and tarsal bones.

Rarely traversing the open growth plate; epiphysis (in children and infants).

RADIOGRAPHIC FEATURES

Plain radiograph

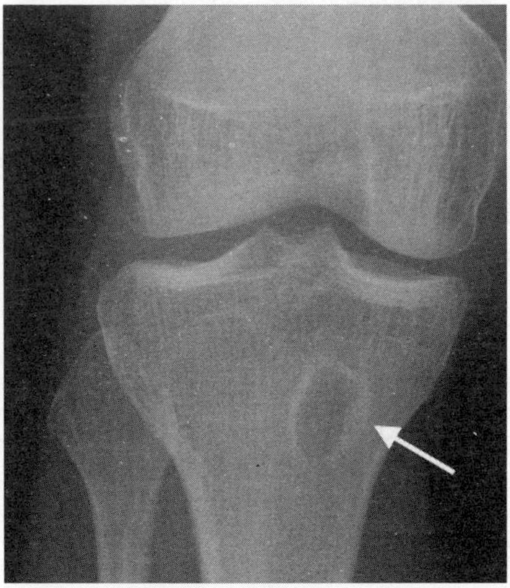

- Lytic lesion often in an oval configuration that is oriented along the long axis of the bone.
- Surrounded by a thick dense rim of reactive sclerosis that fades imperceptibly into surrounding bone.
- Lucent tortuous channel extending toward growth plate prior to physeal closure (pathognomonic).
- Periosteal new-bone formation +/- adjacent soft-tissue swelling.
- May persist for many months.

CT

- Central intramedullary hypodense cystic lesion with thick rim ossification.
- Extensive thick well-circumscribed periosteal reaction and bone sclerosis around the lesion could be seen.

MRI

The "penumbra sign" on magnetic resonance (MR) imaging is useful for discriminating subacute osteomyelitis from other bone lesions. The penumbra sign is a rim lining of an abscess cavity with higher signal intensity than that of the main abscess on T1-weighted images.

Differential Diagnosis

In some situations consider osteoid osteoma.

5. Which is the common site for avascular necrosis in a patient with scaphoid injury?

A. Proximal pole
B. Mid pole
C. Distal pole
D. Waist

Answer: Option A. Proximal pole

Explanation:

Avascular Necrosis

Risk of scaphoid non union and AVN is dependent on the location of the fracture, due to the ***retrograde dorsal arterial supply (from distal to proximal).***

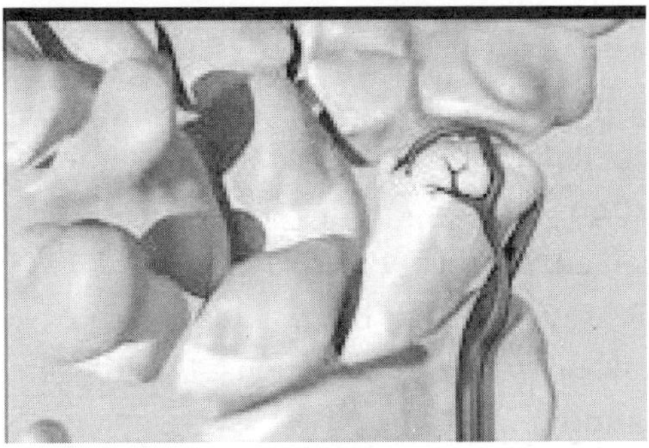

- **Proximal pole** fractures have a high risk of AVN (30%), up to 100% in proximal 1/5 fractures.
- Waist fractures, uncommon.
- Distal pole fractures, rare.
- Occurs in 15-30% of scaphoid fractures.
- Almost always involves proximal pole.
- The more proximal is the fracture line, the risks of avascular necrosis increase.
- The radiographic hallmarks of AVN are collapse and fragmentation.
- MRI may be more sensitive to AVN than conventional radiographs but is not 100% sensitive.

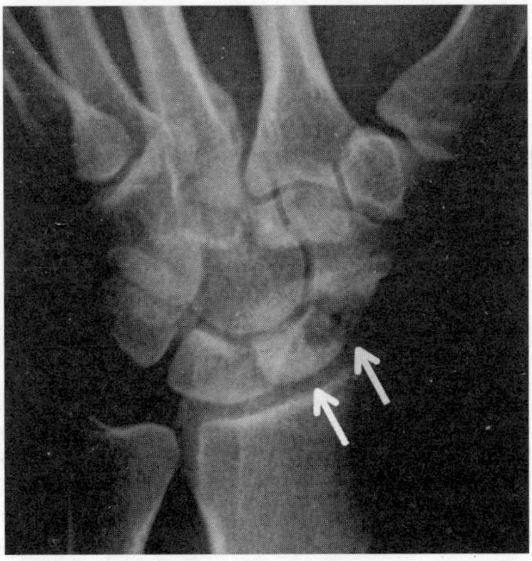

Idiopathic avascular necrosis of the scaphoid: Preiser's disease.

Preiser's disease is commonly associated with avascular necrosis of the scaphoid without fracture or trauma.

Introduction

A condition caused by AVN of scaphoid.

Epidemiology

Rare condition–Average age of onset is 45 years.

Presentation

Symptoms–Dorsoradial wrist pain.

Imaging

Radiographs–show sclerosis and fragmentation of proximal pole without evidence of fracture.

MRI–can further allow classification into complete vs partial involvement.

The scaphoid bone is the most common carpal fracture.

- 65% of all fractures involve the waist /middle third.
- 15% proximal pole.
- 12% distal pole avulsion type fracture is most common fracture type in children.
- 8% tubercle.

Sign – Tenderness in anatomical snuff box. Oblique view important for diagnosis.

- MRI can diagnose occult fractures.
- Treatment is glass holding cast if does not unite or markedly displaced fracture. Headless screw is used.

6. Which is the true regarding patient presented with flexor tenosynovitis?

A. Kanavel's sign is seen in inflammatory flexor tenosynovitis

B. Main affection is at the level of interphalangeal joint

C. There is presence of connection between thumb and little finger

D. Thickening of fibrous tendon sheath mainly at A2 pully

Answer: Option C. There is presence of connection between thumb and little finger

Explanation:

"Horseshoe abscess"

- May develop from spread **pyogenic flexor tenosynovitis.**
- Of many individuals have a **connection between the sheaths of the thumb and little fingers** at the level of the wrist.
- Infection in one finger can lead to direct infection of the sheath on the opposite side of the hand resulting a "horseshoe abscess".

Stenosing Flexor Tenosynovitis Trigger Finger

Due to stenosing tenosynovitis the flexor tendon may become trapped at the entrance to its fibrous digital sheath. The usual cause is thickening of fibrous tendon sheath or constriction of mouth of fibrous digital sheath **(mainly Al pulley) at the level of metacarpophalangeal joint.**

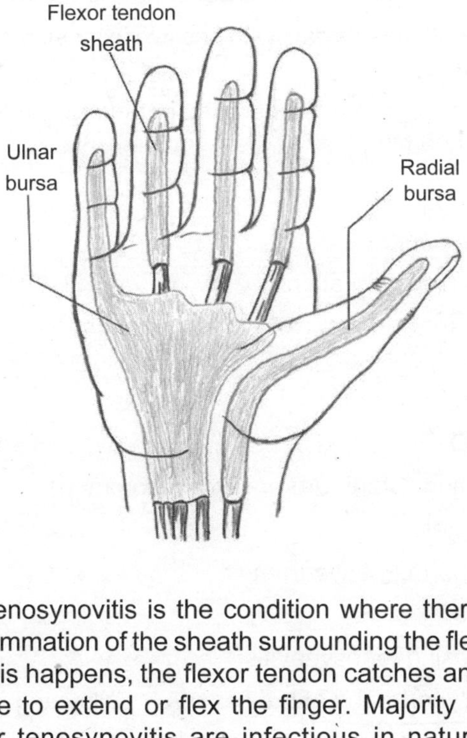

Flexor tenosynovitis is the condition where there is irritation and inflammation of the sheath surrounding the flexor tendons. When this happens, the flexor tendon catches and the patient is unable to extend or flex the finger. Majority of the cases of flexor tenosynovitis are infectious in nature; however, flexor tenosynovitis can also occur due to inflammation from noninfectious causes, such as overuse, diabetes and arthritis.

Clinical Presentation

- Joint swelling.
- Pain in the affected area and pain moving a joint.
- Reddening along the length of the affected tendon.
- Difficulty moving the joint.
- Infectious Flexor Tenosynovitis occurs as a result of trauma or injury occurs due to direct inoculation through a laceration, bite or puncture. Common pathogens seen in trauma are streptococci and staphylococcus aureus.
- **In case of Infectious Flexor Tenosynovitis, patient has the Kanavel's signs which are:**
  – There is fusiform swelling of the finger (sausage finger).
  – The finger is held or bent in a slightly flexed position.
  – Patient feels pain with passive extension of the affected digit.
  – There is tenderness present along the flexor tendon sheath.

Etiology

- Trauma/injury
- Mechanical irritation
- **Rheumatoid arthritis:** Most common to involve extensor carpi ulnaris and flexor carpi radialis
- Gout
- CPPD
- Infection (Staph. Aureus–most common)
- Diabetes
- Compartment syndrome

Subtypes

- Stenosing tenosynovitis:
  ◊ Hypertrophy of the flexor A1 pulley: trigger finger.
  ◊ 1st extensor compartment: De Quervain disease

◊ Flexor hallucis longus in patients with os trigonum syndrome.

RADIOGRAPHIC FEATURES

Plain Radiograph

Plain radiographs are non-diagnostic but may show calcification of one or several **synovial membranes** (this finding orients towards rheumatism for hydroxyapatite or a **condrocalcinosis**) and a **periosteal reaction** in an adjacent bone.

Ultrasound

The synovial membrane is not identified unless there is a pathological swelling. Tenosynovitis is characterized by increased fluid content within tendon sheath, thickening of the synovial sheath with or without increased vascularity which can extend into the tendon sheath, and peritendinous subcutaneous edema. Subcutaneous edema can result in a hypoechoic halo sign and peritendinous subcutaneous hyperaemia on Doppler imaging.

Color Doppler ultrasound is an important part of the tendon sheath assessment; it can differentiate between synovial thickening which is more suggestive of chronic disease and turbid tendon sheath fluid collection–more indicative of acute exudative tenosynovitis. In chronic inactive disease, however, there is synovial thickening with minimal vascularity.

MRI

Increased fluid within tendon sheath:

- **T1:** Low or intermediate if debris within tendon sheath
- **T2:** High
- **T1 C+ (Gd):** Tendon sheath thickening and peritendinous subcutaneous contrast enhancement.

Treatment and Prognosis

Treatments may include non-steroidal anti-inflammatory drugs, bandage or splint, cold therapy, and/or rest. Surgical procedures to release the tendon are very rarely suggested. If there is no infection present, and the tenosynovitis persists after a period of rest, then a steroid injection may be suggested. If the tenosynovitis was caused by infection then a course of antibiotics will likely be offered. Physiotherapy is an option.

7. A 34 years old patient, chronic case of rheumatoid arthritis showing below given image of hand. Currently patient is receiving methotrexate, steroids and NSAIDS for 4 months but activity of disease progression remain same. What is the treatment of this case scenario?

A. Start monotherapy with anti TNF alpha drugs

B. Add sulfasalazine and hydroxychloroquine

C. Continue same treatment

D. Stop oral methotrexate and start parenteral methotrexate

Answer: Option B. Add sulfasalazine and hydroxychloroquine

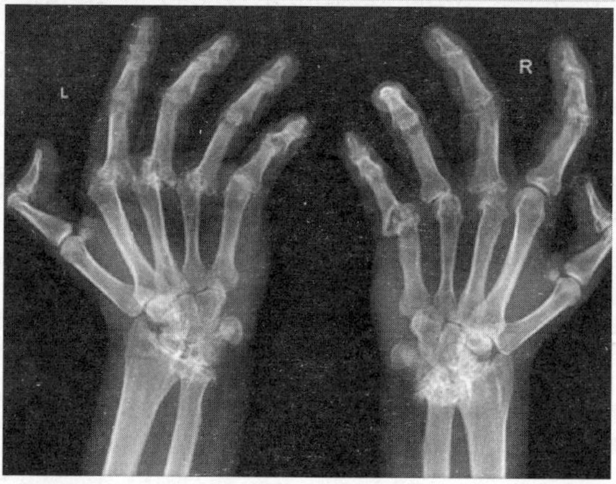

Explanation:

Here, above image is showing changes of severe rheumatoid arthritis with hand deformity. And patient had received 4 months of methotrexate, steroids and NSAIDs. But activity of disease progression remains same. According to Harrison: Failure to achieve adequate improvement with methotrexate therapy calls for a change in DMARD therapy and new treatment must include hydroxychloroquine and sulfasalazine.

Oral triple therapy (hydroxychloroquine, methotrexate and sulfasalazine) is a reasonable first step for the treatment of early RA, including its use as a step-up strategy where treatment is initiated with methotrexate alone and then combined **at 6 months with hydroxychloroquine and sulfasalazine if the disease is not adequately controlled**.

Methotrexate is the DMARD of first choice for initial treatment of moderate to severe RA. Failure to achieve adequate improvement with methotrexate therapy calls for a change in DMARD therapy, usually transition to an effective combination regimen. Effective combinations include: methotrexate, sulfasalazine, and hydroxychloroquine (oral triple therapy); methotrexate and leflunomide; and methotrexate plus a biological.

All of the TNF inhibitors have been shown in randomized controlled clinical trials to reduce the signs and symptoms of RA, slow radiographic progression of joint damage, and improve physical function and quality of life. **Anti-TNF drugs are typically used in combination with background methotrexate therapy.** This combination regimen, which affords maximal benefit in many cases, is often the next step for treatment of patients with an inadequate response to methotrexate therapy. Etanercept, adalimumab, certolizumab pegol, and golimumab have also been approved for use as monotherapy.

Subcutaneous Methotrexate is characterized by higher bioavailability, greater clinical efficacy, and a better tolerability profile than oral methotrexate. But there is lack of evidence for changing the route of administration as mode of therapy in treatment failure.

CHAPTER

16

ANAESTHESIA

1. Which of the following anaesthetic drug does not cause cardiac depression?

A. Ketamine B. Etomidate

C. Thiopentone D. Propofol

Answer: Option A. Ketamine

Explanation:

Ketamine does not cause cardiac depression, instead it stimulates heart.

Induction doses of ketamine typically increase blood pressure, heart rate and cardiac output. The cardiovascular effects are indirect and are most likely mediated by inhibition of both central and peripheral catecholamine reuptake.

Effects of intravenous anaesthetic on vital function

Anaesthetic drug	HR	BP	Resp.	CBF
1. Thiopentone	↑↑	↓↓	↓↓	↓↓↓
2. Propofol	–, ↓	↓↓↓	↓↓↓	↓↓↓
3. Etomidate	–	↓	↓	↓↓↓
4. Diazepan	–, ↑	↓	↓↓	↓↓
5. Ketamine	↑↑	↑↑	↓, –	↑↑↑
6. Fentanyl	↓	↓	↓↓↓	↓

2. Injection of which of the following anaesthetic drug is not painful on intravenous route?

A. Ketamine B. Etomidate

C. Methohexitone D. Propofol

Answer: Option A. Ketamine

Explanation:

Intravenous injection of ketamine does not cause pain.

Pain on injection

Intra arterial injection

Thiopental

Intravenous injection

- **With thrombophlebitis–** Etomidate
- **Without thrombophlebitis**
  - Propofol
  - Methohexital
  - Thiopental

Ketamine

It is pharmacologically related to the hallucinogen phencyclidine. It induces a so called 'dissociative anaesthesia' characterized by profound analgesia, immobility, amnesia with light sleep. The patient appears to be conscious, i.e., opens his eyes, makes swallowing movements and his muscles are stift, but he is unable to process sensory stimuli and does not react to them. Thus, the patient appears to be dissociated from his body and surroundings. The primary site of action is in the cortex and subcortical areas; not in the reticular activating system, which is the site of action of barbiturates. Respiration is not depressed, bronchi dilate, airway reflexes are maintained, muscle tone increases. Non-purposive limb movements occur. Heart rate, cardiac output and BP are elevated due to sympathetic stimulation. A dose of 1–2 (average 1.5) mg/kg I.V. or 3–5 mg/kg I.M. produces the above effects within a minute, and recovery starts after 10–15 min, but patient remains amnesic for 1–2 hr. Emergence delirium, hallucinations and involuntary movements occur in upto 50% patients during recovery; **but the injection is not painful.** Children tolerate the drug better. Ketamine is rapidly metabolized in the liver and has an elimination t1⁄2 of 2–4 hours.

Ketamine has been used for operations on the head and neck, in patients who have bled, in asthmatics (relieves bronchospasm), in those who do not want to lose consciousness and for short operations. It is good for repeated use; particularly suitable for burn dressing. Combined with diazepam, it has found use in angiographies, cardiac catheterization and trauma surgery.

It may be dangerous for hypertensives, in ischaemic heart disease (increases cardiac work), in congestive heart failure and in those with raised intracranial pressure (ketamine increases cerebral blood flow and O_2 consumption), but is good for hypovolemic patients. Clandestinely mixed in drinks, ketamine has been misused as rape drug.

3. Which of the following is used for monitoring the depth of general anaesthesia is?

A. Boyle's apparatus
B. ASA scale
C. Bispectral index
D. Mapleson score

Answer: Option C. Bispectral index

Explanation:

Bispectral index (BIS) is used to monitor depth of anesthesia. BIS monitors are used to supplement Guedel's classification system for determining depth of anesthesia. Titrating anesthetic agents to a specific bispectral index during general anesthesia in adults (and children over 1 year old) allows the anesthetist to adjust the amount of anesthetic agent to the needs of the patient, possibly resulting in a more rapid emergence from anesthesia. Use of the BIS monitor could reduce the incidence of intraoperative awareness during anaesthesia.

BIS cannot be used as the sole monitor of anaesthesia, as it is affected by several other factors, including the anaesthetic drugs used (BIS is relatively insensitive to agents such as ketamine and nitrous oxide), and muscle movement or artefact from surgical equipment. BIS is used as an adjunct to monitoring under anaesthesia – its use has been shown to reduce overall dose of anaesthetic agent used and therefore may improve recovery time from anaesthesia.

The Bispectral Index (BIS)

The BIS monitor displays a real-time electroencephalography (EEG) trace, acquired from a frontotemporal montage. The monitor generates a dimensionless number on a continuous scale of 0-100, with 100 representing normal cortical electrical activity and 0 indicating cortical electrical silence. **Score of 40-60 is related to adequate level of anaesthesia**. The influence of pre-existing neuropathology on BIS values is unknown. As with any EEG signal, BIS is subject to interference and artefact, particularly from electromyographic (EMG) activity, which can artificially elevate the recorded BIS. The display also shows a signal quality index and an indicator of EMG interference.

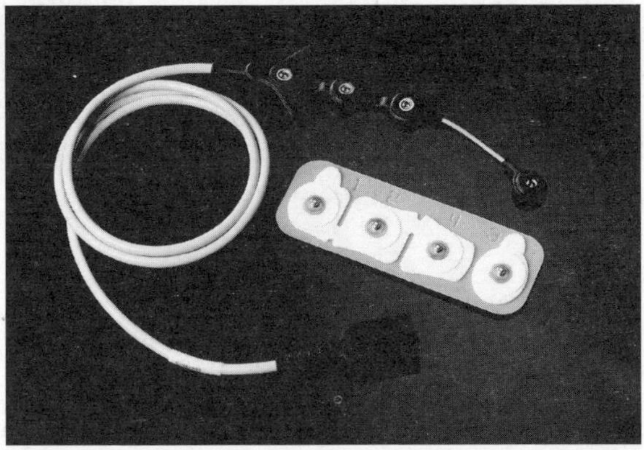

Because there is no 'gold standard' monitor against which to compare BIS, studies have used predictive probability outcome measures–that is, the likelihood of various clinically relevant end-points occurring (loss of consciousness, recovery of consciousness, postoperative recall, suppression of learning) at different BIS values. From these various studies, broad guidelines have emerged to aid the interpretation of BIS values. The probability of postoperative recall is very low when BIS is kept <60 intraoperatively. Studies comparing BIS-titrated anaesthesia with clinical judgement of anaesthetic requirements show reduced anaesthetic consumption and slightly quicker awakening using BIS, supporting the suggestion that, in trying to ensure lack of awareness, we tend towards excessively deep anaesthesia. However, BIS values tend to display considerable variability within study populations, so that, for example, one patient may be unresponsive to command at a BIS of 75, but another may still be responsive at a BIS of 70. This makes it difficult to identify sensitive and specific threshold values that are widely applicable. No BIS value predicts an individual's threshold for loss or recovery of consciousness. BIS values discriminate between awake and asleep states but with considerable overlap of values and no clear-cut transition between awake and asleep values at the end of surgery.

CHAPTER

17 PSYCHIATRY

1. Which of the following disease is associated with Down's syndrome?

A. Parkinson disease B. Alzheimer's disease

C. Carcinoma cervix D. Ulcerative colitis

Answer: Option B. Alzheimer's disease

Explanation:

The patients with Down's syndrome have significantly higher risk for development of Alzheimer's disease. The gene for APP (amyloid precursor protein) is located on chromosome 21.

It is the most common cause of dementia. The prevalence of Alzheimer's disease increases with age, the rates are around 5% for all those aged 65 years and older, increasing to around 20-30% for all those aged above 85 years.

The insight (awareness of illness) is lost relatively early in the course of illness. In the initial phase symptoms include memory disturbances, gradually apraxia, agnosia, aphasia and acalculia develop and executive functions are lost. In the later stages neurological disabilities like tremors, rigidity and spasticity may develop.

Pathophysiology: The classical gross neuroanatomical finding in Alzheimer's disease is diffuse atrophy with flattened cortical sulci and enlarged cerebral ventricles.

The classical microscopic findings are neuritic (senile) plaques and neurofibrillary tangles. **Senile plaques,** also referred to as amyloid plaques are composed of a particular protein Aβ. This protein is derived from amyloid precursor protein (APP) by the action of β- and γ-secretase enzymes. The AP protein combines to form fibrils. The senile plaques are extracellular deposits of Aβ and are found in all cortical areas and also in striatum and cerebellum. The amyloid-β peptide not only deposits in the brain parenchyma in the form of amyloid plaques but also in the vessel walls in the form of cerebral amyloid angiopathy (CAA).

The neurofibrillary tangles (NFTs) are intraneuronal aggregates of tau protein. The tau protein present in tangles is in a highly phosphorylated form and has abnormal functioning. Normally, tau protein binds and stabilizes microtubules, which are essential for axonal transport, however in Alzheimer's this function is deranged. The neurofibrillary tangles are widely distributed in cortical structures and hippocampus, but always spare cerebellum. Multiple studies have established that amount and distribution of NFTs correlates with the duration and severity of dementia.

Granulovacuolar degeneration (GVD) and Hirano bodies (eosinophilic inclusions) are abnormalities seen in the cytoplasm of hippocampal neurons in patients with Alzheimer's disease.

Neurochemistry: Alzheimer's disease is predominantly a disorder of cholinergic neurons'3 and loss of **cholinergic neurons** in nucleus basalis of meynert is a consistent finding. Apart from acetylcholine, norepinephrine and serotonin have also been implicated in some cases.

Genetics: Alzheimer's disease has shown linkage to chromosome 1, 14 and 21. A small number of cases of Alzheimer disease are early onset and familial and are inherited in autosomal dominant fashion. Mutations in three genes, amyloid precursor protein (chromosome 21), presenilin-IQ (chromosome 14) and presenilin-2 (chromosome 1) have been found in most cases with familial Alzheimer's disease. The majority of cases are however sporadic and late onset. ApO E4 gene is associated with the risk of development of Alzheimer's disease,

Risk factors: Age is the most important risk factor. Other risk factors include head injury, hypertension, insulin resistance, depression. Few studies have claimed that smoking is a protective factor against Alzheimer's but this finding has been contradicted by other studies. High education levels and remaining physically and mentally active till late in life are protective factors against Alzheimer's disease.

2. Premature ejaculation occurs during which phase of sexual intercourse?

A. Orgasmic phase
B. Desire
C. Excitement
D. Resolution

Answer: Option A. Orgasmic phase

Explanation:

Premature ejaculation occurs during orgasmic phase of sexual intercourse.

It is also the shortest phase of sexual cycle.

Retarded ejaculation in male or anorgasmia in female also occur during this phase.

Disorders of orgasm phase:

- **Premature ejaculation:** It is characterized by a pattern of persistent or recurrent ejaculation with minimal sexual stimulation before or immediately after the vaginal penetration.

  The cause of premature ejaculation is usually psychogenic.

Treatment

Specific techniques have been described for the management of premature ejaculation.

These include:

a. **Squeeze technique:** When the man gets the feeling of impending ejaculation, the female partner (or the man himself) squeezes the coronal ridge of glans, which results in inhibition of ejaculation.

b. **Stop-start technique (Semans technique):** Here, when the man gets the feeling of impending ejaculation, the sex is stopped for some time and once excitement has decreased, it is restarted.

Apart from these techniques, sex therapy (as described earlier) is also an effective method of treating premature ejaculation.

SSRIs (selective serotonin reuptake inhibitors) are also frequently used as they can delay the ejaculation.

Disorders of Excitement (Arousal) Phase:

Erection disorder occur during Excitement phase of sexual cycle.

Male erectile disorder (erectile dysfunction): It is characterized by recurrent or persistent inability to attain or to maintain the erection required for satisfactory sexual intercourse. Erectile dysfunction is usually caused by psychological factors such as anxiety and poor marital relation.

The presence of early morning erections and erections during REM sleep (nocturnal erections) are suggestive of psychogenic erectile dysfunction. Investigation such as penile plethysmography and nocturnal penile intumescence (NPT) are used to record nocturnal erections.

3. CAM test is useful for which of the screening following disease?

A. Anxiety
B. Delirium
C. Depression
D. Dementia

Answer: Option B. Delirium

Explanation:

CAM (Confusion Assessment Method) is a screening test used for delirium (delirium is also known as acute confusional state).

The Confusion Assessment Method (CAM) Diagnostic Algorithm

Feature 1: Acute Onset and Fluctuating Course

Is there evidence of an acute change in mental status from the patient's baseline? Did the (abnormal) behavior fluctuate during the day, that is, tend to come and go, or increase and decrease in severity?

Feature 2: Inattention

Did the patient have difficulty focusing attention, for example, being easily distractible, or having difficulty keeping track of what was being said?

Feature 3: Disorganized Thinking

Was the patient's thinking disorganized or incoherent, such as rambling or irrelevant conversation, unclear or illogical flow of ideas, or unpredictable switching from subject to subject?

Feature 4: Altered Level of Consciousness

Patient's level of consciousness (alert [normal], vigilant [hyper alert], lethargic [drowsy, easily aroused], stupor [difficult to arouse], or coma [unarousable]).

The diagnosis of delirium by CAM requires the presence of features 1 and 2 and either 3 or 4.

The Confusion Assessment Method Instrument:

1. Acute Onset

2A. Inattention

B. (If present or abnormal)

3. Disorganized thinking
4. Altered level of consciousness
5. Disorientation
6. Memory impairment
7. Perceptual disturbances

8A. Psychomotor agitation

B. Psychomotor retardation

9. Altered sleep-wake cycle.

4. Which of the following is a poor prognosis for OCD?

A. Phasic course

B. Short duration

C. Hoarding

D. Associated with depression as prominent feature

Answer: Option C. Hoarding

Compulsive **hoarding**, also known as **hoarding** disorder, is a behavioral pattern characterized by excessive acquisition of and an inability or unwillingness to discard large quantities of objects that cover the living areas of the home and cause significant distress or impairment.

Certain OCD symptoms have been shown to develop more commonly in this poor response subgroup, including the need for symmetry, ordering, arranging and **hoarding.**

Evidence is increasing that patients in whom **hoarding** is a primary obsessive-compulsive symptom are resistant to traditional behavioral and pharmacologic interventions. In addition, hoarding was the only compulsion associated with a lower probability of remission in pilot study.

Three factors, **hoarding**, contamination/cleaning, and pure obsessions, best explained the variance. Only the first factor was significantly related to OCPD (obsessive-compulsive personality disorder) or a lifetime history of Tourette syndrome.

Intrinsic phenomenological risk factors for poor response to conventional treatment of OCD
Early onset
Content of obsessive-compulsive symptoms
Hoarding
Sexual
Religious
Somatic
Overvalued ideas and poor insight
Sensorial phenomena
Higher symptom severity at onset
Presence of tics
Comorbidities
Schizotypal, borderline and paranoid personality disorders
Anankastic personality disorder

Prognostic factors in OCD	
I. Favourable factors	
(i)	A normal good premorbid personality
(ii)	Mild or atypical symptoms including predominance of phobic symptoms, ruminative ideas and absence of compulsion
(iii)	Short duration of symptoms
(iv)	A phasic course
(v)	Satisfactory resolution of precipitating disturbance
(vi)	Anxiety or depression prominent features
II. Poor prognostic factors	
(i)	Obsessional premorbid personality
(ii)	Early age of onset and
(iii)	A clincial picture showing severe symptoms

Contd.

Contd.

III. Unrelated factors	
(i)	Positive family history
(ii)	Childhood symptoms
(iii)	Sex
(iv)	Intelligence
(v)	Unmarried status
(vi)	Acute versus insidious onset
(vii)	Previous attacks

5. Which of the following is not true about somnambulism?

A. It is also known as sleep walking
B. It is a disorder of sleep arousal
C. Person's conscious remain intact
D. Person has low level of motor skills

Answer: Option C. Person's conscious remain intact

Explanation:

Somnambulism

It is also known as sleep walking.

It is a disorder of sleep arousal.

Person has low level of motor skills as during sleep walking low level of motor activity is required for movement of leg. The patients may carry out a range of activities for which he doesn't have any memory lateron. It may include leaving the bed and walking about and also activities like dressing, moving around or even driving.

Somnambulism is usually seen in NREM III and IV (slow wave sleep).

6. Which of the following term used for morbid fear of darkness?

A. Xenophobia
B. Claustrophobia
C. Nyctophobia
D. Mysophobia

Answer: Option C. Nyctophobia

Explanation:

Nyctophobia is defined as morbid fear of darkness.

Xenophobia is defined as fear of stranger.

Claustrophobia is defined as fear of close space.

Mysophobia is defined as fear of dirt and germs.

Other Specific Types of Phobias

Agoraphobia	–	Fear of places from where escape might be difficult
Acrophobia	–	Fear of heights
Ailurophobia	–	Fear of cats
Hydrophobia	–	Fear of water
Cynophobia	–	Fear of dogs
Pyrophobia	–	Fear of fire
Zoophobia	–	Fear of animals
Thanatophobia	–	Fear of death

7. Which of the following is not true regarding delusional disorder?

A. It may be erotomanic or jealous type

B. Symptoms are usually persistent

C. Early age of onset

D. It is false belief

Answer: Option C. Early age of onset

Explanation:

The mean age of onset is 40 years. Men are more likely than women to develop paranoid delusions; women are more likely than men to develop delusions of erotomania. Associated factors with delusional disorder include being married, being employed, recent immigration status, low socioeconomic status, celibacy (among men), and widowhood (among women).

Delusional disorder is an illness characterized by at least 1 month of delusions but no other psychotic symptoms, according to the American Psychiatric Association's *Diagnostic and Statistical Manual of Mental Disorders, Fifth Edition (DSM-5)*. **Delusions are false beliefs** based on incorrect inference about external reality that persist despite the evidence to the contrary; these beliefs are not ordinarily accepted by other members of the person's culture or subculture.

Delusional disorder: These disorders are characterized by development of either a single delusion or a set of related delusions, **which are usually persistent and sometimes are lifelong.** Other psychotic symptoms like hallucinations, disorganization, negative symptoms are usually absent. If hallucinations occur they are for a very short duration, presence of frequent hallucinations goes against the diagnosis of delusional disorder. The following are the types of delusional disorder:

- **Erotomanic:** The person believes someone is in love with them and might try to contact that person. Often it's someone important or famous. This can lead to stalking behavior.
- **Grandiose:** This person has an over-inflated sense of worth, power, knowledge, or identity. They could believe they have a great talent or made an important discovery.
- **Jealous:** A person with this type believes their spouse or sexual partner is unfaithful.
- **Persecutory:** Someone who has this believes they (or someone close to them) are being mistreated, or that someone is spying on them or planning to harm them. They might make repeated complaints to legal authorities.
- **Somatic type:** Patient may have delusion that he is infested by parasites (delusional parasitosis), that he has misshaped body parts (delusion of dysmorphophobia) or that his body has a foul odor (delusion of halitosis).
- **Nihilistic** (i.e., a conviction that a major catastrophe will occur).
- **Referential** (i.e., belief that gestures, comments, or environmental cues are directed at oneself).
- **Mixed:** These people have two or more of the types of delusions listed above.
- **Unspecified type:** In patients where the above mentioned categories are not applicable. Delusion of misidentification is an example of unspecified type.

Delusion of misidentification can be of many types like:

- **Capgras syndrome:** Patient believes that a familiar person has been replaced by an impostor. For example, a patient believed that his wife has been replaced by a stranger who looks exactly like his wife.
- **Fregoli syndrome:** Patient believes that familiar persons are taking the guise of strangers. For example, a patient saw a beggar, and claimed that his brother is following him in the guise of the beggar.
- **Syndrome of intermetamorphosis:** Patient believes that people can undergo changes in physical and psychological identity and become a different person altogether.
- **Syndrome of subjective doubles:** Patient believes that he has many doubles who are living life of their own.

8. Feeling of guilt, early morning awakening and sadness occurs in which of the following condition?

A. Melancholia B. Schizophrenia

C. Delirium D. Mania

Answer: Option A. Melancholia

Explanation:

Melancholia

Depression with melancholic features (or involutional melancholia) is usually seen in old age.

It is characterized by severe anhedonia, profound guilt feelings, early morning awakening and weight loss, agitation and high suicide risk.

Melancholic depression, or **depression with melancholic features**, is a DSM-IV subtype of clinical depression requiring at least one of the following symptoms:

- Anhedonia (the inability to find pleasure in positive things).
- Lack of mood reactivity (i.e., mood does not improve in response to positive events).

And at least three of the following:

- Depression that is subjectively different from grief or loss

- Severe weight loss or loss of appetite
- Psychomotor agitation or retardation
- Early morning awakening
- Guilt that is excessive
- Worse mood in the morning.

Melancholic features apply to an episode of depression that occurs as part of either major depressive disorder or bipolar disorder I or II.

Melancholic depression is often considered to be a biologically based and particularly severe form of depression. Treatment involves antidepressants, electroconvulsive therapy, or other empirically supported treatments such as cognitive behavioral therapy and interpersonal therapy for depression. A 2008 analysis of a large study of patients with unipolar major depression found a rate of 23.5% for melancholic features. It was the first form of depression extensively studied, and many of the early symptom checklists for depression reflect this. The incidence of melancholic depression has been found to increase when the temperature and/or sunlight are low.

According to the DSM-IV, the "melancholic features" specifier may be applied to the following only:

1. Major depressive episode, single episode
2. Major depressive episode, recurrent episode
3. Bipolar I disorder, most recent episode depressed
4. Bipolar II disorder, most recent episode depressed.

CHAPTER 18 DERMATOLOGY

1. A 2 years child presented with eczematous dermatitis over face showing in below image. His mother has history of bronchial asthma. What is the diagnosis in given scenario?

A. Atopic dermatitis

B. Seborrheic dermatitis

C. Infantile dermatitis

D. Contact dermatitis

Answer: Option A. Atopic dermatitis

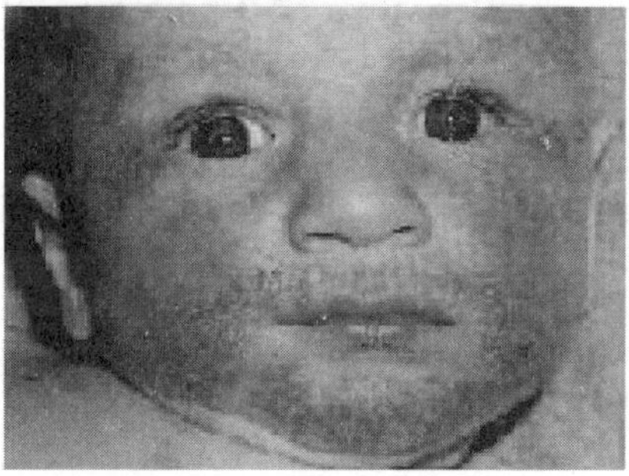

Explanation:

Here, above 2 years child is presented with eczematous dermatitis over face with his mother has history of bronchial asthma and his image of face suggest diagnosis of atopic dermatitis.

Atopic Dermatitis (AD)

It is a chronic, non-contagious, inflammatory skin condition characterized by redness, swollen skin with severe itching.

- Occurs in 10–15% children, often presenting at 2-3 months of age; multifactorial pathogenesis but includes ↑ secretion of TH2 cytokines (IL-4, IL-5).

- **Triad of Atopy:** AD, allergic rhinitis, asthma.
- Few may have allergy to specific foods, which may exacerbate AD (eggs, milk, soybeans, fish, wheat, peanuts).
- Presents with eczematous lesions, xerosis and lichenification.
- Distribution varies with age.

Infants: Face, scalp and extensors.

Children: Antecubital/popliteal fossae, neck, ankles.

Adults: Typically hands (chronic hand eczema).

- **Pityriasis alba:** Hypopigmented patches with minimal scale; may be only manifestation of AD.
- **Complications:** Keratoconus (conical deformity of cornea), eyelid dermatitis, ↑ risk of infection (impetigo, eczema herpeticum, molluscum contagiosum).
- **Treatment:** Topical corticosteroid, topical calcineurin inhibitor, oral corticosteroid (short course), oral antihistamine, phototherapy; if recalcitrant and severe, consider oral immunosuppressant.

Diagnostic criteria (Hanifin and Rajka)

Major features (must have three)	Minor or less specific features
1. Pruritus 2. Typical morphology and distribution • Facial and extensor involvement during infancy and early childhood • Flexural lichenification in childhood or adolescence 3. Chronic or chronically relapsing dermatitis 4. Personal or family history of atopy	• Xerosis • Periauricular fissures • Ichthyosis/Hyperlinear palms/Keratosis pilaris • IgE reactivity (increased serum IgE, RAST, or prick test positivity) • Hand or foot dermatitis • Scalp dermatitis • Susceptibility to cutaneous infections (especially *staphylococcus aureus and herpes simplex)* • Perifollicular accentuation (especially in darkly pigmented races)

2. A 30 years old patient presented with multiple painful blisters with erythematous base along a specific dermatome showing in below image. What is the diagnosis in given scenario?

A. Herpes simplex B. Chickenpox
C. Warts D. Herpes zoster

Answer: Option D. Herpes zoster

Explanation:

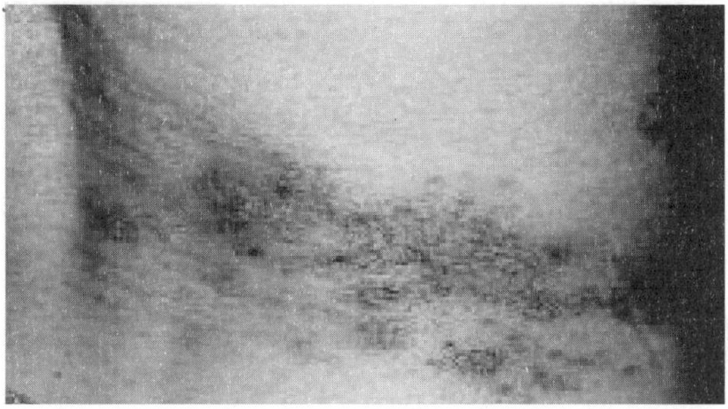

Here patient presented with multiple painful blisters with erythematous base along a **specific dermatome** as showing in above image that suggest diagnosis of herpes zoster.

Other options herpes simplex, chickenpox and warts are not limited to single dermatome.

Varicella-Zoster-Virus (HHV3, VZV, Herpes Zoster)

- Initial infection causes varicella and following resolution, virus lies dormant in spinal dorsal root ganglion until reactivation of latent virus causing localized cutaneous eruption (herpes zoster or shingles).
- Presents with grouped, painful erythematous macules and papules along single sensory dermatome (rarely crossing midline) → vesicles/bullae → rupture forming hemorrhagic crust and become dry over 7-10 days; lesions are infectious until dry; sensory prodrome (pain, pruritus, or paresthesias) in 75% of cases and mild systemic response (headache, malaise, anorexia, etc.) can precede presentation; thoracic dermatome most commonly involved.
- Disseminated zoster, defined as generalized eruption of more than 10-12 extra dermatomal vesicles occurring 7-14 days after onset of classic dermatomal zoster, is seen in 2% of cases in general population and up to 35% in immunocompromised patients; observe these patients

carefully for development of visceral involvement (liver, lung, brain) as pneumonitis and encephalitis can be life-threatening.

- Atypical presentation in AIDS pts: >2 dermatomes affected, may cross midline, may present with verrucous/crusted lesions.
- **Complications:** Post-herpetic neuralgia (PHN), scarring, secondary bacterial infection, meningoencephalitis, Ramsay-Hunt syndrome, ocular blindness, motor paralysis.
- **Postherpetic neuralgia (PHN):** Pain that continues after resolution of the eruption, typically lasting more than 30 days (some experts prefer to reserve the term for pain that lasts more than 90 days); occurs in 10-25% of cases.
- **Ocular involvement:** Lesions on tip of nose signal possible ocular infection (since nasociliary nerve involved, a branch of the ophthalmic nerve).
- **Ramsay-Hunt syndrome:** Infection of geniculate ganglion → ear canal/auricle/tympanic membrane involvement with painful vesicles, facial paralysis/paresis, ipsilateral hearing loss.
- **Treatment:** Antiviral best if within 48-72 hours within appearance of rash (can ↓ PHN risk); of note, concomitant corticosteroid use has no effect on development/duration of PHN; IV acyclovir used in immunocompromised patient if advanced HIV, widespread skin involvement, visceral disease or transplant patients
- Of note, women with varicella infection 5 days before or 2 days after delivery, can result in severe acute infection of newborn (neonatal varicella, mortality of newborn up to 30%); different from VZV embryopathy or congenital varicella syndrome which occurs in first 20 weeks of pregnancy.

3. A 46 years old patient known case of diabetes presented with velvety hyperpigmentation at axillary region as given in below image. What is the diagnosis?

A. Lichen planus B. Seborrheic dermatitis

C. Acanthosis nigricans D. Becker's nevus

Answer: Option C. Acanthosis nigricans

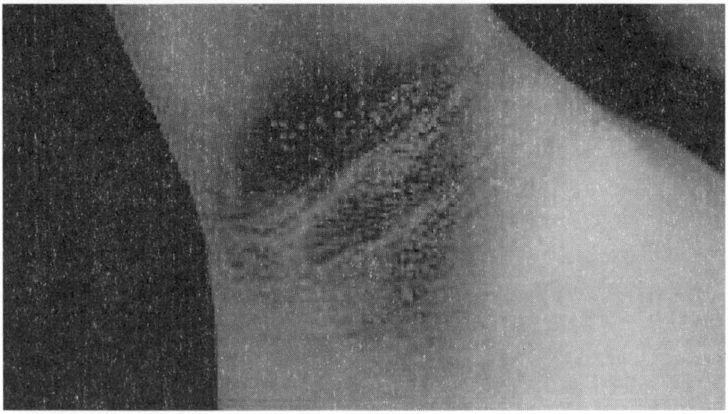

Explanation:

Here, diabetic patient presented with velvety hyper-pigmentation at axillary region (body fold) as given in above image that suggest diagnosis of acanthosis nigricans.

Acanthosis nigricans is a brown to black, poorly defined, velvety hyperpigmentation of the skin. It is usually found in body folds, such as the posterior and lateral folds of the neck, the armpits, groin, navel, forehead and other areas.

- Type I – familial
- Type II – endocrine
- Type III – obesity and pseudoacanthosis nigricans
- Type IV – drug-related
- Type V – malignancy
- Acral acanthotic anomaly.

Classification

Acanthosis nigricans is conventionally divided into benign and malignant forms, although may be divided into syndromes according to cause:

- **Benign:** This may include obesity-related, hereditary and endocrine forms of acanthosis nigricans.
- **Malignant:** This may include forms that are associated with tumour products and insulin-like activity, or tumour necrosis factor.

An alternate classification system still used to describe acanthosis nigricans was proposed in 1994. It delineates acanthosis nigricans syndromes according to their associated syndromes, including benign and malignant forms, forms associated with obesity and drugs, acral acanthosis nigricans, unilateral acanthosis nigricans, and mixed and syndromic forms.

Signs and Symptoms

Acanthosis nigricans may present with thickened, velvety, relatively darker areas of skin on the neck, armpit and in skin folds.

Causes

It typically occurs in individuals younger than age 40, may be genetically inherited, and is associated with obesity or endocrinopathies, such as hypothyroidism, acromegaly, polycystic ovary disease, insulin-resistant diabetes, or Cushing's disease.

Type I – Familial

Familial acanthosis may arise as a result of an autosomal dominant trait, presenting at birth or developing during childhood.

Type II – Endocrine

Endocrine syndromes associated with acanthosis nigricans can develop in many conditions, particularly:

- Starts with insulin resistance, such as diabetes mellitus and metabolic syndrome.
- Excess circulating androgens, particularly Cushing's disease, acromegaly, polycystic ovarian disease.
- Addison's disease and hypothyroidism.
- Rare diseases, including pinealoma, leprechaunism, lipoatrophic diabetes, pineal hyperplasia syndrome, pituitary basophilism, ovarian hyperthecosis, stromal luteoma, ovarian dermoid cysts, Prader-Willi syndrome and Alström syndrome.

Acanthosis nigricans associated with endocrine dysfunction is more insidious in its onset, is less widespread, and the patients are often concurrently obese.

4. A 56 years male patient is suffering from alopecia as in below image, which of the following nail changes are associated with it?

A. Nail pigmentation

B. Whitish discoloration of nails

C. Pterigium of nail

D. Pitting of nail

Answer: Option D. Pitting of nail

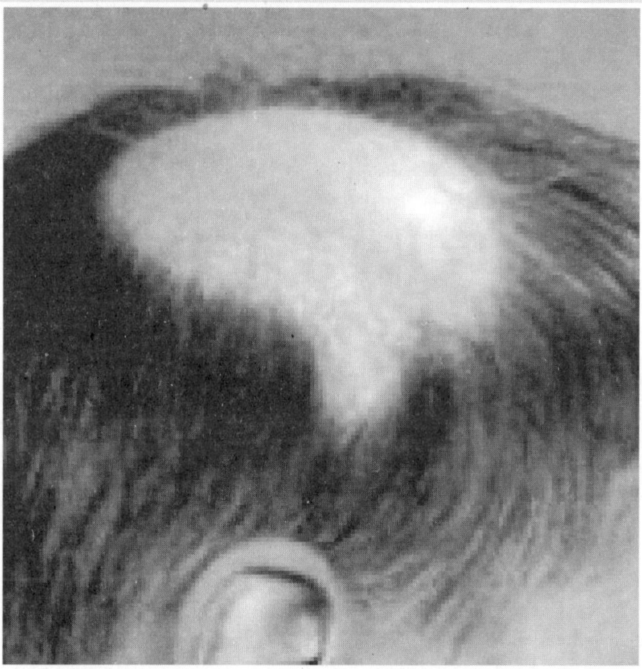

Here, 56 years male patient is suffering from alopecia as in above image suggest diagnosis of alopecia areata. Pitting and trachyonychia (longitudinal striations on the nails) are the most common association of alopecia areata.

Alopecia Areata

- Most common non-scarring alopecia; unknown etiology but likely T cell mediated autoimmune condition in patients with genetic predisposition; upregulation of ULBP3 implicated in pathogenesis.

- Presents with round to oval alopecic non-scarring patches on scalp, 'exclamation mark' hairs; different patterns include patchy (most common), reticular, diffuse with generalized thinning, alopecia totalis (loss of entire scalp hair), alopecia universalis (loss of scalp and body hair), ophiasis pattern (band-like hair loss at periphery of temporal/occipital scalp).
- May have nail involvement (pitting most common).
- **Histology:** Lymphocytes surrounding lower portion of hair follicle resembling 'swarm of bees', ↑ miniature telogen and catagen follicles.

  Trichoscopy **may aid in establishing the diagnosis. In alopecia** areata, trichoscopy shows regularly distributed "yellow dots" (hyperkeratotic **plugs), small exclamation-mark hairs, and "black dots" (destroyed hairs in the hair follicle opening).**
- **Treatment:** Topical/intralesional corticosteroid, other topicals (squaric acid, anthralin, minoxidil), excimer laser, systemic corticosteroid or cyclosporine.
- **Associations:** Thyroid disease, vitiligo, atopy, IBD, IDDM, polyendocrinopathy.

5. Erythema multiforme is associated with:

A. Hodgkin's lymphoma B. Ulcerative colitis

C. Celiac disease D. Antimalarial drug

Answer: Option D. Antimalarial drug

Explanation:

Quinine-antimalarial drug can cause erythema multiforme.

Erythema Multiforme

- Acute, often self-limited skin condition associated with infection (mainly herpes) or medication (less common) and rarely systemic disease; two types: EM minor and EM major.
- Erythema multiforme minor—typical targets or raised, edematous papules distributed acrally.
- Erythema multiforme major—typical targets or raised, edematous papules distributed acrally with involvement of

one or more mucous membranes; epidermal detachment involves less than 10% of total body surface area (TBSiA).

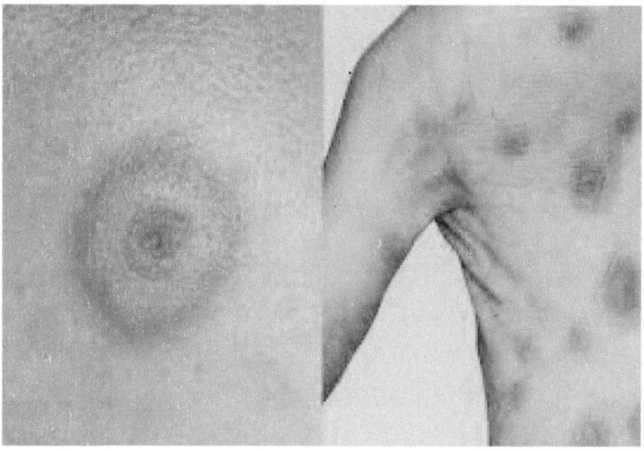

- Presents with abrupt onset of 'target' lesions on face and distal extremities; target lesions often appear as dusky circinate plaques with concentric rings of color, ± bulla, vesicle or crust in center of lesion; may also see atypical papular target lesions; no mucosal or systemic involvement in EM minor.
- **Treatment:** Typically self-limited within 2 weeks, prophylactic antiviral if HSV-related EM with frequent recurrences.

Etiology

Erythema multiforme minor is regarded as being commonly triggered by herpes simplex virus (HSV) (types 1 and 2), and HSV is the most common cause in young adults; in fact, many instances of idiopathic erythema multiforme minor may be precipitated by subclinical HSV infection. Among other infections, *Mycoplasma* species is another common cause.

Bacterial

Bacterial infections that may trigger erythema multiforme include borreliosis, cat scratch disease, diphtheria, hemolytic streptococci, legionellosis, leprosy, *Neisseria meningitidis, Mycobacterium avium* complex, *M pneumoniae,* pneumococci, tuberculosis, *Proteus/Pseudomonas/Salmonella/Staphylococcus/Yersinia* species, *Treponema pallidum*, tularemia, *Vibrio parahaemolyticus,* Vincent disease, and rickettsial infections. Chlamydial infections include lymphogranuloma venereum and psittacosis.

Viral infections, including Adenovirus, coxsackievirus B5, cytomegalovirus (CMV), echoviruses, enterovirus, Epstein-Barr virus (EBV), hepatitis A/B/C viruses (HAV/HBV/HCV), HSV, influenza, measles, mumps, paravaccinia, parvovirus B19, poliomyelitis, varicella-zoster virus (VZV), and variola, are other causes, as well as the virus-drug interactions CMV infection–terbinafine and EBV infection–amoxicillin.

Other

Fungal infections such as coccidioidomycosis, dermatophytosis, and histoplasmosis and some parasitic infections, including *Trichomonas* species and *Toxoplasma gondii*, may trigger erythema multiforme.

Drugs

More than 50% of cases of erythema multiforme major are related to medication use, but no test reliably proves the link between a single case and a specific drug.

Regarding medications, sulfa drugs are the most common triggers (30%). The second most commonly involved agents are the anticonvulsants, including barbiturates, carbamazepine, hydantoin, phenytoin and valproic acid.

Causative antibiotics include penicillin, ampicillin, tetracyclines, amoxicillin, cefotaxime, cefaclor, cephalexin, ciprofloxacin, erythromycin, minocycline, sulfonamides, trimethoprim-sulfamethoxazole and vancomycin.

Antituberculoid agents such as rifampicin, isoniazid, thiacetazone and pyrazinamide are also known offenders. Antipyretic agents as triggers include analgesics, especially aspirin as well as phenylbutazone, oxyphenbutazone and phenazone.

Others drugs that may cause erythema multiforme include acarbose, albendazole, alendronate, allopurinol, arsenic, bromofluorene, quinine (Chinine).

6. All of the following statements are true about anatomy of skin, except:

A. 90 percent of cells in epidermis are keratinocytes

B. Epidermis is derived from ectoderm and dermis from mesoderm

C. Skin weighs about 15 percentage of body weight

D. Dermal collagen 1 and 3 are in ratio of 3:2 in dermis

Answer: Option D. Dermal collagen 1 and 3 are in ratio of 3:2 in dermis

Explanation:

More than 70% of the dry weight of the normal dermis consists of collagen. The major collagens are Type I and Type III. **Type I collagen** has a molecular mass of about 290 KDa and accounts for **approximately 80%** of the total amount of collagen in the dermis. Type I collagen is arranged in a dense orthogonal meshwork of bundles in the reticular dermis. **Type III collagen** makes up approximately **10% of dermal collagen**, it being called also fetal collagen because it is noted first in embryonic dermis where it serves as a framework on which Type I collagen subsequently is synthesized.

Epidermis – Keratinocytes

- **Ectodermal derivation**; **keratinocytes comprise approximately 80–85% of epidermal cells.**
- **Total epidermal turnover time:** Average 45–60 days (30–50 days from stratum basale to stratum corneum and approximately 14 days from stratum corneum to desquamation).

DERMIS

- **Mesoderm-derived components.**
- Divided into superficial papillary dermis and deep reticular dermis (latter with larger collagen bundles and mature branching elastic fibers).

Collagen

- Family of fibrous proteins, 20+ genetically distinct types identified; provides structural stability and accounts for 70–80% dry weight of dermis; major dermal constituent.
- Composed of 3 chains combined into a triple helix configuration; contains Gly-x-y repeats (glycine always 3rd residue, x frequently proline, y often hydroxylysine or hydroxyproline).
- Collagen degraded by interstitial collagenases (metallo-proteinases or MMPs).
- Collagen synthesis stimulated by: Retinoic acid.

- Collagen synthesis inhibited by: IL-1 (↑ MMP expression), glucocorticoids, IFNγ, TNFα, D-penicillamine, UV irradiation.

"The skin is the largest organ in the body: ***12-15% of body weight***, with a surface area of 1-2 [square] meters." The human skin is the body's largest organ. The skin of an average adult weighs 8-10 pounds and averages an area of about 22 square feet.

7. A young female having history of oral ulcers and fever, presented with erythematous lesions over cheeks as shown in below image. She also had photophobia, what is the diagnosis?

A. Rosacea

B. Systemic lupus erythematosis

C. Dermatomyositis

D. Purpura

Answer: Option B. Systemic lupus erythematosis

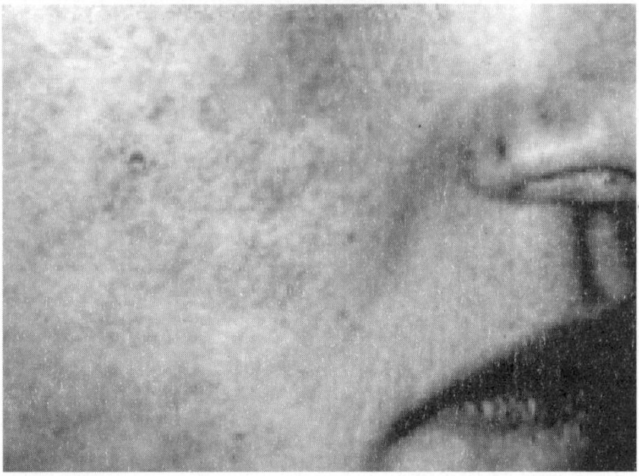

Explanation:

Here, young female having history of oral ulcers and fever, presented with erythematous lesions over cheeks and photophobia so her diagnosis is SLE with lesion as shown in above image is typical malar rash or butter fly rash involving cheeks and nasal bridge sparing the **nasolabial folds** (involved in dermatomyositis) of the face that confirms diagnosis of **systemic lupus erythematosis**.

Lupus Erythematosus (LE)

- **Spectrum with three major forms:** Systemic LE (SLE), subacute LE (SCLE) and chronic cutaneous LE (CCLE).
- **Chronic cutaneous LE (discoid LE)**
  - Chronic cutaneous form with involvement typically of face/scalp in young women; ↑ incidence in African American patients.
  - Presents with indurated erythematous thin papules with adherent scale and follicular plugging on face, scalp and/or ears (concha bowl), 'carpet tack' sign (follicular plugs with removal of scale); subsequent atrophy, telangiectasias, dyschromia, scarring (SCC may develop in scars); ¼ with oral involvement; no systemic symptoms or extracutaneous involvement; rarely may see widespread discoid involvement (↑ serologic abnormalities have ↑ likelihood to develop SLE).
  - Variants.
- **Tumid lupus:** Deeper, more nodular lesions with erythema and induration mainly involving face and trunk, no scaling or follicular plugging; dermis with mucin and intense inflammatory infiltrate.
- **Lupus panniculitis or profundus:** Tender subcutaneous nodules with typical DLE surface changes involving buttocks, chest, shoulder, face; heals with deep atrophy; 10-15% meet SLE criteria.
- **Hypertrophic or verrucous LE:** Hyperkeratotic or verrucous papules/plaques over extensor arms, ± face/ trunk, may appear similar to warts.
- **Chillblain LE:** Acral dusky purple papules and plaques associated with acrocyanosis, minimal atrophy/scarring.
  - *Histology:* Atrophic epidermis with plugged follicles, vacuolar degeneration of basal layer, thickened basement membrane, melanin incontinence, perivascular/ periadnexal lymphocytic infiltrate, ↑ mucin between collagen bundles; 90% of lesional biopsies show diffuse irregular band of IgG/C3 at BMZ (lupus band).

  - *Labs:* ¼ with +ANA (low titer); 5-10% with DLE may develop SLE over time.
  - *Treatment*: Sun avoidance, topical/IL corticosteroids, antimalarial, topical calcineurin inhibitors.
- **Neonatal LE:** Autoimmune disease caused by transplacental passage of maternal autoantibodies against Ro/SS-A (>90%), La/SS-B and less commonly U1-RNP associated with high mortality and morbidity.
  - Can present in infants born to mothers with above autoantibodies; presents within first few months with annular scaly red plaques involving head and extremities and lesions resolve spontaneously within 6 months without scarring; associated with congenital heart block (may be only manifestation), thrombocytopenia and transaminitis.
  - *Labs:* Anti-Ro positive (maternal autoantibodies)

    Of note, C2 deficiency increases susceptibility to autoimmune conditions, especially lupus (DLE, SCLE, SLE).
- **Subacute cutaneous LE (SCLE)**
  - Overlap between DLE and SLE with photosensitivity.
  - Presents with papulosquamous or annular/polycyclic erythematous scaly patches/plaques on shoulders, trunk, extensor arms; face typically spared; heal without scarring but telangiectasia common; fatigue and arthralgias common but limited organ involvement.
  - *Histology:* Atrophic epidermis, some vacuolar change of BMZ, sparse inflammatory infiltrate.
  - *Labs:* 60-80% with + ANA, anti-Ro (60-90%).
  - *Course:* Persistent with intermittent flares, up to 50% will eventually meet SLE criteria (but milder disease).
  - *Treatment:* Sun protection, antimalarial, oral corticosteroid, dapsone or other immunosuppressive agent (topical corticosteroids rarely sufficient alone).
  - *Associations:* HLA-B8 (strongest), HLA-DR3, HLA-DRw52, HLA-DQ1.
- **Systemic LE (SLE)**
  - Systemic multi-organ involvement typically in young adults; ↑ incidence in African American patients.

- Need 4 out of 11 criteria for diagnosis (see below).
- Cutaneous lesions include bilateral malar erythema following sun exposure, discoid lesions, oral ulcerations, photosensitivity, patchy to diffuse nonscarring alopecia with lupus hairs (along frontal scalp line), Raynaud's phenomenon, livedo reticularis, acrocyanosis, cutaneous signs of antiphospholipid syndrome, urticarial vasculitis, red lunulae, multiple dermatofibromas.
- *Histology:* Modest vacuolar change, perivascular and periadnexal lymphocytic infiltrate, ↑ dermal mucin
- *Labs:* > 95% with + ANA, anti-dsDNA and anti-Sm are both highly specific for SLE.
- *Treatment:* Antimalarial, oral/topical corticosteroid, steroid-sparing immunosuppressive agent.
- *Associations:* HLA-DR2, HLA-DR3.

- **Criteria (need 4 out of 11):** Malar erythema, Discoid LE + ANA Arthritis, Hematologic disorder, Immunologic (dsDNA, Sm), Neurologic disorder, Serositis, Photosensitivity, Nephropathy, Oral ulcers.
- **Drug-induced SCLE:** Hydrochlorothiazide, terbinafine, diltiazem, ACEI, NSAIDs, griseofulvin, antihistamines, IFN, PUVA, TNFα.
- **Drug-induced SLE:** Hydralazine, procainamide, chlorpromazine, INH, quinidine, practolol, D-penicillamine, PUVA, minocycline.

MD SOAP BRAIN:

***M**alar rash, **D**iscoid rash, **S**erositis, **O**ral ulcers, **A**rthritis, **P**hotosensitivity, **B**lood (heme), **R**enal, **A**NA, **I**mmuno abnormality, **N**eurologic.*

8. A 6 years child presented with erythematous lesion at region between intertriginous folds of neck, as shown in below given image. What is the diagnosis?

A. Contact dermatitis

B. Seborrheic dermatitis

C. Candidal intertrigo

D. Atopic dermatitis

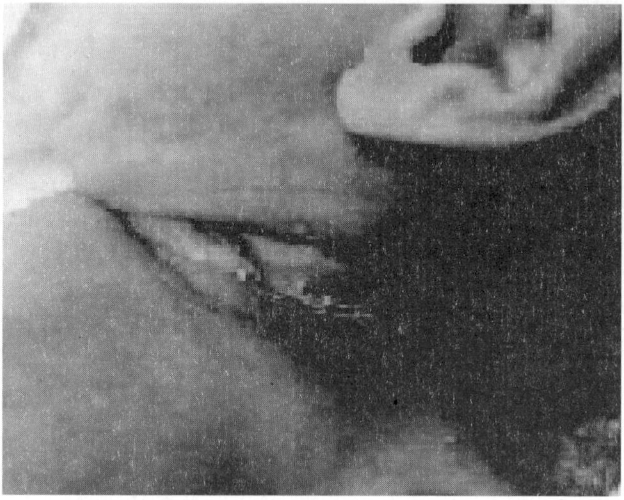

Answer: Option C. Candidial intertrigo

Explanation:

6 years child presented with erythematous lesion at region between intertriginous folds of neck. Here only condition from above given options commonly affects skinfold is Candidal intertrigo.

Candidal intertrigo refers to superficial skinfold infection caused by the yeast, candida.

Candidal intertrigo is triggered by a combination of the following factors:

- The hot and damp environment of skinfolds, which is conducive to the growth of candida species, particularly Candida albicans.
- Increased skin friction.
- Immunocompromise.

Factors that increase an individual's risk of developing candidal intertrigo include:

- Occlusive clothing, gloves and footwear
- Obesity
- Excessive sweating (hyperhidrosis)
- Incontinence causing irritant contact dermatitis

- Diabetes mellitus
- Immune deficiency conditions, such as human immunodeficiency virus infection (HIV) or immune suppression by medications (chemotherapy, systemic corticosteroids).

Candidal intertrigo classically presents as erythematous and macerated plaques with peripheral scaling. There are often associated superficial satellite papules or pustules.

Affected areas may include:

- Skinfolds below the breasts or under the abdomen
- Armpits and groin
- Web spaces between the fingers or toes (erosio interdigitalis blastomycetica).

Other Cutaneous Features of Candidiasis

- C. albicans common inhabitant of skin, GU and GI tract.
- Opportunistic organism, can become pathogen in skin, nails and mucous membranes.
- Frequently infects intertriginous areas.

Thrush (Moniliasis)

Presents as gray-white plaques on mucous membranes with reddish macerated base and/or smooth-surfaced bright red tongue (atrophic papillae).

Vulvovaginitis

Overgrowth of candida causes burning, itching, discharge; associated with diabetes mellitus, antibiotic use, pregnancy.

Candidal paronychia

Redness, tenderness, edema of nailfold; associated with chronic exposure to moisture and irritants.

Perleche (Angular cheilitis)

Transverse fissuring and maceration of oral commissures.

Diaper candidiasis

Erythematous patches in groin, ± satellite papules/pustules.

Perineal candidiasis

Perianal dermatitis with erythema, maceration, burning and pruritus (due to mechanical chafing ± incontinence).

Erosio interdigitalis blastomycetica

Maceration between webspace of fingers (nearly always third web space), similar in toes but usually fourth webspace affected.

9. What is the diagnosis based on given below image?

A. Contact leukoderma
B. Vitiligo
C. Inverse psoriasis
D. Albinism

Answer: Option A. Contact leukoderma

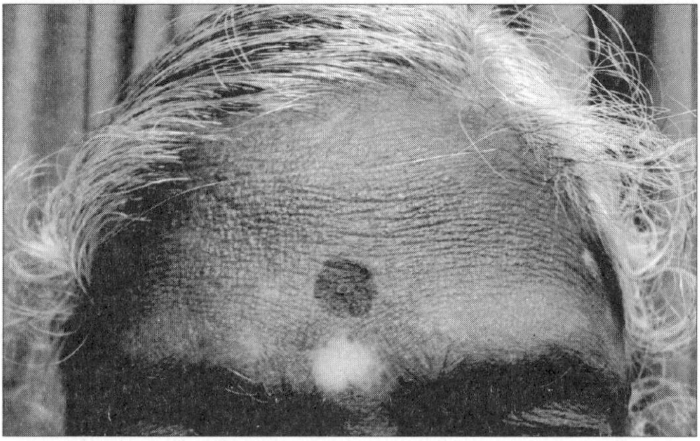

Explanation:

Here, above image is showing focal rounded area of loss of skin color at the site of bind at forhead region, so diagnosis here is contact leukoderma.

Contact leukoderma is the loss of skin colour (whitening of skin) following contact with chemicals known to destroy the skin pigment cells (melanocytes). It is usually due to chemicals found in the workplace, but it can also follow the use of certain cosmetic products. It is also known as chemical leukoderma and may be spelt leucoderma.

Contact leukoderma may develop in the setting of pre-existing idiopathic **vitiligo**, suggesting a genetic predisposition. This genetic susceptibility may explain why only some people will get leukoderma upon contact with certain chemicals. Liver and thyroid disease have been reported in some patients. However, in the majority of patients, there is neither a personal nor family history of vitiligo nor other autoimmune disease.

The main chemicals that have been known to cause contact leukoderma include aromatic or aliphatic derivatives of phenols and catechols. Monobenzylether of hydroquinone (MBH) was the first identified chemical to cause leukoderma in leather manufacturing workers who wore rubber gloves cured with MBH. Other chemicals that are known to cause occupational leukoderma include the phenolic compounds, para-tertiary butylphenol, para-tertiary octylphenol and para-tertiary butylphenolformaldehyde.

The most common cause of contact leukoderma from cosmetics is **para-phenylenediamine (PPD)** in hair dyes. The hair dye may have been used by the patient or they may have applied it to someone else. As PPD can also be found in black socks and footwear, the leukoderma may also affect the feet. Sensitization to PPD may have followed the application of a temporary **black henna tattoo**, also leaving a white mark. Frequent use of hair dye has also been associated with an increased risk of developing vitiligo.

Contact leukoderma due to the azo dyes has been reported with the use of facial cosmetics in the following products:

- Lipsticks
- Lipliner
- Eyeliners.

Contact leukoderma can also be caused by para-tertiary butyl phenol (PTBP) in deodorants and spray-on perfumes.

A series of cases followed the use of skin lightening cream containing **monobenzylether of hydroquinone** on the hands. **Monobenzylether of hydroquinone** has also been deliberately applied to pigmented areas to reduce the unsightliness of extensive vitiligo.

A skin lightening cream containing rhododendrol (another phenolic compound) resulted in localised contact leukoderma and widespread vitiligo in about 18,000 users in Japan in 2013.

Methylphenidate patches (used to treat attention-deficit/hyperactivity disorder) may rarely cause permanent loss of skin colour at the site of application.

In addition, it has been reported with cultural practices, particularly in India, related to the use of alta, an azo dye painted on the feet. The specific azo dye identified in alta was solvent yellow 3. Contact leukoderma has also been reported in Asian women with an adhesive bindi, the coloured spot applied to the forehead. The chemical associated with bindi leukoderma is PTBP in the adhesive.

Contact leukoderma presents as a white patch(es) of skin, initially at the site(s) of application but can spread beyond the area of known contact in approximately one-quarter of patients. A single lesion occurs in approximately one-third of patients; multiple patches are more common. Contact leukoderma is never present at birth.

Contact leukoderma due to cosmetics occurs most frequently on the face. The eyelids are particularly involved. Contact leukoderma due to hair dyes applied to the patient usually affects the hair margin rather than the scalp skin. It can subsequently lead to white patches in distant sites, i.e., vitiligo.

Typically there are small confettisized flat spots of white skin with a sharply defined margin seen under magnification. The skin is not scaly.

Wood lamp examination shows an accentuation of the pigment loss although this is not always as shows an accentuation of the pigment loss although this is not always as clear as in vitiligo.

Listed below is suggested diagnostic criteria for contact leukoderma (Ghosh S, Mukhopadhyay S. 2009). A patient should have three of the four criteria.

- Acquired vitiligo-like depigmented lesions.
- History of repeated exposure to specific chemicals.
- A pattern of flat vitiligo-like macules at the site of exposure to the chemical.
- Confetti macules.

10. What is the diagnosis based on given below image?

A. Sebaceous cyst

B. Dermoid cyst

C. Epidermoid cyst

D. Meningeoma

Answer: Option A. Sebaceous cyst

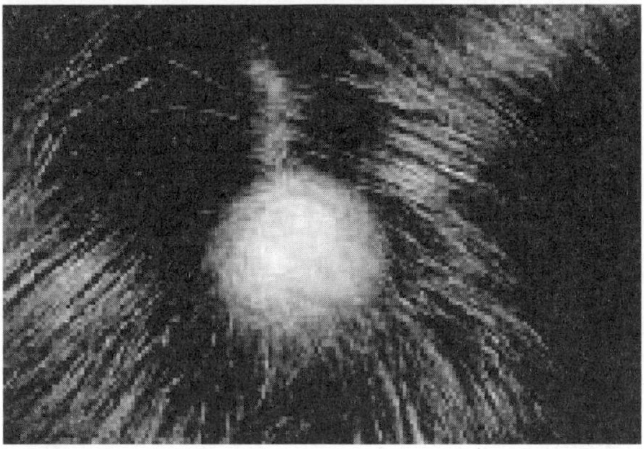

Explanation:

Here above given image is showing cystic scalp swelling which slightly reddish in color. Here it is probably originate from scalp hair that suggest diagnosis of sebaceous cyst.

Other options dermoid cyst and epidermoid cysts are usually present on parts of the body with relatively little hair. Meningioma usually seen as intra cranial or intra spinal region.

A **sebaceous cyst** is a term commonly used to refer to either:

- Epidermoid cysts (also termed *epidermal cysts*, *infundibular cyst*), or
- Pilar cysts (also termed *trichelemmal cysts*, *isthmus-catagen cysts*).

Both of the above types of cyst contain keratin, not sebum, and neither originates from sebaceous glands. Epidermoid cysts originate in the epidermis and pilar cysts originate from hair follicles. Therefore, technically speaking they are not sebaceous cysts. True sebaceous cysts, cysts which originate from sebaceous glands and which contain sebum, are relatively rare and are known as steatocystoma simplex or, if multiple, as steatocystoma multiplex.

A **pilar cyst, trichilemmal cyst**, also known as a **wen**, or **isthmus-catagen cyst**, is a common cyst that forms from a hair follicle. They are most often found on the scalp. The cysts are smooth, mobile and filled with keratin, a protein component found in hair, nails, skin and horns. They are, however, clinically and histologically distinct from trichilemmal horn, which are much more rare and not limited to the scalp. Trichilemmal cysts may run in families and they may or may not be inflamed and tender, often depending on whether they have ruptured. Rarely, these cysts may grow more extensively and form rapidly multiplying trichilemmal tumors, also called proliferating trichilemmal cysts, which are benign but may grow aggressively at the cyst site. Very rarely, trichilemmal cysts can become cancerous.

Sebaceous cysts generally do not require medical treatment. However, if they continue to grow, they may become unsightly, painful, infected, or all of the above.

Surgical

Surgical excision of a sebaceous cyst is a simple procedure to completely remove the sac and its contents.

There are three general approaches used: traditional wide excision, minimal excision, and punch biopsy excision.

11. A 6 years old child having infective lesion over neck region as shown in below image. His slide shows gram-positive cocci in long chains. What is the diagnosis in below given image?

A. Scrofuloderma
B. Folliculitis
C. Erthrasma
D. Impetigo contagiosa

Answer: Option D. Impetigo contagiosa

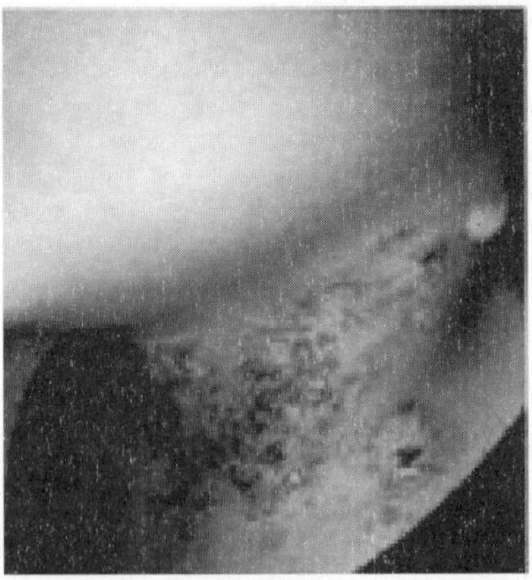

Explanation:

Here, 6 years old child having infective lesion over neck region with slide shows gram-positive cocci in long chains–suggest streptococcal infection. From above given options impetigo contagiosa is only streptococcal infection and skin lesion is showing golden crust in an erythematous lesion, so diagnosis here is impetigo contagiosa.

Nonbullous **impetigo**, also known as **impetigo contagiosa**, is the most common skin infection in children, accounting for approximately 10% of all cutaneous problems in pediatric clinics. It is more contagious than the bullous type.

Impetigo Contagiosa

- Highly contagious infection seen primarily in children

  This acute, highly contagious infection of the superficial layers of the epidermis is primarily caused by *Streptococcus pyogenes* or *Staphylococcus aureus*.

  Erythematous macule → pustule/vesicle → erosion with golden crust (+ culture from exudate under crust)

  Children with nonbullous impetigo commonly have multiple coalescing lesions on their face (perioral, perinasal) and extremities or in areas with a break in the natural skin defense barrier. The initial lesions are small vesicles or pustules (< 2 cm) that rupture and become a honey-colored crust with a moist erythematous base. Pharyngitis is absent, but mild regional lymphadenopathy is commonly present. Nonbullous impetigo is usually a self-limited process that resolves within 2 weeks.

  Bullous impetigo also differs from nonbullous impetigo in that bullous impetigo may involve the buccal mucous membranes, and regional adenopathy rarely occurs.

- **Erythrasma** is a bacterial infection that affects the skin. It usually appears in the folds of the skin. It's more commonly seen in warm or humid climates, and is usually caused by the bacteria Corynebacterium minutissimum.
- **Bacterial Folliculitis**

  Superficial infection of hair follicle usually due to *S. aureus.*

Presents with pustules in follicular distribution associated with hairs.

- **Scrofuloderma** (also known as "**Tuberculosis cutis colliquativa**") is a skin condition caused by tuberculous involvement of the skin by direct extension, usually from underlying tuberculous lymphadenitis.

CHAPTER

19

RADIOLOGY

1. Identify the white arrow structure in following given image:

A. Fornix
B. Basal ganglia
C. Corpus callosum
D. Internal capsule

Answer: Option A. Fornix

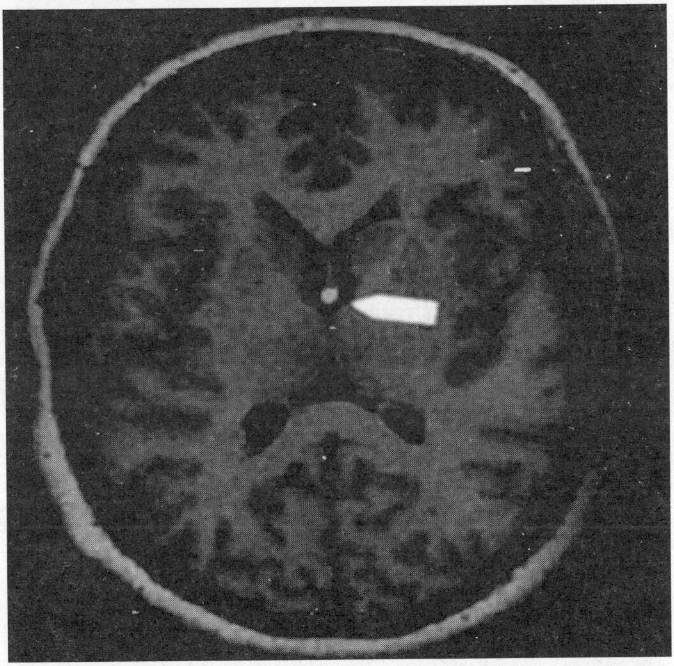

Explanation:

Above image is T1 weighted axial image. Arrow structure is fornix.

The **fornix** is the main efferent system of the hippocampus and an important part of the limbic system.

It is one of the commissural fibers connecting the cerebral hemispheres.

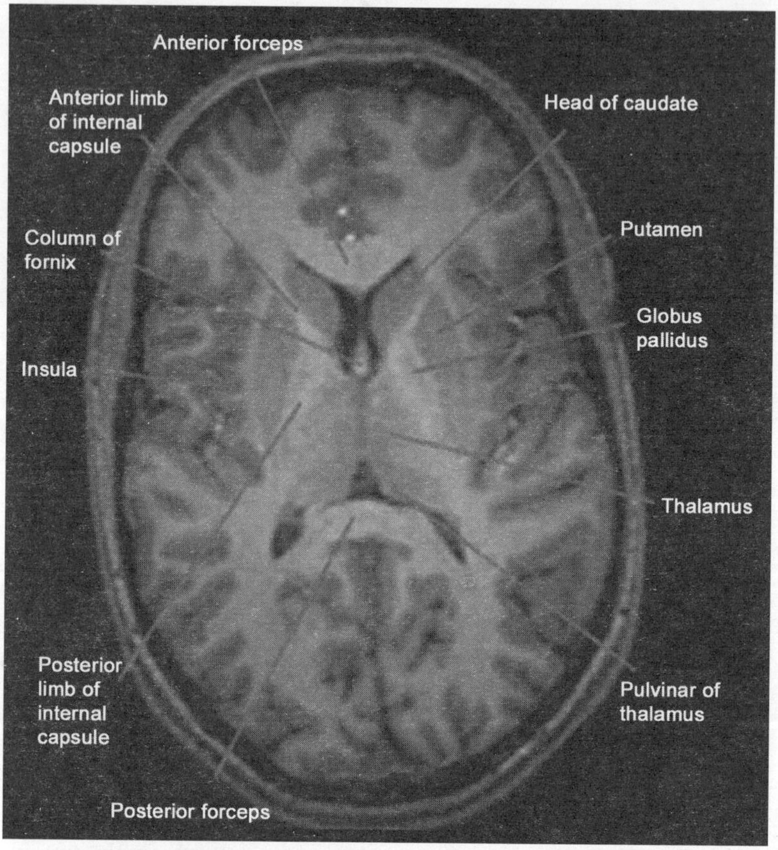

Gross Anatomy

Roughly C-shaped, the fornix extends from the hippocampus to the mammillary bodies of the hypothalamus and the anterior nuclei of the thalamus.

It is a curvilinear bundle of white matter fibers that begins as a group of myelinated fibers called the alveus.

The alveus joins to form the fimbria of the hippocampus.

The fimbria of each hippocampus thickens and then splits off from the hippocampus to form the crus (leg) of the fornix.

The fornix is composed of four parts:

1. **Crura:** Best seen at the splenium of the corpus callosum at the level of the superior colliculus on coronal images.
2. **Commissure:** Connects the crura.

3. **Body:** From the merging of the crura, provides one of two major paths through which the hippocampi communicate with each other.
4. **Columns (anterior pillars):** Curves anteriorly and dives into the hypothalamus (mammillary bodies).

2. Identify the following image:

A. Acute lacunar infarct at left basal ganglia
B. Sub arachnoid hemorrhage
C. Intra ventricular hemorrhage
D. Intra parenchymal hemorrhage

Answer: Option A. Acute lacunar infarct at left basal ganglia

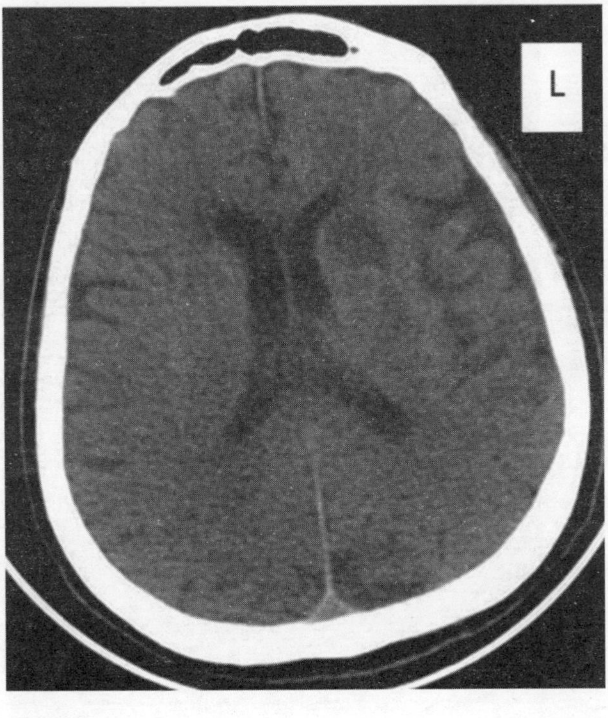

Explanation:

Above CT axial image is at level of basal ganglia showing two small hypodense areas involving left sided basal ganglia (caudate and putamen).

Now, infarct appears as hypodense on CT scan while acute hemorrhage appear as hyper dense on CT scan.

In our case, CT brain shows hypodense areas, therefore answer would be **Acute lacunar infarct at left basal ganglia (lacunar means small-around 10 mm size).**

3. Identify following given image:

A. Urinary bladder calculus

B. Bilateral ureterocele

C. Vesico-ureteric reflux

D. VUJ calculus

Answer: Option B. Bilateral ureterocele

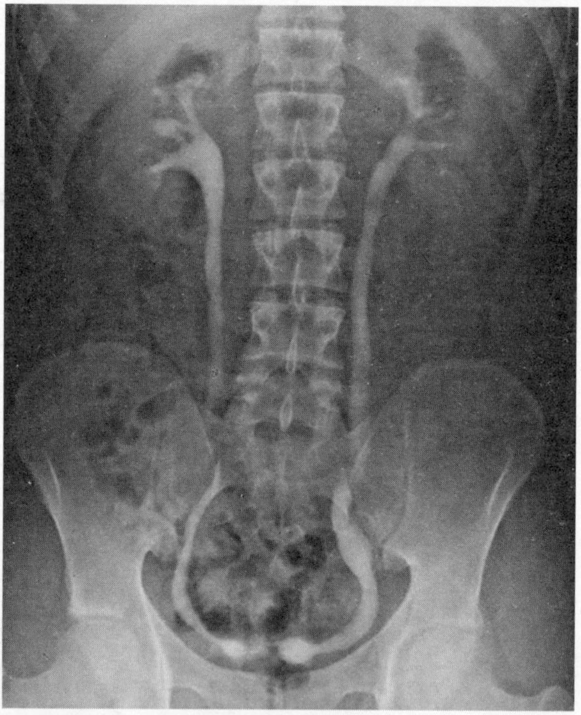

Explanation:

Image is of IVP study, showing normal excretion of both kidneys with opacification of both ureter.

Now, distal end of both ureters are dilated near its opening into bladder (vesico-ureteric junction) which is called as ureterocele.

Different types of ureteroceles classified by their association with the renal unit.

1. **Single system ureteroceles** are those associated with a single kidney, a single collecting system, and a solitary ureter.
2. **Duplex system ureteroceles** are associated with kidneys that have a completely duplicated collecting system and two ureters.
3. **Orthotopic ureterocele** is a ureterocele whose orifice is located in a normal anatomic position within the bladder. These are commoner in adults.
4. **Ectopic ureterocele** refers to those ureteroceles whose orifices are located in an ectopic position, such as the bladder neck or urethra. They typically arise from the upper pole moiety of a duplicated collecting system and are more common in the pediatric population.

IVP Signs of Ureterocele

- Hydronephrotic upper pole displacing the lower pole moiety laterally and inferiorly (i.e., the “drooping lily” sign).
- Ureteral displacement by the hydroureter or hydronephrotic upper pole moiety.
- **“Cobra-head” or “Adder-head”** extension of the distal ureter (seen in adults) is classical and is diagnostic.

The **cobra head sign**, also known as the **spring onion sign**, refers to dilatation of the distal ureter, surrounded by a thin lucent line, which is seen in patients with an adult type ureterocoele. The cobra head appearance indicates an uncomplicated ureterocele.

4. Identify structure in following given image:

A. Cerebrum B. Cerebellum

C. Basal ganglia D. Brainstem

Answer: Option B. Cerebellum

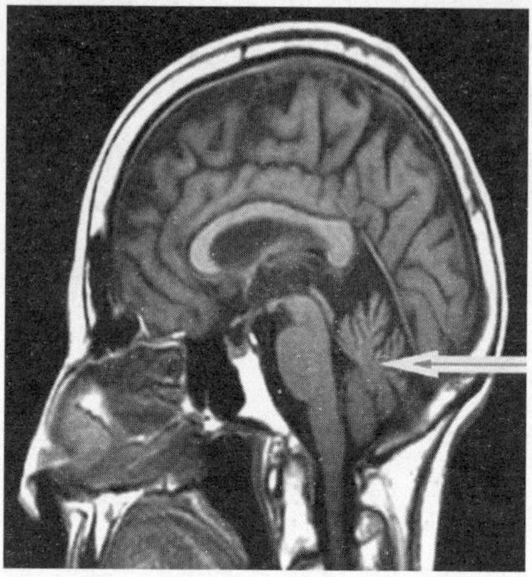

Explanation:

This is a sagittal image of MRI brain FLAIR sequence at mid sagittal level. The arrow marked structure is cerebellum characterized by its typical location at posterior fossa, posterior to brainstem having multiple cerebellar folia.

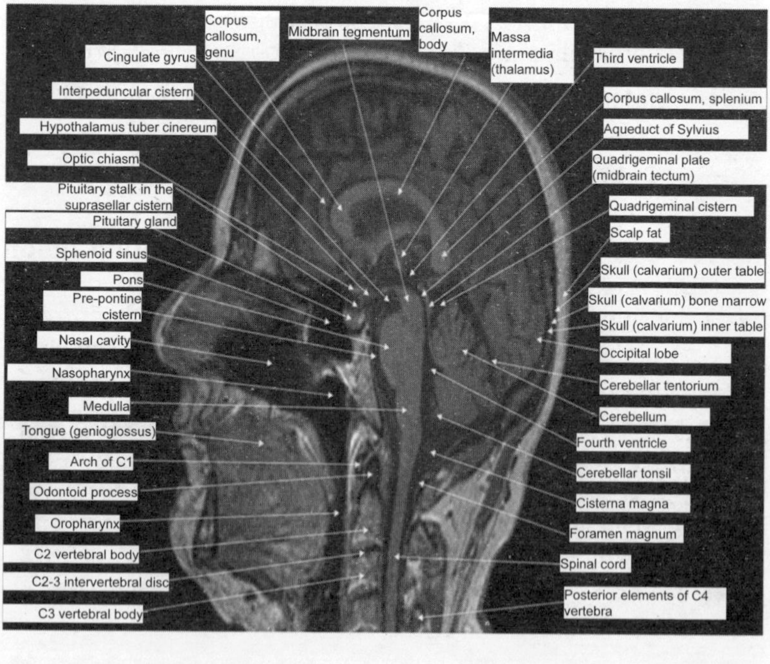

5. Clinical image and plain CT skull image are given for a patient with history of diplopia.

Find out diagnosis:

A. Blow-out fracture
B. Fracture of nasal bone
C. Fracture of zygomatic bone
D. Fracture of sphenoid bone

Answer: Option A. Blow-out fracture

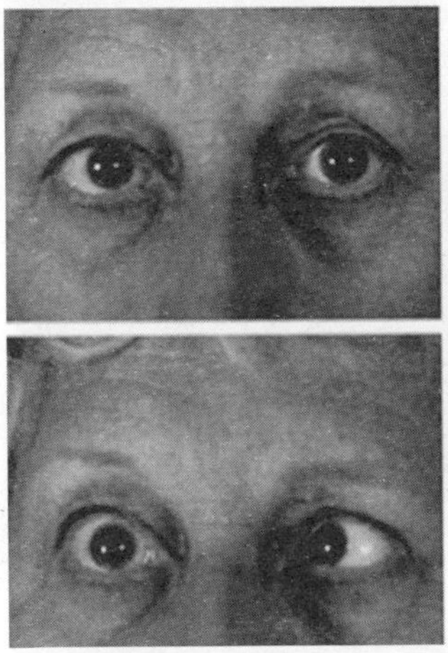

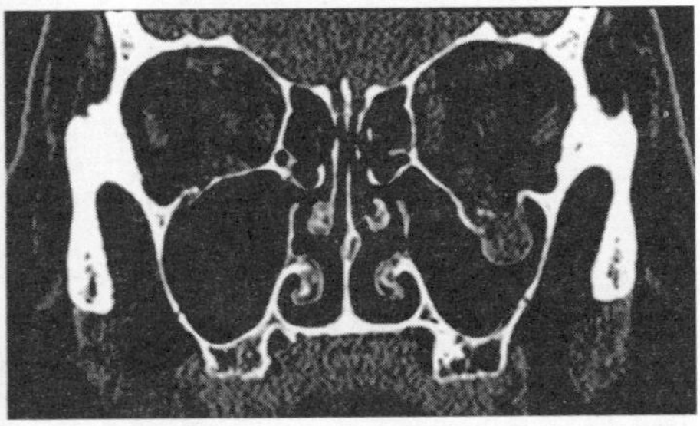

Explanation:

Here coronal CT scan image of orbit is showing fracture of inferior wall of left orbit with herniation of orbital soft tissue through it–which is called as blow-out fracture/tear drop fracture.

Another clinical image of eye is showing diplopia which is a presentation of this blow-out fracture.

- **Orbital blow-out fractures** occur when there is a fracture of one of the walls of orbit but the orbital rim remains intact. This is typically caused by a direct blow to the central orbit from a fist or ball.
- The blow-out fracture is the most common type of orbital fracture and is usually the result of trauma. This is reflected in the demographics: it is more prevalent in young men.

Clinical Presentation

- Orbital blow-out fractures are usually the result of a

direct blow to the orbit, which causes a sudden increase in intraorbital pressure. Decompression then occurs by fracture of one or more of the bounding walls of the orbit.

- Although the causative trauma is usually substantial, presentation and diagnosis may be delayed in the setting of extensive soft tissue swelling and (by definition) an intact orbital rim. In particular, clinical findings of diplopia and restricted ocular motion may be temporarily masked by intraorbital swelling which can compensate for the traumatically-expanded osseous orbital volume.

Clinical Findings

- **Enophthalmos:** Due to increased orbital volume
- **Diplopia:** Due to extraocular muscle entrapment
- **Orbital emphysema:** Especially when the fracture is into an adjacent paranasal sinus
- **Malar region numbness:** Due to injury to the inferior orbital nerve
- Hypoglobus.

Types of Blow-out Fracture

- Inferior (floor)
- Medial wall (lamina papyracea)
- Superior (roof)
- Lateral wall
- Inferior blow-out fracture

Inferior blow-out fractures are the most common. Orbital fat prolapses into the maxillary sinus and may be joined by prolapse of the inferior rectus muscle. In children, the fracture may spring back. Most fractures occur in the floor posterior and medial to the infraorbital groove. In ~50% of cases, inferior blow-out fractures are associated with fractures of the medial wall.

6. Coronal NCCT image of para nasal sinus is given below. Find out the sign in given image.

A. Ground glass B. Double density

C. Honeycombing D. Onion peel

Answer: Option B. Double density

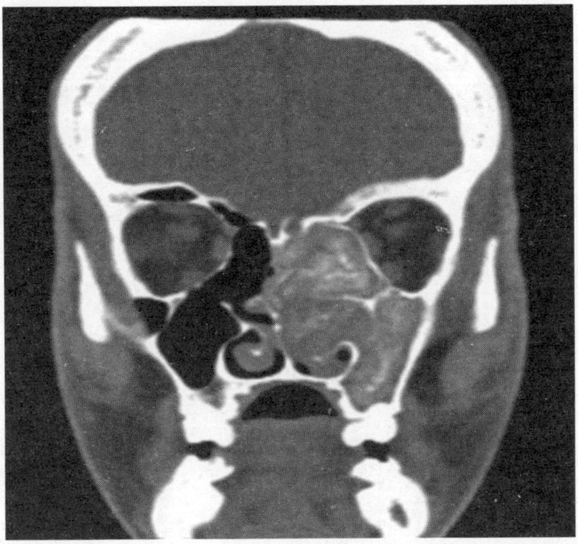

Explanation:

Here above coronal CT image of face shows soft tissue density areas within left maxillary and ethmoid sinus which has central serpiginous **hyperdensity** and peripheral **hypodensity–Double Density sign.**

Allergic fungal sinusitis is the most common form of fungal sinusitis and is common in warm and humid climates.

The ethmoid sinus is the most common location, followed by the maxillary, frontal and sphenoid sinuses.

Associations

- Asthma in 65% of cases.

CT

The majority of sinuses show near complete opacification.

On unenhanced CT, the sinuses are typically opacified by centrally (often serpiginous) hyperdense material with a peripheral rim of hypodense mucosa.

Approximately 40% of patients may have each of the following features:

- Expansion of an involved sinus
- Remodeling and thinning of the bone sinus walls
- Erosion of the sinus wall

7. Identify the disease in following given image:

A. Pneumonia B. ILD
C. Miliary TB D. Collapse

Answer: Option C. Miliary TB

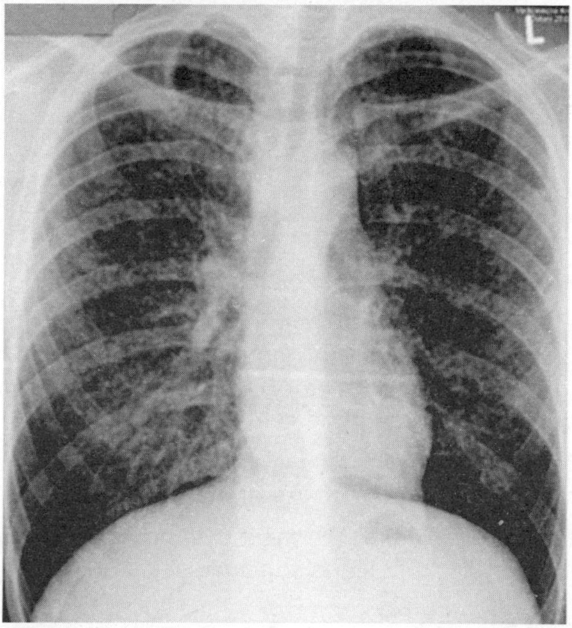

Explanation:

Above PA chest X-rays demonstrate widespread small (2-4 mm) nodular opacities distributed throughout both lungs. This pattern is called as miliary pattern.

Etiology

The causes can be broadly sub-grouped dependent on whether or not the patient is febrile.

Afebrile

- Infection

- **Tuberculosis (often febrile but may be afebrile)**
  - ◊ Miliary tuberculosis
- **Fungal (often febrile)**
  - ◊ Immunocompromised or elderly patients may be afebrile
- Healed varicella pneumonia

- Miliary metastases
  - Thyroid carcinoma
  - Renal cell carcinoma
  - Breast carcinoma
  - Malignant melanoma
  - Pancreatic neoplasms
  - Osteosarcoma
  - Trophoblastic disease
- Others
  - **Sarcoidosis:** Miliary sarcoidosis
  - Pneumoconioses
    - ◊ Silicosis
    - ◊ Coal workers pneumoconiosis
  - Pulmonary hemosiderosis
  - BCGosis
  - Hypersensitivity pneumonitis
  - Langerhans cell histiocytosis (LCH)
  - Multifocal micronodular pneumocyte hyperplasia (MMPH)
  - Diffuse pulmonary meningotheliomatosis
  - Pulmonary alveolar proteinosis
    - ◊ Small acinar opacities can mimic a miliary pattern.

Febrile

- Infection
  - Tuberculosis
  - Fungal
  - Viral pneumonitis

- Nocardiosis
- Salmonella

- Hypersensitivity pneumonitis.

Miliary tuberculosis is an uncommon pulmonary manifestation of tuberculosis.

It represents haematogeneous dissemination of uncontrolled tuberculous infection and carries a relatively poor prognosis.

It is seen both in primary and post-primary tuberculosis and may be associated with tuberculous infection in numerous other tissues and organs.

RADIOGRAPHIC FEATURES

Plain Radiograph

Miliary deposits appear as 1-3 mm diameter nodules, which are uniform in size and uniformly distributed.

8. Identify the investigation in following given image:

A. Barium swalllow

B. Barium meal

C. Barium meal follow through

D. Barium enema

Answer: Option C. Barium meal follow through

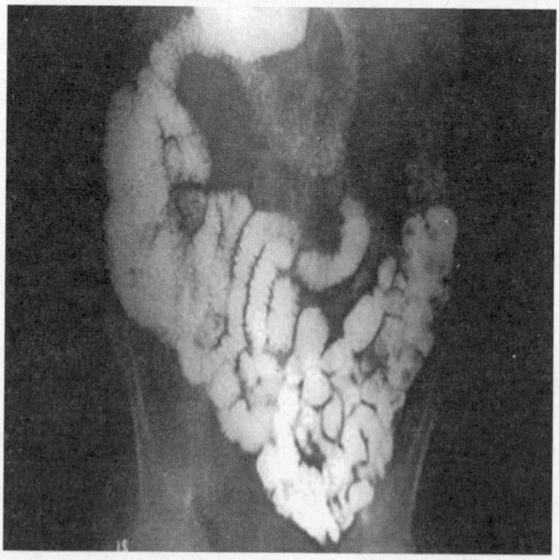

Explanation:

Here above mentioned image is showing opacification of small bowel, which is called as barium meal follow through study.

Barium swallow is a dedicated test of the pharynx, esophagus and proximal stomach.

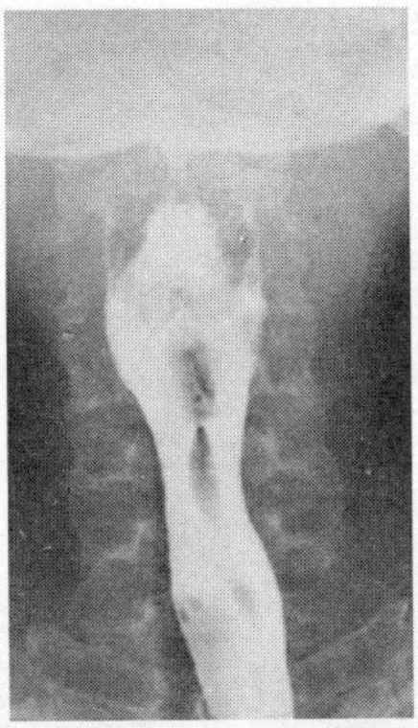

Barium meal is a dedicated test of the whole stomach.

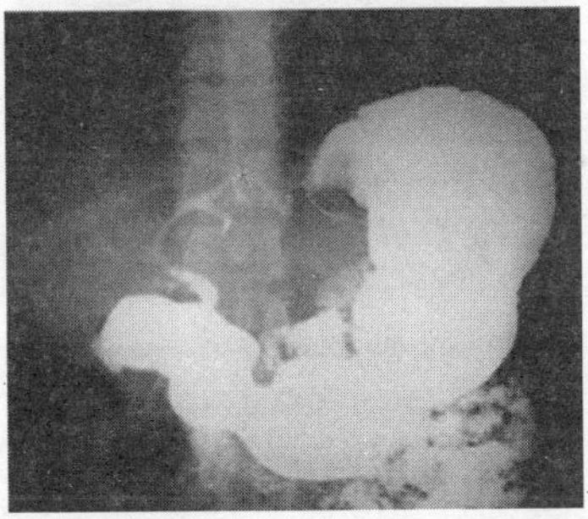

Barium enema is a dedicated test of the large bowel and rectum.

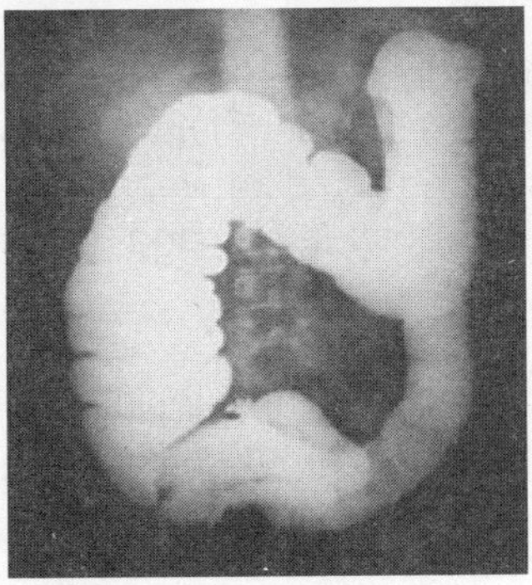

9. Find out false statement regarding following given image of a patient with 25 years old.

A. Eccentric location

B. Having distinct margin

C. Involves epiphyseal and metaphyseal region

D. Chemotherapy is treatment of choice

Answer: Option D. Chemotherapy is treatment of choice

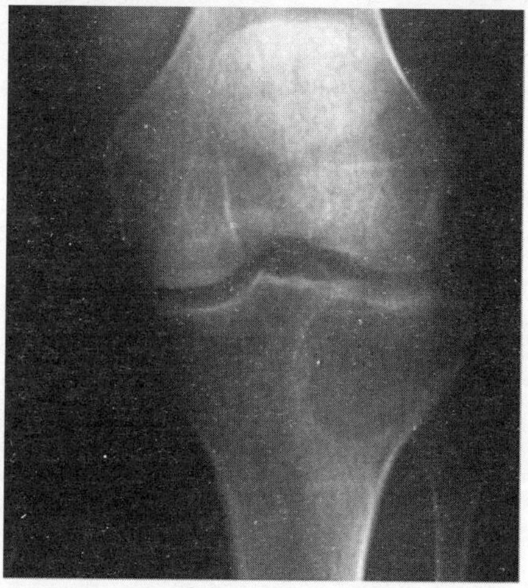

Explanation:

Giant cell tumors of bone, also known as **osteoclastomas**, are relatively common bone tumors and are usually benign. They typically arise from the metaphysis of long bones, extend into the epiphysis adjacent to the joint surface, and have a narrow zone of transition.

They almost invariably (97-99%) occur when the growth plate has closed and are therefore typically seen in early adulthood. 80% of cases are reported between the ages of 20 and 50, with a peak incidence between 20 and 30 years.

Location

They typically occur as single lesions. Although any bone can be affected, the most common sites are:

- **Around the knee:** Distal femur and proximal tibia: 50-65%.

- **Distal radius:** 10-12%
- **Sacrum:** 4-9%
- **Vertebral body:** 7%
  - Thoracic spine most common, followed by cervical and lumbar spines.

Multiple locations: ≈1% (multiple lesions usually occur in association with Paget disease).

RADIOGRAPHIC FEATURES

Classic Appearance

There are four characteristic radiographic features when a giant cell tumor is located in a long bone:

- Occurs only with a closed growth plate
- **Abuts articular surface:** 84-99% come within 1 cm of the articular surface.
- Well-defined with non-sclerotic margin (though <5% may show some sclerosis).
- **Eccentric:** If large this may be difficult to assess.

TREATMENT AND PROGNOSIS

Classically, treatment is with curettage and packing with bone chips or polymethyl methacrylate (PMMA).

Local recurrence is from the periphery of the lesion and has historically occurred in up to 40-60% of cases.

Newer intraoperative adjuncts such as thermal or chemical treatment of the resection margins have lowered the recurrence rate to 2.5-10%.

Wide local excision is associated with a lower recurrence rate but has greater morbidity.

10. Which of the following is a cause of "Gasless abdomen"?

A. Ulcerative colitis

B. Acute pancreatitis

C. Intussusception

D. NEC

Answer: Option B. Acute pancreatitis

Explanation:

Common causes of 'Gasless abdomen' include:

- Small bowel obstruction–most common cause.
- Bowel ischemia
- Congenital atresia
- Ascites
- **Pancreatitis**
- Gastroenteritis
- Large abdominal mass – due to displacement.
- Post surgery following total colectomy, esophagogastrectomy, gastrectomy and low anterior resection.
- A paucity of small bowel gas may be a normal finding in some adults.

11. Which of the following is the water soluble contrast media?

A. Gadolinium B. Barium

C. Iodine D. Chloride

Answer: Option C. Iodine

Explanation:

Iodinated contrast media are water soluble contrast agents that contain iodine atoms used for X-ray-based imaging modalities such as computed tomography (CT), although they are also used in fluoroscopy, angiography and venography, and even occasionally, plain radiography.

Barium is used in form of barium sulfate as contrast agent. **Barium sulfate is insoluble in water and therefore very little of the toxic barium metal is absorbed into the body**.

Water-soluble iodinated contrast media can be classified by osmolality.

High Osmolality Contrast Media

High osmolality contrast media (HOCM) are approximately five to eight times the osmolality of serum.

HOCM remain used for gastrointestinal and cystourethral administration, including the following agents:

- **Diatrizoate** sodium/meglumine (Gastrografin, MD-Gastroview, Cystografin).
- Iothalamate sodium/meglumine (Conray, Cysto-Conray).

Low Osmolality Contrast Media

Low osmolality contrast media (LOCM) are less than three times the osmolality of human serum and preferred for intravascular and intrathecal administration.

LOCM in current use include the following:

- Iopamidol (Isovue)
- Iohexol (Omnipaque)
- Iopromide (Ultravist)
- Ioversol (Optiray)
- Ioxilan (Oxilan).

The LOCM category also includes iso-osmolal contrast media (IOCM), which are approximately the same osmolality as serum. The only IOCM in current use is a non-ionic dimer, which is composed of two covalently bound tri-iodinated benzene rings:

- Iodixanol (Visipaque).

Water-insoluble

Water-insoluble iodinated contrast media have limited uses.

The only currently approved agent is ethiodized poppyseed oil (Lipiodol), which is used for embolo/sclerotherapy and hysterosalpingography.

A historically-popular but now discontinued water-insoluble iodinated agent was **iophendylate (Pantopaque/Myodil)**, which was used for myelography.

12. In a patient with Tetralogy of Fallot, Boot shaped heart is due to:

A. Left ventricular hypertrophy

B. Right ventricular hypertrophy

C. Left atrial hypertrophy

D. Right atrial hypertrophy

Answer: Option B. Right ventricular hypertrophy

Explanation:

Chest radiographs may classically show a "boot-shaped" heart with an upturned cardiac apex due to right ventricular hypertrophy and concave pulmonary arterial segment.

Tetralogy of Fallot is classically characterized by four features, which are:

1. Ventricular septal defect (VSD)
   - May be multiple in ~5% of cases
2. Right ventricular outflow tract obstruction (RVOTO) due to:
   - Infundibular stenosis, or
   - Hypoplastic pulmonary valve annulus, or
   - Bicuspid pulmonary valve, and/or
   - Hypoplasia of pulmonary artery
3. Overriding aorta
4. Right ventricular hypertrophy: Only develops after birth.

13. A 70 years female patient, known case of hypertension and diabetes presented with left sided hemiparesis. Find out diagnosis in given image:

A. Intraparenchymal hemorrhage

B. Acute infarct

C. Intraventricular hemorrhage

D. Subarachnoid hemorrhage

Answer: Option B. Acute infarct

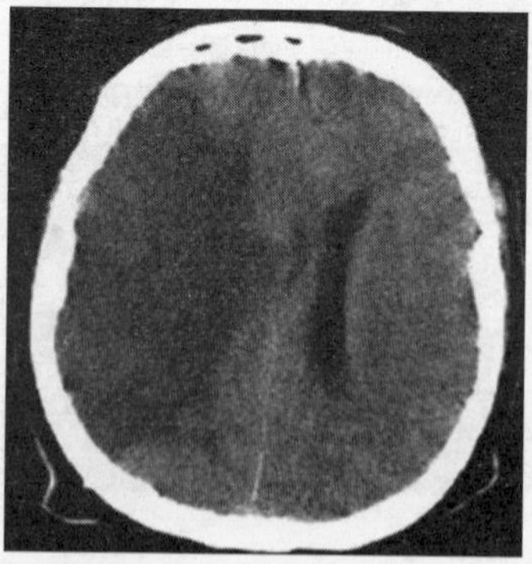

Explanation:

Here patient with hypertension and diabetes presented with left sided hemiparesis. Her CT brain shows a large hypodense area at right cerebral region (fronto-parietal lobe, insular cortex and basal ganglia-capsular region).

Now acute infarct appears as hypodense areas and acute hemorrhage appear as hyperdense on CT scan. Therefore in our case CT brain shows acute infarct (hypodense area) in right cerebrum.

CT

Non-contrast CT of the brain remains the mainstay of imaging in the setting of an acute stroke.

The goals of CT in the acute setting are:

1. Exclude intracranial hemorrhage, which would preclude thrombolysis
2. Look for any "early" features of ischemia
3. Exclude other intracranial pathologies that may mimic a stroke, such as tumor.

Immediate

The earliest CT sign visible is a hyperdense segment of a vessel, representing direct visualization of the intravascular thrombus / embolus and as such is visible immediately.

It is most often observed in the middle cerebral artery (see hyperdense middle cerebral artery sign and middle cerebral artery dot sign).

Early Hyperacute

Within the first few hours, features include:

- Loss of grey-white matter differentiation, and hypoattenuation of deep nuclei:
  - Lentiform nucleus changes seen as early as 1 hour after occlusion, visible in 75% of patients at 3 hours.
- Cortical hypodensity with associated parenchymal swelling with resultant gyral effacement.
  - Cortex which has poor collateral supply (e.g., insular ribbon) is more vulnerable.

Acute

With time the hypoattenuation and swelling become more marked resulting in a significant mass effect.

Subacute

As time goes on the swelling starts to subside and small amounts of cortical petechial hemorrhages result in elevation of the attenuation of the cortex. This is known as the CT fogging phenomenon .

Chronic

Later still the residual swelling passes, and gliosis sets in eventually appearing as a region of low density with negative mass effect.

14. A patient present with acute abdominal pain at emergency department with given image of X-ray abdomen. What is the best management?

A. Conservative management

B. Laparotomy

C. Ventilator therapy

D. Intubation

Answer: Option B. Laparotomy

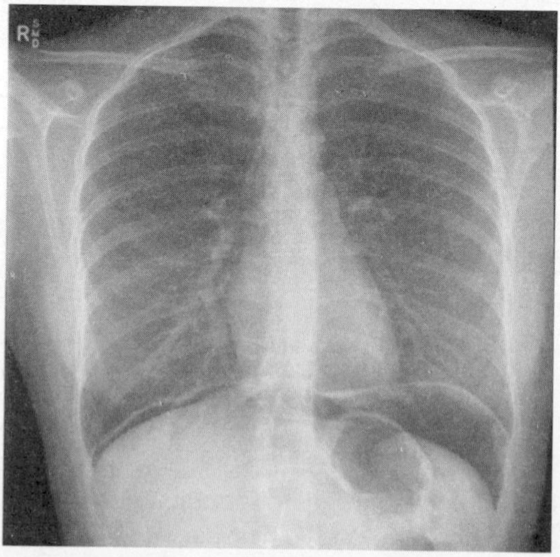

Explanation:

Here patient presents with acute abdominal pain with X-ray chest showing gas under diaphragm suggest pneumoperitoneum. Now Pneumoperitoneum in the presence of acute abdominal pain is an indication for laparotomy.

RADIOGRAPHIC FEATURES OF PNEUMOPERITONEUM ON PLAIN RADIOGRAPH

Chest radiograph

- Subdiaphragmatic free gas
- Cupola sign (on supine film)

Abdominal radiograph

- Double wall sign (also known as Rigler sign or bas-relief sign).
- Telltale triangle sign (also known as the triangle sign or telltale triangle).
- Peritoneal ligament-related signs
  - Football sign
  - Falciform ligament sign
  - Lateral umbilical ligament sign (also known as inverted "V" sign)
  - Urachus sign
- Right upper quadrant signs
  - Cupola sign
  - Fissure for ligamentum teres sign
  - Hepatic edge sign
  - Lucent liver sign
  - Morison pouch sign (doge cap sign)
  - Periportal free gas sign

15. A 56 years male alcoholic patient with acute pancreatitis developed acute onset dyspnoea. On auscultation he had crepitation. Find out diagnosis based on his X-ray chest.

A. ARDS
B. Pneumonia
C. ILD
D. Collapse

Answer: Option A. ARDS

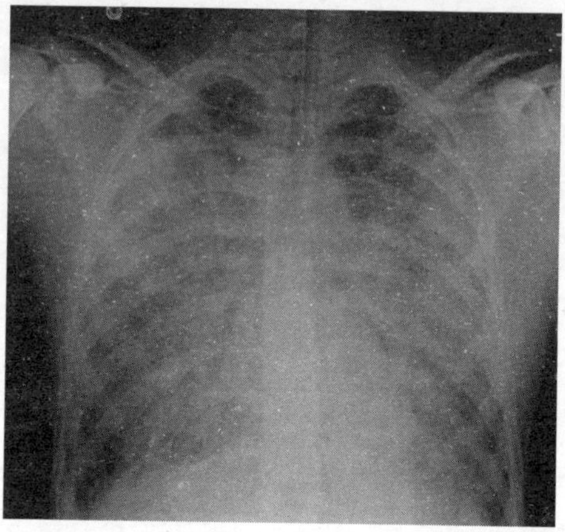

Explanation:

Here, male alcoholic patient with acute pancreatitis has developed acute onset dyspnea and his X-ray chest is showing diffuse bilateral coalescent opacities–suggestive of ARDS.

In case of pneumonia opacity is in form of consolidation–air bronchogram pattern.

ILD appears as reticulonodular thickening on CXR.

Collapse generally shows homogenous opacity on chest X-ray.

ARDS

Etiology:

Pulmonary causes	Extra-pulmonary causes
• Fat embolism	• **Pancreatitis**
• Near-drowning	• Burns
• Viral pneumonia	• Trauma
• Oxygen toxicity	• **Septicaemia**
• Smoke inhalation	• Hypovolemic shock
• Disseminated intravascular coagulopathy	• Head injury
• Aspiration of gastric contents	• Transfusion reaction
• Lung contusion	• Cardiopulmonary bypass

RADIOGRAPHIC FEATURES

Plain Radiograph

Chest radiographic findings of ARDS are non-specific and resemble those of typical pulmonary edema or pulmonary hemorrhage.

There are diffuse bilateral coalescent opacities (the only radiological criterion defined by the Consensus Conference).

Chest X-ray features usually develop 12-24 hours after initial lung insult as a result of proteinaceous interstitial edema.

Within one week, alveolar pulmonary edema (hyaline membrane) occurs due to type 1 pneumocyte damage.

In contrast to cardiogenic pulmonary edema, which clears in response to diuretic therapy, ARDS persists for days to weeks.

16. A 67 years old female patient presented with backache. Now based on below given radiograph of spine which of the following will be diagnosis?

A. Spondylolisthesis

B. Spodylolysis

C. Osteoporosis

D. Discovertebral osteomyelitis

Answer: Option C. Osteoporosis

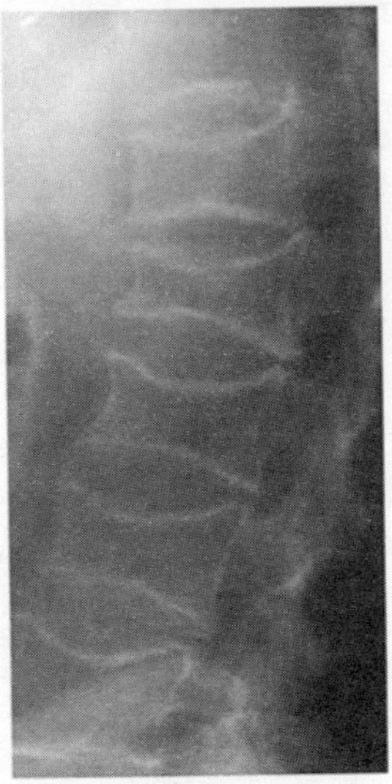

Explanation:

Here above image is showing biconcave appearance of lumbar vertebrae, also called fish vertebra/ codfish vertebra, which is seen in osteoporosis.

Osteoporosis is a metabolic skeletal disease defined as a reduction of bone mineral density below a defined lower limit of normal.

The World Health Organization (WHO) defines osteoporosis as a T-score less than -2.5 SD. However, Z-scores are more reliable than T-scores (which are defined against adult white females) as they compare with normal people of same age and gender – see dual-energy X-ray absorptiometry (DEXA) for additional discussion of T and Z scores.

Clinical Presentation

Osteoporosis per se is asymptomatic and is most often diagnosed when individuals are evaluated on the basis of risk factors or following presentation with fragility fracture.

Pathology

Osteoporosis is essentially decreased bony tissue per unit volume of bone. There is no microstructural and biochemical change as occurs in osteomalacia or rickets. Hence the mineral-to-osteoid ratio is normal (cf. osteomalacia in which the mineral-to-osteoid ratio is decreased).

Osteoporosis can be localized or diffuse and be divided into:

- **Primary:** No cause is identifiable.
  - *Postmenopausal (type 1):* Occurs in 50-65-year-old females; disproportionate loss of cancellous bone as compared to cortical bone resulting in more involvement of cancellous bone-rich areas, like vertebrae and ends of long bones.
  - *Senile (type 2):* Occurs in the elderly; proportionate loss of cortical and cancellous bones affecting long bones.
  - Idiopathic juvenile osteoporosis.
- **Secondary (type 3):** Occurs due to a range of causes including:
  - Endocrine disease (e.g. Cushing syndrome, hyperthyroidism, hyperparathyroidism, diabetes mellitus).

- Chronic illness (e.g. COPD, chronic liver disease, multiple sclerosis, celiac disease).
- Inflammation.
- Medications (e.g. steroids, phenytoin).
- Thalassemia major.
- Nutritional disturbances (e.g. malnutrition, anorexia).

Radiographic Features

Decreased bone density can be appreciated by decreased cortical thickness and loss of bony trabeculae in the early stages in radiography. Bones like the vertebra, long bones (proximal femur), calcaneum and tubular bones are usually looked at for evidence of osteoporosis.

Plain Radiograph

- Not a sensitive modality, as more than 30-50% bone loss is required to appreciate decreased bone density on a radiograph.
- Vertebral osteoporosis manifests as:
  - Pencilling of vertebrae.
  - Loss of cortical bone (picture frame vertebra) and trabecular bone (ghost vertebra).
  - Compression fractures and vertebra plana.
- Loss of trabeculae in proximal femur area, which is explained by Singh's index (and can also be seen in the calcaneum).
- In tubular bones (especially metacarpals), there will be thinning of the cortex.
  - Cortical thickness <25% of the whole thickness of metacarpal signifies osteoporosis (normally 25-33%).

Bone Mineral Density Measurement

Bone mineral density (BMD) measurement is the method of estimation of calcium hydroxyapatite. Multiple X-ray based, gamma-ray based and ultrasonic methods are available:

- Radiographic absorptiometry (RA).

- Single photon and X-ray absorptiometry (SPA).
- Dual energy X-ray absorptiometry (DEXA)–most commonly-used and most reliable.
- Quantitative computed tomography can be used.

MRI

Bone marrow signal takes on a heterogeneous appearance with rounded focal fatty lesions replacing normal marrow with coalescence often occurring:

- **T1:** Heterogeneously hyperintense.
- **T2:** Variable signal.

Treatment and Prognosis

As osteoporosis decreases bone strength, patients are at an increased risk of fracture, often with minimal trauma, and commonly at the pelvis, hip and wrist.

Oral bisphosphonates are the most commonly prescribed medications and are effective in reducing the risk of further osteoporotic fracture. There are a range of other medications that can also be used, including intravenous bisphosphonates, selective estrogen receptor modulators (e.g. raloxifene), denosumab, strontium ranelate, calcitonin, and parathyroid hormone-based treatments (e.g. teriparatide).

Complications

Bisphosphonates and denosumab have been associated with rare, but serious, side effects including bisphosphonate-related atypical femoral fractures and bisphosphonate-related osteonecrosis of the jaw.

17. A 56 years old patient with HIV infection presented with cough and dyspnea. His CD4 count is < 200/mm³. Which of the following organism causes this infection based on his chest X-ray?

A. Tuberculosis

B. Pneumocystis Jirovecii

C. CMV

D. Mycoplasma

Answer: Option B. Pneumocystis Jirovecii

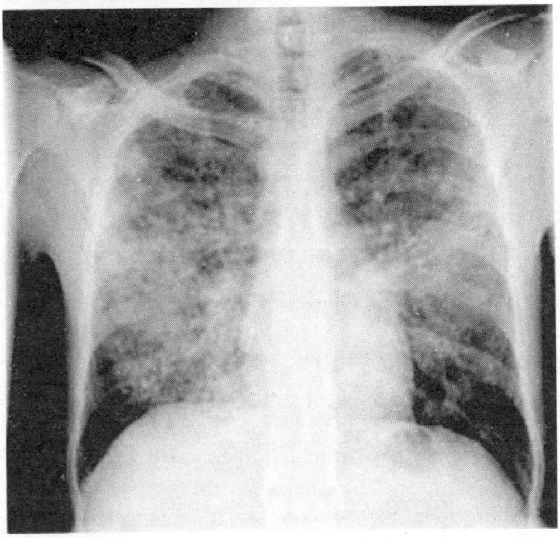

Explanation:

Here above patient's chest X-ray is showing fluffy opacities mainly at bilateral perihilar region with K/C/O AIDS and CD4 count is below 200/mm^3, presented with dyspnea and cough. These features are in favor of infection with pneumocystis jirovecii/carini.

Plain Radiograph

Although up to 90% of chest radiographs in patients with PCP are abnormal, appearances are often non-specific. Between 10-15% of patients with PCP have normal chest radiographs and close to 30% have non-specific or inconclusive findings.

Features which are highly suggestive of PCP in patients with CD4 counts below 200/mm^3 include:

- Small pneumatoceles
- Subpleural blebs
- Fine reticular interstitial changes
- Predominantly perihilar in distribution
- Nodular densities, cavitary lesion, Pneumothorax can also occur

Pleural effusions are normally not a feature, seen in less than 5% of cases.

– ↑ Frequency of upper lobe infiltrate in patient who take aerosolized pentamidine. Reduced arterial O_2 pressure (PaO_2); increase alveolar arterial O_2 gradient.
– (PAO_2- PaO_2); Respiratory alkalosis.

CT

High-resolution computed tomography is more sensitive and may be used to exclude PCP in patients with clinical suspicion for PCP but normal or inconclusive chest radiographs.

Features include:

- Ground-glass pattern
  - Considered a principal finding
  - Predominantly involving perihilar or mid zones
    - ◊ There may be a mid, upper or lower zone predilection depending on whether the patient is on prophylactic aerosolised medication.
    - ◊ If they are, then the poorly ventilated upper zones are prone to infection, whereas in those who are not, the lower zones are more frequently involved.
    - ◊ There may be a relative preservation of previously irradiated areas.
    - ◊ May show some peripheral sparing in a considerable number of patients (~40%).
- Reticular opacities or septal thickening may also be present; a crazy paving pattern may, therefore, be seen when both ground-glass opacities and septal thickening are superimposed on one another.
- Pneumatoceles
  - Varying shape, size, and wall thickness
  - Are seen in up to 30% of cases
- Pleural effusions are rare
- Lymphadenopathy is uncommon (10%).

Especially in patients treated prophylactically, features are more frequently atypical including:

- **Consolidation:** Can be more common in patients without HIV infection and tends to develop more rapidly, reflecting pulmonary damage from the host immune response.

- Nodules (granulomas)
  - May cavitate.
  - Small nodules and tree-in-bud opacities are uncommon in patients with AIDS and PCP and usually indicate the presence of infectious bronchiolitis from other organisms.
- Lymphadenopathy.
- Pleural effusions are also more frequently encountered in this group of patients.

A cystic form of PCP is also recognized, again more frequently in patients receiving aerosolized prophylaxis. In this pattern, features include:

- Thin walled cysts: In most cases these are pneumatoceles
- Upper lobes
- May be bilateral
- Increased risk of pneumothorax.

PNEUMOCYSTIS INFECTION

- Opportunistic fungal pulmonary pathogen, lacks ergosterol so not susceptible to antifungal which inhibit ergosterol synthesis.
- Human isolate – P. jiroveci; P.carnii is found in rats.
- **Most prominent antigen:** Major surface glycoprotein which shows antigenic variation and facilitates its adherence.
- Other important antigen is 35-55kDa–which acts as marker of infection.

Pathogenesis and Pathology

- Defects in CMI and humoral immunity predispose for its infection, e.g., In HIV infection occur when CD4 + <200.
- Principal host effector cells – alveolar macrophage.
- Transmission – Airborne; person to person.
  - In alveoli:
    - ◊ It attach to type I cells (extracellular), damage it.
    - ◊ Hypertrophy of type II cells occur causing, surfactant abnormalities.

  - ◊ Increase IL-8 and neutrophil in BAL fluid.
  - ◊ Alveoli filled with typical foamy vacuolated exudate.
- – Severe disease:
  - ◊ Mild mononuclear cell (ever plasma cell) interstitial infiltrate seen so called Interstitial plasma cell pneumoniae.
  - ◊ Risk factors for Pneumocystis Pneumonia.
  - ◊ HIV.
- – Immunosuppressive therapy particularly glucocorticoids for cancer.
- – Organ transplantation and other disorders.
- – Children with primary immunodeficiency disease and premature malnourished infants.

Clinical Features

- Symptom: Dyspnea, fever, non-productive cough.
- Sign: Tachypnea tachycardia and cyanosis but lung auscultation reveals few abnormalities.
- Risk for extrapulmonary spread increase with: Administration of aerosolized pentamidine.
- Most common extrapulmonary site: Lymph node, spleen, liver, bone marrow.
- Most widely used prognostic factor is degree of hypoxemia.

Diagnosis

1. Definitive diagnosis by histopathologic detection by:
   a. Staining
      - Methenamine silver, toludine blue stain cell wall while Wright-Giemsa stain the nuceli.
      - Immunofluorescence with monoclonal antibodies; more sensitive.

   b. DNA amplification by PCR
      - Most sensitive.
2. Specimen collection
   a. Fiberoptic bronchoscopy with BAL which is more sensitive than sputum induction, is the mainstay of diagnosis.

b. Transbronchial biopsy and open lung biopsy – only when diagnosis can't be made by BAL.

Treatment

- DOC cotrimoxazole for all forms of pneumocystosis including extrapulmonary disease.
- Alternative for mild to moderate case – Trimethoprim + dapsone and clindamycin + primaquine.
- Alternative for moderate to severe – Pentamidine slow IV.
- Adjunctive therapy – Glucocorticoid in HIV patient with moderate to severe pneumocystosis whose pulmonary function deteriorates on taking anti-pneumocystis drugs.

Prophylaxis

- DOC for HIV primary and secondary (both HIV and Non-HIV) prophylaxis is cotrimoxazole.
- Alternative Dapsone.
- In HIV prophylaxis given when:– CD4 + <200. History of oropharyngeal candidiasis.

18. Which of the following is not useful as personal protective device against radiation exposure?

A. Gloves
B. Glasses
C. Lab coat
D. Face shield

Answer: Option C. Lab coat

A white coat or laboratory coat (often abbreviated to lab coat) is a knee-length overcoat/smock worn by professionals in the medical field or by those involved in laboratory work. The coat protects their street clothes and also serves as a simple uniform. It has no protective effect against radiation exposure. So it is not useful as personal protective device against radiation exposure.

Its lead apron that is used as personal protective device against radiation exposure.

Exposure to the primary beam of radiation could be of the operator's fingers; these would then be seen on the monitor if they are being exposed, and **protective gloves** should be worn. Using an under couch tube is obviously preferable in terms of staff doses, both finger and whole body.

The employer has to provide personal protective equipment. In the case of X-rays, this might include lead aprons, thyroid shields, and **leaded glasses** or goggles.

Universal **Face Shields** cover a broad area of the face and head for more complete protection. Lead impregnated, acrylic face shields are suspended from an adjustable headpiece. Adjust shield to any angle over face with temple dials to minimize scatter radiation passing under the shield.